Psychology in Diabetes Care

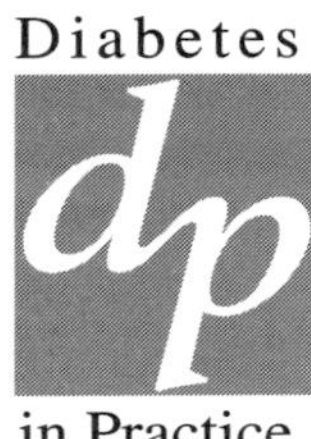

Other titles in the Wiley *Diabetes in Practice* Series

Diabetes in Old Age
Paul Finucane and Alan J. Sinclair (Editors)

Prediction, Prevention and Genetic Counseling in IDDM
Jerry P. Palmer (Editor)

Diabetes and Pregnancy:
An International Approach to Diagnosis and Management
Anne Dornhorst and David R. Hadden (Editors)

Diabetic Complications
Ken M. Shaw (Editor)

Childhood and Adolescent Diabetes
Simon Court and Bill Lamb (Editors)

Hypoglycaemia in Clinical Diabetes
Brian M. Frier and B. Miles Fisher (Editors)

Exercise and Sport in Diabetes
Bill Burr and Dinesh Nagi (Editors)

Psychology in Diabetes Care

Edited by

Frank J. Snoek
Vrije Universiteit, Amsterdam, The Netherlands

T. Chas Skinner
University Hospital Lewisham, London, UK

JOHN WILEY & SONS, LTD
Chichester • New York • Weinheim • Brisbane • Singapore • Toronto

Baffins Lane, Chichester,
West Sussex PO19 1UD, England

National 01243 779777
International (+44) 1243 779777
e-mail (for orders and customer service enquiries): cs-books@wiley.co.uk
Visit our Home Page on http://www.wiley.co.uk
or http://www.wiley.com

Other Wiley Editorial Offices

John Wiley & Sons, Inc., 605 Third Avenue,
New York, NY 10158-0012, USA

WILEY-VCH Verlag GmbH, Pappelallee 3,
D-69469 Weinheim, Germany

Jacaranda Wiley Ltd, 33 Park Road Milton,
Queensland 4064, Australia

John Wiley & Sons (Asia) Pte Ltd, 2 Clementi Loop #02-01,
Jin Xing Distripark, Singapore 129809

John Wiley & Sons (Canada) Ltd, 22 Worcester Road,
Rexdale, Ontario M9W 1L1, Canada

Library of Congress Cataloging-in-Publication Data

Psychology in diabetes care/edited by Frank J. Snoek, T. Chas Skinner.
p.; cm — (Wiley diabetes in practice series)
Includes bibliographical references and index.
ISBN 0-471-97703-9 (cased : alk. paper)
1. Diabetes—Psychological aspects. I. Snoek, Frank J. II. Skinner, T. Chas. III. Diabetes in practice
[DNLM: 1. Diabetes Mellitus—psychology. 2. Behaviour Therapy. 3. Diabetes Mellitus—therapy. WK 810 P974 2000]
RC660 .P79 2000
616.4′62′0019—dc21 99-089083

British Library Cataloguing in Publication Data

A catalogue record for this book is available from the British Library

ISBN 0-471-97703-9

Typeset in 10/12pt Palatino from the authors' disks by Techset Composition Ltd, Salisbury.
Printed and bound in Great Britain by Biddles Ltd, Guildford and King's Lynn.
This book is printed on acid-free paper responsibly manufactured from sustainable forestry, in which at least two trees are planted for each one used for paper production.

MEDICAL LIBRARY
AILSA HOSPITAL
DALMELLINGTON ROAD
AYR KA6 6AB

Contents

Contributors

Barbara Anderson *Joslin Diabetes Center, 1 Joslin Place, Boston, MA 02215, USA*

Robert Anderson *Department of Medical Education, 0201 Towsley Center, University of Michegan Medical School, Ann Arbor, MI 48109-0201, USA*

Julienne Bracket *Joslin Diabetes Center, 1 Joslin Place, Boston, MA 02215, USA*

Anita Carlson *LUCD, Karolinska Hospital, Stockholm S-171 76, Sweden*

Sue Channon *Psychology Department, Children's Centre, Heath Hospital, Cardiff CF4 7XW, UK*

Marlène Chatrou *Ignatius Ziekenhuis, Department of Medical Psychology, PO Box 90158-4800, RK Breda, The Netherlands*

William Clarke *Behavioral Medicine Center, Box 223, University of Virgina Health Sciences Center, Charlottesville, VA 22908, USA*

Daniel Cox *Behavioral Medicine Center, Box 223, University of Virgina Health Sciences Center, Charlottesville, VA 22908, USA*

Sue Cradock *Diabetes Centre, Queen Alexandria Hospital, Cosham, Portsmouth PO6 3LY, UK*

Yvonne Doherty *Fife Primary care, NHS Trust, Dunfermline KY12 0SU, UK*

Elizabeth G. Eakin *AMC Cancer Research Center, 1600 Pierce Street, Denver, CO 80214, USA*

Martha Funnell *University of Michigan Diabetes Research and Training Center, Charlottesville, VA 22908, USA*

Russel E. Glasgow *AMC Cancer Research Center, 1600 Pierce Street, Denver, CO 80214, USA*

Linda Gonder-Frederick *Behavioral Medicine Center, Box 223, University of Virgina Health Sciences Center, Charlottesville, VA 22908, USA*

Lesley Howells *Department of Child Health, Ninewells Hospital Medical School, Dundee DD1 9SY, UK*

Peter James *Department of Clinical Psychology, North Tyneside Hospital, Rake Lane, North Shields NE29 8NH, UK*

Diana Julian *Behavioral Medicine Center, Box 223, University of Virgina Health Sciences Center, Charlottesville, VA 22908, USA*

Adele McEvilly *Diabetes Home Care Unit, Birmingham Children's Hospital, Steelhouse Lane, Birmingham B4 6NH, UK*

Sue Roberts *Diabetes Center, North Tyneside Hospital, Rake Lane, North Shields NE29 8NH, UK*

Richard R. Rubin *Johns Hopkins University School of Medicine, 500 West University Parkway, Suite 1-M, Baltimore, MD 21210, USA*

Nuha Saleh-Statin *LUCD, Karolinska Hospital, Stockholm S-171 76, Sweden*

T. Chas Skinner *Research Centre, University Hospital Lewisham, Lewisham High Street, London SE13 9LH, UK*

Frank J. Snoek *Vrije Universiteit, Medical Psychology, Diabetes Research Group, Van der Boechorststraat 7, 1081 BT Amsterdam, The Netherlands*

Nicole C. W. van der Ven *Vrije Universiteit, Medical Psychology, Diabetes Research Group, Van der Boechorststraat 7, 1081 BT Amsterdam, The Netherlands*

Foreword

Diabetes is a very human condition. Even to those of us with many years of clinical practice in diabetes, the infinite diversity of individual response to diabetes is a constant source of amazement but also professional enhancement. People are different and behave differently, and often unexpectedly. That is what makes involvement in diabetes care such a three-dimensional experience. Diabetes and its consequences have a fundamental physical basis, but these are deeply intertwined with complex psychosocial issues. Such interrelationships are considerable, sometimes subtle; sometimes overwhelming.

Awareness of these issues is crucial to enabling people with diabetes to lead a healthy and fulfilled life. Empathy and appreciation of the psychosocial needs of patients are essential requirements for those involved in diabetes care, and indeed most do seem to acquire that intuitive understanding of patient–professional relationships so fundamental to good clinical care. But the world of psychology has progressed; much more is known and the evidence base of psychological management in diabetes care is becoming clearer.

Despite the widespread and increasing prevalence of diabetes in the population, the diagnosis at a personal level can still be a considerable shock and source of distress to the individual and family concerned. Suddenly a label is applied that seemingly sets them aside from others; that invokes dire consequences to both current well-being and to future health. Such initial fears and misgivings may result from misunderstandings and ignorant, albeit well intentioned, advice from others. The misguided term "mild diabetes" may be used inappropriately to allay fears and anxieties, but in so doing it undermines the essential need to manage diabetes with due consideration and respect.

Recent published studies and clinical experience indicate that future prospects for people with diabetes should be very positive and encouraging, but despite the substantial improvements in treatments and technology, a demanding daily discipline is still required.

Realistic information and education needs to be very much geared to the individual, taking into account the very diversity of such individual needs and perspectives. Necessary messages should be understood, but balancing the immediate influences on quality of life with longer term objectives on future health. Living with diabetes is a lifelong educational exercise and a similar experience for those involved in diabetes care. No amount of theoretical knowledge can match this constant learning through daily encounters with diabetes, but it is this experience that can be used to interpret and reassure. It is about achieving the right balance, and for this psychological awareness is essential.

Although the concept of a specific diabetes personality has been irrevocably refuted, diabetes will inevitably affect individuals emotionally in different ways. Both at diagnosis and in subsequent years a complex interaction between the physical consequences of diabetes and its psychological demands is constantly contributing to the vicissitudes of diabetes well-being. Even the term diabetes control carries psychological undertones, but it is the term we use most frequently. Poor control may refer to inadequate achievement of good blood glucose levels, but it will also contribute to poor quality of life and often loss of personal confidence. It is the model of a vicious cycle. In contrast for others, particularly those with type 2 diabetes, the "silent" nature of the condition can be deceptive and deflect away from the need to maintain discipline and diligence.

Steering the narrow gap between Scylla and Charybdis is never easy, but there are now many new aids to assist the person with diabetes along the right pathway. No longer are treatments so rigid and set in tablets of stone; improved education and understanding do offer more flexibility adapted to the individual's needs.

The person with diabetes should equally contribute to discussions and decisions concerning care and best treatment, fully informed and in collaboration with the clinician. Understanding the psychosocial issues of this partnership is fundamental to success. The expert and well-respected contributors to this book offer a valuable and necessary insight into the interaction between psychology and diabetes care, and in so doing provide guidance on psychological interventions to further minimise the daily demands of living with diabetes.

Professor K.M. Shaw
March 2000

Preface

Psychosocial issues are increasingly recognized as being of primary importance in diabetes care. This is illustrated by the burgeoning number of publications on behavioural and social issues in both psychological and medical journals. In addition, an increasing number of international conferences and symposia on diabetes are beginning to address cognitive, emotional and behavioural issues surrounding diabetes, its complications and management. With this growing awareness of the importance of psychology in diabetes care, health care professionals experience an increasing need for easily accessible background information and practical guidelines on behavioural issues. However, only a handful of books are available for clinicians who wish to know what to do about the psychological aspects of diabetes care, from supporting patients and families coping with diagnosis and following the treatment regimen, through to complex psychological problems such as the diagnosis and management of depression and eating disorders. These are the issues this book hopes to begin to address. It seeks to bridge the gap between psychological research on the self-care and management of diabetes and the delivery of care and services provided by the diabetes care team. As such, this book is seen as an accompaniment to Clare Bradley's *Handbook of Psychology and Diabetes* (1994), which focuses on psychological assessment in diabetes. The content of this book is targeted at all individuals involved in the delivery of diabetes, including our fellow psychologists.

When considering who to ask to contribute to this book, we were acutely aware of two groups of psychologists. The largest, and most well-established group is the Council of Behavioural Medicine and Psychology of the American Diabetes Association (ADA). To date, these North American behavioural scientists have generated the overwhelming majority of psychological research and publications, and have compiled an excellent how-to-do-it book under the editorship of Barbara Anderson and Richard Rubin (1996). Fortunately, we can see steadily increasing European work in this field, facilitated by the EASD Study Group, Psychosocial Aspects of Diabetes (PSAD). This group continues to develop and bring a distinctly European perspective to the psychology of diabetes care. Therefore, when seeking contributors for this compilation, we have endeavoured to reflect the work of both groups of researchers, thereby offering a true international perspective on psychology in diabetes care.

This book also seeks to provide a broad, evidence-based approach to behavioural intervention in diabetes care. Based on reviews of empirical and theoretical work, each chapter will make practical recommendations for diabetes care provision and future research. The authors of the nine chapters were asked to explore different approaches to intervention with children, adolescents and adults with diabetes. The first chapter is by Barbara Anderson and Julienne Brackett (USA), on Diabetes during childhood, addressing developmental and family issues. Chas Skinner, Sue Chanon, Lesley Howells and Adele McEvilly (UK) then discuss the abundance of psychological literature on adolescents with diabetes, with special reference to the beliefs and attitudes of adolescents with diabetes and how these affect their self-care behaviours. Research on the psychological impact of pregnancy in diabetes is reviewed in Chapter 3 by Frank Snoek (The Netherlands), with special focus on pre-conception counselling programmes. In Chapter 4, a truly international group of authors from the USA (Bob Anderson and Martha Funnell), Sweden (Anita Carlson and Nuha Saleh-Stattin) and the UK (Sue Cradock and Chas Skinner), discuss the background and implications of the empowerment approach to diabetes education and self-management, taking into account ethnic and cultural factors. The rich potential of motivational interviewing as a vehicle for behaviour change in diabetes patients is reviewed by Yvonne Doherty, Peter James and Sue Roberts (UK) in Chapter 5. This clearly sets the stage for Russell Glasgow and Elizabeth Eakins (USA) chapter on medical office-based interventions and how these can significantly contribute to the behaviour change process in diabetes. Chapters 7 and 8 expand on two different psychoeducational group programmes that were developed specifically for diabetes patients: Blood Glucose Awareness Training (BGAT), by Linda Gonder-Frederick, Daniel Cox, William Clarke and Diana Julian (USA), and Cognitive-Behavioural Group Training (CBGT), by Nicole van der Ven, Marlène Chatrou and Frank Snoek (The Netherlands). The last chapter, by Richard Rubin (USA), building on rich experience as a psychologist involved in diabetes care, reviews the indications and benefits of psychotherapy and counselling in diabetes, with reference to adaptional problems, depression, anxiety and eating disorders.

In conclusion, this book offers a comprehensive summary of current psychological knowledge and thought as it relates to the delivery of diabetes care and how to support professionals and individuals with diabetes to achieve their goals. We hope this book is a worthy start to this endeavour. Albeit incomplete, we sincerely hope you will find it informative, that it helps you reflect on your practice, whatever your professional role, and that it enables you to develop a more thoughtful approach to those individuals you are striving to care for.

We would like to thank the authors for their willingness to contribute to this volume and their considerable efforts to meet the editorial demands. We also thank Deborah Reece and Colleagues from John Wiley & Sons Ltd, Chichester, UK, for their initiative, efficiency and support.

Frank Snoek and Chas Skinner

1

Diabetes During Childhood

BARBARA ANDERSON and JULIENNE BRACKET
Joslin Diabetes Center, Boston, MA, USA

INTRODUCTION

The results of the Diabetes Control and Complications Trial[1,2] focused the attention of the medical community on the importance of maintaining blood glucose levels as close to the normal range as possible in order to prevent or delay the devastating complications of diabetes. However, translating this message to families coping with this disease in a child presents many challenges and requires a multi-disciplinary team to care for each family[3,4]. Type 1 (insulin-dependent) diabetes is frequently singled out from many other chronic childhood diseases because its successful treatment demands much self-care and family responsibility for implementing a complex treatment regimen[5]. When a child is diagnosed with diabetes, the critical tasks of decision-making concerning the child's daily survival and treatment are transferred from health care professionals to the family. Immediately following diagnosis, the family is responsible for carefully balancing multiple daily insulin injections and food intake with physical activity in order to prevent large fluctuations in blood glucose levels, which can interfere with the child's normal growth and development. Frequent blood glucose monitoring is also required to assess this tenuous balance between insulin, food and activity.

In the psychosocial literature on paediatric diabetes, it is well-documented that this complex daily regimen impacts on every aspect of the child's development and family life[4,6,7]. With respect to psychological development, 'good emotional adjustment' is strongly related to better glycaemic control[6,8,9]. Sufficient studies comparing groups of children with diabetes to non-diabetic comparison samples have been conducted using standard-

Psychology in Diabetes Care. Edited by Frank J. Snoek and T. Chas Skinner.

ized, objective measures that we can confidently conclude that children with diabetes are not a psychologically 'deviant' group[8,10,11]. However, such global studies have not provided much information about what it is about diabetes that affects the developing child and almost every aspect of family life.

Therefore, this chapter will focus on identifying and understanding the specific stresses of living with diabetes, which the child and parent must confront at each developmental stage between infancy and the eleventh year, and the coping responses that lead to healthy psychological and physical outcomes. Because each developmental stage presents different challenges, we will divide the discussion into: (a) diabetes in infancy (0–2 years of age); (b) diabetes in toddlers and preschoolers (2–5 years); and (c) diabetes in the school-age child (6–11 years). For each section, we will briefly review the central milestones of normal psychological development and then examine how the treatment demands of diabetes impact on the developmental tasks of each period. Next, we will discuss how diabetes impacts on the family and vice versa. We will also translate research findings into brief recommendations for health care providers to assist in developing services that best meet the changing psychosocial needs of their paediatric diabetes patients and their families in each of these developmental periods. The final section of the chapter will review some of the risk factors for poor adjustment and diabetes control that have been identified across all of childhood.

DIABETES IN INFANCY

PSYCHOLOGICAL DEVELOPMENT AND THE IMPACT OF DIABETES IN INFANCY

Diabetes diagnosed during infancy has a profound effect on the parent–child relationship. For the first 2 years of life, the central psychological task is the establishment of a mutually strong and trusting emotional attachment between the infant and the primary caregivers[12,13]. The infant's psychological well-being depends on the predictable presence of an adult who meets the infant's physical needs, provides a stable environment, and responds to his/her social advances.

Because type 1 diabetes is relatively rare in infants and toddlers, and symptoms may vary from those commonly seen, young children with diabetes are often misdiagnosed initially[14]. The child may present with acute vomiting and marked dehydration, which is often attributed to gastroenteritis The diagnosis of type 1 diabetes in infants is often delayed because it is more difficult for parents to detect classic symptoms of diabetes, such as frequent urination, which would signal the need to seek medical attention. Due to such delays and misdiagnoses at diagnosis, infants and toddlers are more likely than older children to be in diabetic ketoacidosis (DKA) and require hospitalization in an intensive care unit. When hospitalized, infants endure disruptions of expected home routines and are often subjected to invasive medical procedures. Once home, the 'trusted' caregivers are required to give injections and perform painful fingersticks on infants who lack the cognitive ability to understand that the procedures are beneficial[15]. Therefore, the diagnosis of diabetes may threaten the infant's development of a trusting relationship with caregivers. In a qualitative study by Hatton and colleagues[16], mothers of infants and toddlers with diabetes reported feeling a diminished bond with their children and a loss of the ideal mother–child relationship.

Because young children with diabetes are totally dependent on their parents to manage their disease and to recognize dangerous fluctuations in blood glucose, parents must be constantly vigilant. Due to the stress of the day-to-day management of diabetes, many parents are too exhausted and fearful to leave their child in the care of another[16]. In addition, finding 'relief' caregivers who are competent and comfortable caring for a young child with diabetes is often extremely difficult, if not impossible[3,4]. Therefore, diabetes may put the infant–parent relationship at risk for overdependency and may restrict the positive separation and reunion experiences that are necessary during infancy.

FAMILY ISSUES: CARING FOR AN INFANT WITH DIABETES

When a child is diagnosed with IDDM during the first 2 years of life, the parent(s) or caregiver(s) become the real 'patient'. The grief experienced by parents of infants after diagnosis is often stronger and more emotionally disruptive than when a child is diagnosed at an older age because parents of young infants have more recently celebrated the birth of a 'healthy, perfect' child. In addition, infants are more often critically ill at diagnosis, and the parents may have witnessed their child being cared for in an intensive care unit. This heightens the trauma already experienced by the parents, and emphasizes the vulnerability of their child, as well as the seriousness of diabetes. After the acute crisis abates, the parents of a very small child are now faced with the reality and implications of the diagnosis. They may find it extremely difficult, both psychologically and physically, to inject insulin into or to take a drop of blood from their infant's tiny body. Parents described feeling 'riveted to a totally inflexible regimen that ruled their very existence'[16] (p. 572). Parents not only grieve for the loss of a 'healthy' child, but also for the loss of spontaneity, flexibility and freedom to which they may have been accustomed. In order to ensure that the infant's medical needs are constantly monitored, major lifestyle changes are frequently required[16]. For all of these reasons, the diagnosis of IDDM during infancy is emotionally devastating and extremely stressful to parents. Many parents report that the diagnosis of diabetes increased strain in their marriages and heightened miscommunication between spouses, as well as leading to feelings of depression[16]. However, with time and knowledge, parents in the study by Hatton *et al.*[16] felt greater confidence and found more flexibility in the management regimen, which contributed to adaptation. Even as they felt more adapted, the many stresses of diabetes continued to evoke emotional responses[16].

DIABETES IN TODDLERS AND PRESCHOOLERS

PSYCHOLOGICAL DEVELOPMENT AND THE IMPACT OF DIABETES: AGES 2–5 YEARS

Diabetes during the second through fourth years of life continues to have a profound effect on the parent–child relationship. At this developmental period, the toddler's two central psychological tasks are: (a) to separate from the parent or primary caregiver and to establish him/herself as a separate person, by developing a sense of autonomy, with more clearly defined boundaries between the child and the parent; and (b) to develop a sense of mastery over the environment and the confidence that he/she can act upon and produce results in the environment, including the people making up his/her social environment[12,13].

The restrictions of diabetes management and parental fear stemming from diabetes stress the normal drive of toddlers to explore and master their environments. The toddler's sense of autonomy can be threatened by overprotective caregivers, who may be unable to let the child out of their sight. Out of fear, the parents may scold toddlers for exploring, which can lead to feelings of guilt and shame[17]. The autonomy that a child does develop is often reflected in refusals to cooperate with injections or blood glucose monitoring, as well as in conflicts over food. Toddlers can learn to use food to manipulate their parents who are afraid of hypoglycaemia, causing the dinner table to become a battleground. Although the diabetes management tasks must be carried out, parents can help foster the developing sense of autonomy by allowing the toddler to choose between two injection sites or fingers for blood samples[17].

As the child reaches the preschool years, the central developmental task becomes the use of the newly established sense of autonomy to investigate the world outside the home. The child is involved in gaining a sense of gender identity, in developing new cognitive abilities which allow more cause–effect thinking, and in separating successfully from parents for the first 'school' experience[12,13]. At this developmental stage, the child must learn to adapt to the expectations of other adults, to trust these adults to provide for his/her needs, and to begin to form relationships with peers and adults outside the family. The child takes increasing initiative to explore and master new skills in environments outside of the home.

For preschool-aged children with diabetes, meeting their peers may lead to the first awareness that they are 'different' from other children, in terms of eating, checking blood glucose levels, or wearing medical identification jewelry. As children with diabetes recognize that they are somehow different from others, it is common for them to believe that diabetes is a form of punishment. During this developmental stage, the child is developing his/her own explanations and perceptions of the world. Because diabetes plays a large role in the child's life, the child uses developing, but limited, ideas of causality to reason that diabetes and its painful treatment are the result of his/her bad behaviour[15].

Given the toddler's and preschooler's normal developmental tasks of establishing his/her independence from the parent, diabetes only fuels the parent–child conflicts so typical of these stages. Unfortunately, in previous research studies, infants and toddlers with diabetes have been grouped with children under 6 years of age, and studied as a 'preschool sample', yielding little data on these stages specifically. One empirical research study by Wysocki and colleagues[11] has studied the psychological adjustment of very young children from the mothers' perspective, with a sample of 20 children, 2–6 years of age, with a mean age of approximately 4 years. The authors indicated that mothers reported that their children showed significantly more 'internalizing' behaviour problems on the standardized Child Behaviour Checklist (CBCL)[18], such as symptoms of depression, anxiety, sleep problems, somatic complaints, or withdrawal. However, the authors emphasize that mothers did not rate their toddler and preschool children with diabetes in the clinically deviant range, as measured on this standardized instrument[11]. In contrast to the findings of Wysocki *et al.*, Northam and colleagues[19] found no significant deviations from normative scores on any scale of the CBCL at diagnosis or 1 year later in a sample of 18 children under 4 years of age. In both studies, there were no assessments made of the children's behaviour independent of maternal report. This is important to note in light of the other major finding by Wysocki and colleagues, that mothers of very young children with diabetes reported more overall stress in their families when contrasted with a non-diabetic standardization sample, citing the child with diabetes as the source of that stress[11]. Despite the cautious interpretation both authors gave to their findings, it is possible that a non-diabetic standardization sample is an inappropriate comparison group. Both Eiser[20] and Garrison and McQuiston[21] have suggested that these types of behavioural changes in the young child and changes in parental perceptions are to be expected when *any* chronic illness is present in the child. Therefore, it is important not to conclude from these findings that it is diabetes *per se* that causes the behavioural adjustment problems or that all mothers of preschoolers with diabetes see their families as severely stressed. Clearly, more research into the psychological adjustment of very young children with diabetes is needed. In addition, independent assessments of adjustment need to be used, rather than relying solely on parental report, which can be affected by feelings of guilt or pity[19].

FAMILY ISSUES: PARENTING TODDLERS AND PRESCHOOLERS WITH DIABETES

As is true for infants with diabetes, when a toddler or preschooler has diabetes, the parent(s) or caregiver(s) is the real 'patient'[3]. Parents continue to be responsible for making complex, clinical decisions, and for vigilantly monitoring the child for symptoms of hypoglycaemia. As the child experiences growth spurts, parents often struggle to maintain the child's blood sugar within a safe and acceptable range—a struggle made more difficult by the child's inability to understand the importance of the regimen, and the toddler's inability to verbalize symptoms of high or low blood glucose. Compared to findings from a sample of older children and adolescents with diabetes, mothers of very young children report more concerns about identifying hypoglycaemia, and perceive greater family disruption from diabetes[11,22]. Adding to the parents' stress, toddlers and preschoolers, who are getting physically stronger, may actively resist and refuse insulin injections, blood monitoring or needed meals and snacks. Restraining the squirming child at injection time or forcing the child to eat may be necessary but extremely stressful for parents who begin to feel that they are 'feeding the insulin, not the child' (p. 573)[16]. The children can now also verbalize their fear and anger about invasive procedures, which can devastate parents as these emotions are usually directed at them[16].

Once children begin to test their autonomy, it is important for parents to set limits and discipline their children appropriately. Temper tantrums are common among young children, hence the phrase 'terrible twos', but they may also signal hypoglycaemia in children with diabetes. Many parents report difficulty in distinguishing diabetes-related mood swings from normal toddler behaviour[16]. Once hypoglycaemia has been ruled out through blood glucose monitoring, parents need to set limits and have clear expectations for the child, as they would for a child without diabetes. Unfortunately, feelings of guilt or pity about the child's disease may interfere with such limit-setting[17,23].

Hatton and colleagues report that anticipation of a child entering preschool and being entrusted to another's care can cause much anxiety and concern for parents[16]. Overprotectiveness and pity for a child suffering from separation anxiety can tempt parents to cancel or delay plans for preschool education or daycare, but doing so can thwart the child's growing sense of independence and development of social skills[17].

TREATMENT ISSUES FOR CHILDREN UNDER 6 YEARS OF AGE

Once diagnosed, the basic goals of diabetes therapy for children under the age of 6 years are similar to those recommended to all children and adolescents and include the avoidance of high and low blood glucose levels and the maintenance of normal growth and development. However, due to the continued development of the central nervous system, young children are particularly vulnerable to the debilitating consequences of recurrent hypoglycaemia.

There is a growing body of evidence supporting the negative consequences—mild cognitive deficits—resulting from overly aggressive attempts to normalize metabolism in young children. Ack *et al.*[24] reported modest cognitive deficits in patients with a younger onset of type 1 diabetes. Others also reported brain damage as a result of severe hypoglycaemia, particularly in young children[25,26]. A series of studies by Ryan *et al.*[27–29], using a battery of neurobehavioural tests, identified significant differences between youths with diabetes compared with control subjects on measures of verbal intelligence, visual–motor coordination and critical flicker threshold. Additionally, children diagnosed with diabetes under 5 years of age manifested significant cognitive deficits when evaluated during the adolescent years, probably resulting from symptomatic or asymptomatic hypoglycaemia occurring earlier in life, before final maturation of the central nervous system. In another study by Rovet *et al.*[30], children diagnosed under 4 years of age scored lower than other children with diabetes diagnosed later in childhood, and lower than non-diabetic sibling controls on tests of visual–spatial orientation, but not on verbal ability. Hypoglycaemic seizures were found to occur in greater frequency in the group of children diagnosed under 4 years of age compared to those diagnosed at older ages, suggesting that severe hypoglycaemia may impair later cognitive functioning[30].

Golden and colleagues[31] collected longitudinal data on the frequency of hypoglycaemia from the time of diagnosis in a sample of 23 children with diabetes onset prior to the age of 5 years. Correlating this data with subscale scores on the Stanford–Binet Intelligence Scale yielded no significant findings between frequency of severe hypoglycaemia and any of the subscales. Importantly, it was the frequency of asymptomatic and mildly symptomatic hypoglycaemia that was significantly correlated with lower scores on the abstract/visual reasoning scale, indicating that even mild or asymptomatic episodes of hypoglycaemia can have a negative cumulative effect on cognitive functioning.

In the previously described studies, no measurements of neurocognitive functioning were made near the time of diagnosis to rule out the possibility that the metabolic decompensation of diabetes onset affected such functioning. Two studies have followed children with diabetes prospectively from diagnosis using neuropsychological assessments. The preliminary findings of Rovet and colleagues[32] indicated no evidence of neurocognitive impairment in these children at diagnosis or 1 year later, but the authors reported that they may not have followed subjects long enough to observe any impairment. Northam and colleagues[33] compared the performance of children with IDDM with the performance of control subjects on standardized measures of general intelligence, attention, speed of processing, memory, learning and executive skills. At 3 months post-diagnosis, there were no differences between the groups, but at 2 years post-diagnosis, children with diabetes demonstrated smaller gains, particularly in the areas of information-processing speed, acquisition of new knowledge and conceptual reasoning skills. The subset of the diabetes sample that performed worst were those children with early onset of diabetes, which further suggests an early onset effect[33].

In light of these findings, suggesting that even asymptomatic hypoglycaemia in young children with developing nervous systems can be deleterious, prevention of severe and recurrent hypoglycaemia needs to be of paramount importance. In addition, infants and toddlers are unable to verbalize when they are suffering from hypoglycaemia, which can lead to delayed treatment and unconsiousness and/or seizures. The current trend of intensive insulin therapy, as advocated by the Diabetes Control and Complications Trial,[1,2] for persons over 13 years of age must be aggressively avoided in these vulnerable young patients[14,34–36]. Therefore, age-specific blood glucose target ranges, with the provision for wide glycaemic excursions, should be the rule rather than the exception.

Achieving optimal glycaemic control in this age range is further complicated by the finicky eating habits, erratic physical activity and rapid growth of young children. Treatment goals, therefore, must be individualized to provide safe and effective medical treatment yet also permit the young child to master the normal developmental tasks of childhood. For example, the toddler who is a picky, pokey eater may be best suited to rapid-acting insulin analogue (Humulog) injections after meals, rather than prior to the meals, in order to avoid frantic parents who are unable to 'force their child to eat'.

PSYCHOSOCIAL RECOMMENDATIONS TO HEALTH CARE PROVIDERS

It is essential that health care providers who work in paediatric diabetes appreciate and address the many stresses and demands confronting parents of infants, toddlers and preschoolers with diabetes by promoting the development of clinical services, childcare referral sources, educational materials and support groups for families living with diabetes at these earliest developmental periods. Parents have reported a need for understanding from and collaboration with a health care team[16,22]. Managing diabetes in young children requires an integrated multi-disciplinary team approach in order to address adequately the complex physiological and psychosocial needs of the children and their families[3]. Support groups and educational materials targeted towards families of very young children can also help parents feel less alone and can normalize feelings of guilt, anxiety and fear[3]. The health care team must create a supportive environment by providing 24-hour on-call coverage to help parents cope with unexpected problems, especially as they adjust to life with diabetes outside of the hospital[3,6]. Reassurance and non-judgemental support for all members of the family is of great value, given the emotional challenges of adapting to post-diagnosis life[16].

DIABETES IN SCHOOL-AGED CHILDREN

PSYCHOSOCIAL DEVELOPMENT AND DIABETES IN THE SCHOOL-AGED CHILD

The primary developmental tasks of the child during the elementary school years include: making a smooth adjustment from the home to the school setting; forming close friendships with children of the same sex; obtaining approval from this peer group; developing new intellectual, athletic and artistic skills; and evaluating him/herself positively when comparing his/her abilities to those of the peer group[12,13].

Psychological development in school-aged children is assessed primarily with respect to the child's sense of self-esteem and the development of peer relationships. In a careful review of the early empirical psychosocial literature on children with diabetes, Johnson concluded that: 'most youngsters with diabetes do not have psychological problems, but among those who do, peer relationship difficulties are quite common... Among all of the personality traits assessed, the evidence for peer or social relationship problems seems the strongest' (p. 101)[8].

Studies of self-esteem in school-aged children with diabetes have consistently linked low self-esteem and poor social-emotional adjustment to poorly-controlled diabetes[8,9]. Herskowitz-Dumont and colleagues[37] found a significant association between recurrent diabetic ketoacidosis (DKA) over 8 years post-diagnosis and higher ratings of behaviour problems and lower levels of social competence, as measured by psychological testing in the first year after diagnosis. Similarly, Liss *et al.*[38] found that children who had been hospitalized with DKA in the preceding 12 months reported lower levels of self-esteem and social competence than children who had no episodes of DKA in the same period. In addition, a significantly larger proportion of the DKA group met the diagnostic criteria for at least one psychiatric disorder (88% vs. 28%).

Because the development of peer relationships is an important aspect of the school-age years, it is crucial to examine how diabetes interferes with social development. Several older interview studies have shed light on this topic. Bregani *et al*[39]. emphasized that during this developmental period, children with diabetes often begin to feel a heightened sense of frustration and of social stigma from their dietary restrictions. The authors pointed out that the child's emerging self-awareness and ability to reflect on his/her diabetes and to compare him/herself with peers made the child very vulnerable to feelings of inadequacy. Similarly, Zuppinger *et al.*[40], in interviews with 23 children with diabetes at this age, found that half of the sample identified teasing from peers and difficulty in accommodating meal schedules to school activities as the major difficulties in following the diabetic diet. Leaverton[41] also suggested that the most common resentment of the child with diabetes in the elementary school years is following a planned diet because it gives an obvious sign to peers that the child is different. In addition to food restrictions and regularity of meal timing, the need for frequent blood glucose monitoring and insulin injections can emphasize differences and make peer acceptance more difficult[15].

Kovacs and colleagues[42] found in a longitudinal study of school-aged children newly diagnosed with diabetes that 25% of their sample of school-aged children reported being teased by peers about their diabetes. When asked about the most difficult aspects of diabetes, insulin injections and dietary issues were most commonly cited. Despite the difficult regimen and challenges to peer acceptance, children's self-ratings indicated good self-esteem and few signs of emotional distress in the first year of life with diabetes. Children in this study also reported showing their diabetes supplies to their friends and demonstrating glucose testing, which suggested that the children were actively trying to integrate diabetes into their lives.

SCHOOL ISSUES

Because the school environment presents many opportunities for building self-esteem and developing socialization skills, it is important for the school-aged child with diabetes to participate fully in all activities, with as few restrictions as possible, in order to facilitate a normal school experience. Children need to understand that, although they have diabetes, they are not 'sick' or 'abnormal'[15]. Participation in school activities helps to minimize the child's sense of being different from peers. Some modifications in a typical school day may need to be made to accommodate diabetes safely, such as the scheduling of lunch and gymnastics classes to prevent hypoglycaemia, but restricting the child from gymnastics classes or school outings only emphasizes differences and may foster a sense of inferiority[43].

Children with diabetes should also be encouraged to participate in as many extracurricular activities and sports as they chose and as scheduling permits. For all children, such activities can boost self-esteem and feelings of competence. This effect may be particularly important for children with chronic diseases, such as diabetes[44].

Participation in school is disrupted if the child has unusually high or low blood sugars or if the child uses diabetes to avoid particular classes[44]. In addition, poorly controlled diabetes can lead to frequent or prolonged absences. Such events may result in educational setbacks and interfere with peer relationships, which may contribute to lower self-esteem[15].

Minimizing the occurrence of hypoglycaemia during the school day is crucial in light of findings by Puczynski and colleagues[45], which indicated that memory and concentration may continue to be impaired even after the physical symptoms of hypoglycaemia have subsided. These findings have important implications for classroom functioning, because many students return to their studies after recovering from the physical symptoms when they may not be able to function cognitively as usual. Unfortunately, this study did not determine the length of time cognitive abilities remained impaired, but it did suggest that teachers should consider whether an episode of hypoglycaemia may have affected a student's performance.

In order for children with diabetes to have a normal school experience while maintaining optimal diabetes control, it is necessary for parents and health care providers to provide information and guidance to school personnel to outline expectations for the child's care during the school day. Holiday parties, for instance, can be particularly difficult for the child with diabetes, who may feel left out if not allowed to eat the same foods. Teachers need to be informed of parental preferences relating to what the child is permitted to eat and if substitute foods will be provided from home. School personnel must also be informed about the treatment of out-of-range blood glucose levels, the need for snacks during physical activity, and the frequency of blood glucose monitoring and insulin administration, if such procedures are deemed necessary during school hours. It is essential that families meet with teachers and school nurses before the start of school to provide such information and guidelines and to facilitate cooperation between the school and the family. By communicating with the school regularly throughout the year, families can prevent conflicts, clarify expectations and feel more confident that their child is safe at school[44].

FAMILY ISSUES

Because studies suggest that participation with peers, positive self-image and regimen flexibility (especially nutritional flexibility) are critical and interrelated goals for the school-aged child with diabetes, parents should avoid unrealistic demands for adherence to a meal, insulin or monitoring schedule that restricts the elementary-school child from active participation in age-appropriate school and peer activities. The newer, revised nutritional guidelines permitting more liberal carbohydrate intake[46] may obviate the social stigmatism previously experienced by these school-aged children.

FAMILY FACTORS RELATED TO GLYCAEMIC CONTROL AND ADHERENCE

Due to the relatively small number of children under the age of 6 with diabetes, there have been few, if any, studies on how family environment variables relate to glycaemic control and adherence. For school-aged children, this area has received more attention. One of the first empirical studies of families with children with diabetes under the age of 12 years was conducted by Waller and colleagues[47]. These authors concluded that for school-aged patients, more diabetes-related family guidance and control was linked to better metabolic outcomes, and that diabetes-related parental warmth and caring were important for optimal outcomes. Liss *et al.*[38] had similar findings in her study of children hospitalized with DKA, who also reported lower levels of parental diabetes-related warmth and caring.

Non-diabetes-specific family factors, such as conflict, stress and family cohesion, have also been linked to glycaemic control and adherence[48–54]. Viner and colleagues[54] found that high levels of family stress were correlated with poorer glycaemic control in children under 12 years of age. In addition, the authors found that social support was found to buffer the impact of general family stress on the children's glycaemic control. The authors emphasized that the relationship between family stress and glycaemic control is '...bi-directional, with poor diabetic control producing family stress, as well as family stress inducing poor control in the child' (p. 420)[54].

In contrast, other investigations have not found relationships between general family factors and metabolic control or treatment adherence in school-aged children[55–57]. Various methodological and sampling issues have been used to explain these different findings with respect to the link between family stress and metabolic outcomes in school-aged children. Kovacs *et al.*[57], in a longitudinal study of school-aged children newly diagnosed with diabetes, found no relationship between metabolic control and two general measures of family life—parental perceptions of the quality of family life and the quality of the marriage. These authors speculate that 'metabolic control of children may be affected by aspects of family functioning that are too subtle to have been captured by the measures of general functioning used in this study' (p. 413)[57]. Moreover, Kovacs and her colleagues also suggest that a link between metabolic control and family factors in school-aged children may be shown by studying other variables that 'mediate the relationship of family life to metabolic control' (p. 413)[57], variables such as family behaviour with respect to regimen tasks. These authors also reported that for a small subset (approximately 7%) of their research families, poorer ratings of the family environment at diagnosis were related to subsequent poor metabolic control[57].

A second longitudinal study of school-aged children with newly-diagnosed diabetes by Jacobson, Hauser and colleagues[49,58] revealed that the child's perception of family conflict, as measured by a general family measure given at diagnosis, was the strongest predictor of poor adherence to insulin administration, meal planning, exercise and blood glucose monitoring tasks over a 4-year follow-up period[49]. The relationship between family factors and metabolic control was not examined in this report. This connection between conflict, adherence, and glycaemic control was also examined by Miller-Johnson *et al.*[51] In this study, parent–child conflict was a significant correlate of both adherence and glycaemic control. In multivariate analyses, the relationship between conflict and glycaemic control was non-significant when adherence was entered into the model. These results indicate that conflict may interfere with glycaemic control by disrupting treatment adherence.

FAMILY INVOLVEMENT IN THE DIABETES MANAGEMENT OF A SCHOOL-AGED CHILD

One area of importance for families and health care providers concerns issues of transferring diabetes care responsibilities from the parent to the child[59]. The expanding skills and increased cognitive abilities of the elementary school child make it seem reasonable to transfer more and more daily diabetes care responsibilities. However, there is a growing consensus among recent empirical studies that children and adolescents given greater responsibility for their diabetic management make more mistakes in their self-care, are less adherent and are in poorer metabolic control than those whose parents are more involved[60–65]. Studies using diabetes-specific instruments have consistently found that older children assuming greater responsibility for the tasks of the treatment regimen are in poorer metabolic control than those who assumed less responsibility[62,66–68].

In her important review of the empirical literature on family responsibility sharing in diabetes, Follansbee[69] concluded: 'Cumulatively, these studies yield important information about the role of parent–child interaction in influencing youngsters' assumption of diabetes management. It seems that interdependence, rather than independence, is a worthwhile goal' (p. 350)[69].

From these studies, it has become increasingly clear that parental involvement in diabetes management is required throughout the school-age developmental period. Each family needs to negotiate its own acceptable pattern of parent–child teamwork, based on factors such as child temperament and parent availability. By identifying *shared responsibility* rather than *child independence* as the expectation for school-age children with diabetes, the health care team can help make parent involvement seem less inappropriate to the child or family. It is imperative that the family hears a clear message that diabetes management tasks must be protected from the child's normal drive to achieve independent mastery.

TREATMENT ISSUES FOR SCHOOL-AGED CHILDREN

The goals of diabetes therapy for school-aged children are to: avoid severe metabolic decompensation (diabetic ketoacidosis); maintain normal height and weight; minimize the debilitating symptoms of either severely high or severely low blood glucose levels; establish and maintain a healthy psychosocial environment for the child and family; and maintain the involvement of family members in carrying out daily injections and blood sugar monitoring. At this age, children may be more able developmentally and intellectually to recognize and appropriately treat hypoglycaemia. Thus, as the child exits the preschool period, the diabetes team can now work together with the family towards improved glycaemic control, with lower target blood glucose values. While attempting to improve glycaemic control, it is important for the health care providers to develop treatment regimens that are minimally interruptive to the child's school day. For instance, lunchtime blood glucose monitoring and insulin administration should be prescribed only when necessary.

Overall, the diabetes treatment team must try to teach problem-solving skills to the parent(s) and child to allow flexibility in the diabetes treatment plan. Similar to the preschool period, diabetes management therapy for the school-aged child is often reactive rather than predictive. During the elementary school years the family continues to be the 'patient'. Parents are an important part of every medical office visit, and parents maintain telephone communication for follow-up at home. At the same office visit, the child and family may see more than one member of the diabetes care team. Because the child grows rapidly during this developmental period, frequent adjustments are needed in the meal plan. Therefore, school-aged children should see the nutritionist at least once each year. The mental health specialist on the team can be especially important in the prevention and negotiation of conflicts over diabetes care issues between the parents and others (such as school personnel) while the child is away from home.

To ensure a safe school environment for the child, members of the health care team must be willing to help families communicate guidelines and expectations to school personnel. Diabetes information sheets, with the telephone number of the team, should be available for families to provide to the schools

DISEASE COURSE AND RISK FACTORS: IMPLICATIONS FOR CLINICAL PRACTICE

The groundwork for understanding stages of the disease course in diabetes has been laid by three major longitudinal investigations which have followed school-aged children recently-diagnosed with IDDM over the early years of their disease. Two research teams followed recently-diagnosed children and families over their first decade of life with diabetes[49,58,70–73]. The third investigation, by Grey and colleagues[74] studied a newly diagnosed cohort of children carefully over their first 2 years of living with diabetes.

The longitudinal study by Kovacs *et al.*[71–72] followed patients from 2–3 weeks after diagnosis for 6 years. At the end of the first year, the initial emotional distress of both parents and children seemed to have resolved[75,76]. However, results from yearly evaluations indicated that as IDDM duration increased, patients' emotional distress about diabetes management again increased. Children rated the management regimen as more difficult the longer they had diabetes[71]. This result contrasted with the finding that mothers of these children found it easier to cope with IDDM as duration increased[72]. The finding that the mothers found it easier to cope with diabetes as duration increased 'could reflect that the children had to take increasing responsibility for (their own) diabetes care' (p. 630)[71]. Despite finding it easier to cope with diabetes, the level of emotional symptomatology in mothers also increased slightly after the first year. In addition, these longitudinal studies provided much evidence that initial emotional distress in both children and parents predicted later levels of such distress[71,72]. These studies indicate that clinicians may need to closely monitor children and their parents for signs of emotional distress as disease duration increases, in order to intervene early, especially if the family was initially unusually distressed.

Kovacs *et al.*[73] also examined 'non-compliance with medical treatment' and demonstrated that 50% of patients will become non-compliant to the point of endangering their health. Non-compliance or non-adherence emerged at an average of 3.5 years post-diagnosis and at an average age of l5 years, indicating that years 3 and 4 following the diagnosis of IDDM, as well as the adolescent period, may be particularly high-risk times for non-compliance. The authors suggest that the period of time between diagnosis and the onset of adherence problems may reflect a critical period of adaptation of IDDM, and that because a low recovery rate was found with non-compliance, interventions to prevent its development are needed during the early period of adaptation.

Adherence to the treatment regimen was also a focus of the longitudinal studies of Jacobson, Hauser and colleagues[49,58,70], in which patients were followed from within the first 9 months of diagnosis. Jacobson *et al.*[58] reported that within this patient cohort of newly-diagnosed children and adolescents, patients who were school-age at diagnosis (<13 years) had better adherence over a 4 year follow-up period than did patients who were older (>12 years) at diagnosis. Similarly, Jacobson *et al.*[70] found that initial child reports of self-esteem and social functioning and adjustment predicted subsequent adherence. Data from this longitudinal study revealed that 'patterns of adherence established early in year 1 are maintained over time' (p. 523)[58], although deterioration in adherence occurred as duration increased. In addition, they found that the strongest predictor of treatment adherence 4 years after diagnosis was the child-reported level of family conflict near the time of diagnosis[49].

Data from this prospective study also indicate that early in the course of the disease, youths with IDDM establish a pattern of glycaemic level and regularity of medical appointment-keeping[77]. Youths with the best glycaemic control in the first 4 years of IDDM who also maintained regular medical follow-up had the lowest incidence of retinopathy outcomes 10–12 years after diagnosis. Assessments of family psychosocial variables, such as cohesiveness , conflict and expressiveness, taken near diagnosis, indicated that a more favourable family environment (i.e. more cohesive and less conflicted) was associated with less deterioration in glycaemic control and fewer acute complications of diabetes, such as DKA and severe hypoglycaemia[37,52]. Based on such findings, family environment at the time of diagnosis and early clinic attendance and adherence should be considered when assessing a child's risk for complications and need for services.

Grey *et al.*[74] studied a cohort of 8–14 year-old children newly diagnosed with diabetes and a non-diabetic peer comparison group. The researchers reported that children's adjustment problems at diagnosis disappeared at 1 year post-diagnosis but reappeared at 2 years post-diagnosis, a pattern similar to that found by Kovacs *et al.*[71,72,75,76]. Grey *et al.* argued that, while previous studies have suggested that the period immediately after diagnosis is the most crucial, their data suggest that a second period of adjustment occurs in the second year after diagnosis, and that intervention is important during the critical second year of life with diabetes for prevention of psychosocial deterioration[74].

These longitudinal studies over the course of diabetes in children have revealed three important points for health care providers. First, a period of difficulty in adjusting to diabetes appears to occur at diagnosis and also during the second year. Secondly, treatment adherence patterns seem to be established in the early years, 2–4 years post diagnosis. Third, family functioning and adjustment assessments may be important predictors of later adherence and diabetes control. The results of these studies indicate that interventions should be carried out after diagnosis and before poor adherence patterns can be established. The logical point for multidisciplinary family-centred interventions, which will support adherence to the rigorous treatment regimen by children and families, is, therefore, in the early years post-diagnosis.

Several other important risk factors for poor diabetes control have been investigated in cross-sectional studies. Auslander and colleagues[78,79] found that African–American youths are in significantly poorer glycaemic control than Caucasian youths. Lower levels of adherence in African–American youths contributed to this difference, as did a higher prevalence of single-parent homes. Single-parent families have been linked to poorer diabetes outcomes in several studies[78–80]. In a study of correlates of illness severity at diagnosis, children from single-parent homes tended to have more severe symptoms of diabetes, such as DKA, than those living in two-parent families, suggesting that the stress of single parenting and insufficient resources or support may prevent some single parents from seeking medical attention earlier in the disease onset[81]. In a single-parent household, the entire burden of diabetes management falls on one parent, who may have less time to devote to his/her family due to the necessity to work. Financial resources are also typically more limited. Therefore, stress levels in such households may be higher than in two-parent homes. As discussed earlier, family stress has been correlated to glycaemic control in several studies[48–54]. Auslander *et al.*[50] found that levels of family resources were also strongly related to glycaemic control. Furthermore, lower socio-economic levels have been implicated as a risk factor for poor glycaemic control and recurrent hospitalizations[78,82]. In light of the findings of these studies, it is crucial for health care providers to assess, at diagnosis and on an ongoing basis, the resources (financial, social and emotional) of the family of a child with diabetes. Although other minority groups need to be studied in relation to diabetes control, it seems reasonable to suggest that children from single-parent, low socio-economic status and/or minority homes be closely followed to assure early intervention if diabetes control deteriorates.

CONCLUSIONS

As we enter the twenty-first century, it is possible to have a more *optimistic* viewpoint about the prospects, progress and problems of children with type 1 diabetes. In the context of improvements in treatment technologies[83] and treatment recommendations[1,2], we confront a future in which the acute and the chronic physical complications of IDDM for children can be more readily prevented. In addition, two decades of behavioural research with children with IDDM and their families have helped to make it possible to identify some of the 'predictable crises'[84] that occur as the child moves through the stages of normal growth and development and the phases of diabetes, as well as to identify critical family environment variables that signal potential problems.

We have been encouraged by these recent treatment and research advances, and therefore, in this chapter, we have attempted to identify the intersection between research focused on behavioural and family issues in children with diabetes and diabetes treatment, with the goal of illustrating the potential for prevention of certain behavioural and family 'complications' in childhood diabetes. Armed with a more comprehensive, developmental understanding of the impact of diabetes and its treatment on growing children and their parents, diabetes health care teams can work to prevent problems or to intervene before problems overwhelm families, and thereby improve the quality of life for children and families living with diabetes. Above all, health care providers must strive to provide a family-based model of care, recognizing the impact that diabetes has on *all* members of the family.

In our era of competition for health care resources, it becomes even more critical to ensure that the prevailing philosophy of 'doing less' does not move us backwards in the diabetes care of children and adolescents. Now, more than ever before, a multidisciplinary team is critical for the appropriate translation of advances such as the DCCT recommendations and for the prevention of problems—such as severe hypoglycaemia in the preschool period or premature responsibility for diabetes management by older children—that have plagued previous cohorts of children and families. Now that we can offer hope for a healthy future to young patients, as health care providers and investigators, we must discover the energy and vision to create feasible health care systems to deliver this improved, more advanced and comprehensive treatment to children and their families.

REFERENCES

1. Diabetes Control and Complications Trial Research Group. The effect of intensive treatment of diabetes on the development and progression of long-term complications in insulin-dependent diabetes mellitus. *N Engl J Med* 1993; **329**: 977–86
2. Diabetes Control and Complications Trial Research Group. Effect of intensive diabetes treatment on the development and progression of long-term complications in adolescents with insulin-dependent diabetes mellitus: Diabetes Control and Complications Trial. *J Pediat* 1994; **125**: 177–88
3. Kushion W, Salisbury PJ, Seitz KW, Wilson BE. Issues in the care of infants and toddlers with insulin dependent diabetes mellitus. *Diabetes Educ* 1991; **17**: 107–10
4. Wolfsdorf JI, Anderson BA, Pasquarello C. Treatment of the child with diabetes. In Kahn CR, Weir G (eds) *Joslin's Diabetes Mellitus*, 13th edn. Philadelphia: Lea and Febiger, 1994; 430–51
5. Anderson BJ, Auslander WF. Research on diabetes management and the family: a critique. *Diabetes Care* 1980; **3**: 696–702
6. Silverstein JH, Johnson S. Psychosocial challenge of diabetes and the development of a continuum of care. *Pediat Ann* 1994; **23**: 300–305
7. Faulkner MS, Clark FS. Quality of life for parents of children and adolescents with type 1 diabetes. *Diabetes Educ* 1998; **24**: 721–7
8. Johnson SB. Psychological factors in juvenile diabetes: a review. *J Behav Med* 1980; **3**: 95–116
9. Ryden O, Nevander L, Johnsson P, Hansson K, Kronvall P, Sjoblad S, Westbom L. Family therapy in poorly controlled juvenile IDDM: effects on diabetes control, self-evaluation, and behavioral symptoms. *Acta Paediat* 1994; **83**: 285–91
10. Jacobson AM, Hauser ST, Wertlieb D, Wolfsdorf JI, Orleans J, Vieyra M. Psychological adjustment of children with recently diagnosed diabetes mellitus. *Diabet Care* 1986; **9**: 323–9
11. Wysocki T, Huxtable K, Linscheid TR, Wayne W. Adjustment to diabetes mellitus in pre-schoolers and their mothers. *Diabet Care* 1989; **12**: 524–9

12. Erikson EH. *Childhood and Society*. New York: Norton, 1950
13. Erikson EH. *Identity: Youth and Crisis*. New York: Norton, 1968
14. Bland GL, Wood VD. Diabetes in infancy: diagnosis and current management. *J Natl Med Assoc* 1991; **83**: 361–5
15. Pond JS, Peters ML, Pannell DL, Rogers CS. Psychosocial challenges for children with insulin-dependent diabetes mellitus. *Diabet Educ* 1995; **21**: 297–9
16. Hatton DL, Canam C, Thorne S, Hughes AM. Parents' perceptions of caring for an infant or toddler with diabetes. *J Adv Nurs* 1995; **22**: 569–77
17. Lipman TH, Difazio DA, Meers RA, Thompson RL. A developmental approach to diabetes in children: birth through preschool. *MCN Am J Matern Child Nurs* 1989; **14**: 255–9
18. Achenbach TM, Edelbrock CS. *Manual for the Child Behavior Checklist and Revised Child Behavior Profile*. Burlington, VT: University of Vermont Press, 1983
19. Northam E, Anderson P, Adler R, Werther G, Warne G. Psychosocial and family functioning in children with insulin-dependent diabetes at diagnosis and one year later. *J Pediat Psychol* 1996; **21**: 699–717
20. Eiser C. *Chronic Childhood Disease: An Introduction to Psychological Theory and Research*. New York: Cambridge University Press, 1990
21. Garrison WT, McQuiston S. *Chronic Illness during Childhood and Adolescence*. Newbury Park, CA: Sage, 1989
22. Banion CR, Miles MS, Carter MC. Problems of mothers in management of children with diabetes. *Diabetes Care* 1983; **6**: 548–51
23. Yoos L. Chronic childhood illness: developmental issues. *Pediat Nurs* 1987; **13**: 25–8
24. Ack M, Miller I, Weil WB. Intelligence of children with diabetes mellitus. *Pediatrics* 1961; **28**: 764–70
25. Bale RN. Brain damage in diabetes mellitus. *Br J Psychiat* 1973; **122**: 337–91
26. Holmes CS, Hayford JT, Gonzalez JL, Weydert JA. A survey of cognitive function in different glucose levels in diabetic persons. *Diabet Care* 1983; **6**: 180–83
27. Ryan C, Vega A, Longstreet C, Drash A. Neuropsychological changes in adolescents with insulin-independent diabetes. *J Consult Clin Psychol* 1984; **52**: 335–42
28. Ryan C, Longstreet C, Morrow L. The effects of diabetes mellitus on the school attendance and school achievement of adolescents. *Child Care Health Dev* 1985; **11**: 229–40
29. Ryan C, Vega A, Drash A. Cognitive deficits in adolescents who developed diabetes early in life. *Pediatrics* 1985; **75**: 921–7
30. Rovet JF, Ehrlich RM, Hoppe M. Intellectual deficits associated with early onset of insulin-dependent diabetes mellitus in children. *Diabet Care* 1987; **10**: 510–15
31. Golden MP, Ingersoll GM, Brack CJ, Russell BA, Wright JC, Huberty TJ. Longitudinal relationship of asymptomatic hypoglycaemia to cognitive function in IDDM. *Diabet Care* 1989; **12**: 89–93
32. Rovet JF, Ehrlich RM, Czuchta D. Intellectual characteristics of diabetic children at diagnosis and one year later. *J Pediat Psychol* 1990; **15**: 775–88
33. Northam EA, Anderson PJ, Werther GA, Warne GL, Adler RG, Andrewes D. Neuropsychological complications of IDDM in children 2 years after disease onset. *Diabet Care* 1998; **21**: 379–84
34. Golden MP, Russell BP, Ingersoll GM, Gray DL, Hummer KM. Management of diabetes in children younger than 5 years of age. *Am J Dis Child* 1985; **139**: 448–52

35. Drash AL. The child, the adolescent, and the Diabetes Control and Complications Trial. *Diabet Care* 1993; **16**: 1515–16
36. Brink SJ, Moltz K. The message of the DCCT for children and adolescents. *Diabet Spectrum* 1997; **10**: 259–67
37. Herskowitz Dumont R, Jacobson AM, Cole C, Hauser ST, Wolfsdorf JI, Willett JB, Milley JE, Wertlieb D. Psychosocial predictors of acute complications of diabetes in youth. *Diabet Med* 1995; **12**: 612–18
38. Liss DS, Waller DA, Kennard BD, McIntire D, Capra P, Stephens J. Psychiatric illness and family support in children and adolescents with diabetic ketoacidosis: a controlled study. *J Am Acad Child Adolesc Psychiat* 1998; **37**: 536–44
39. Bregani P, Della Porta V, Carbone A *et al.* Attitude of juvenile diabetics and their families towards dietetic regimen. *Pediat Adolesc Endocrinol* 1979; **7**: 159–63
40. Zuppinger K, Schmid E., Schutz B. Attitude of juvenile diabetics, his family and peers toward a dietetic regimen. *Pediat Adolesc Endocrinol* 1979; **7**: 153–8
41. Leaverton DR. The child with diabetes mellitus. In Noshpitz JD (eds) *Basic Handbook of Child Psychiatry*, vol I. New York: Basic Books, 1979; 452
42. Kovacs M, Brent D, Steinberg TF, Paulauskas S, Reid J. Children's self-reports of psychologic adjustment and coping strategies during first year of insulin-dependent diabetes mellitus. *Diabet Care* 1986; **9**: 472–9
43. Lipman TH, Difazio DA, Meers RA, Thompson RL. A developmental approach to diabetes in children: school-age through adolescence. *MCN Am J Matern Child Nurs* 1989; **14**: 330–32
44. Balik B, Haig B, Moynihan PM. Diabetes and the school-aged child. *MCN Am J Matern Child Nurs* 1986; **11**: 324–30
45. Puczynski MS, Puczynski SS, Reich J, Kaspar JC, Emanuele M. Mental efficiency and hypoglycaemia. *J Dev Behav Pediat* 1990; **11**: 170–74
46. Franz MJ, Horton ES Sr, Bantle JP, Beebe CA, Brunzell JD, Coulston AM, Henry RR, Hoogwerf BJ, Stacpoole PW. Nutrition principles for the management of diabetes and related complications. *Diabet Care* 1994; **17**: 490–518
47. Waller D, Chipman JJ, Hardy BW, Hightower MS, North AJ, Williams SB, Babick AJ. Measuring diabetes-specific family support and its relation to metabolic control: a preliminary report. *J Am Acad Child Psychol* 1986; **25**: 415–18
48. Marteau TM, Bloch S, Baum JD. Family life and diabetic control. *J Child Psychol Psychiat* 1987; **28**: 823–33
49. Hauser ST, Jacobson AM, Lavori P, Wolfsdorf JI, Herskowitz RD, Milley JE, Bliss R, Gelfand E, Wertlieb D, Stein J. Adherence among children and adolescents with insulin-dependent diabetes mellitus over four-year longitudinal follow-up. II. Immediate and long-term linkages with the family milieu. *J Pediat Psychol* 1990; **15**: 527–42
50. Auslander WF, Bubb J, Rogge M, Santiago JV. Family stress and resources: potential areas of intervention in children recently diagnosed with diabetes. *Health Soc Work* 1993; **18**: 101–13
51. Miller-Johnson S, Emery RE, Marvin RS, Clarke W, Lovinger R, Martin M. Parent–child relationships and the management of diabetes mellitus. *J Consult Clin Psychol* 1994; **62**: 603–10
52. Jacobson AM, Hauser ST, Lavori P, Willett JB, Cole CF, Wolfsdorf JI, Dumont RH, Wertlieb D. Family environment and glycemic control: a four-year prospective study of children and adolescents with insulin-dependent diabetes mellitus. *Psychosom Med* 1994; **56**: 401–9

53. Goldston DB, Kovacs M, Obrosky S, Iyengar S. A longitudinal study of life events and metabolic control among youths with insulin-dependent diabetes mellitus. *Health Psychol* 1995; **14**: 409–14
54. Viner R, McGrath M, Trudinger P. Family stress and metabolic control in diabetes. *Arch Dis Child* 1996; **74**: 418–21
55. Chase HP, Jackson GG. Stress and sugar control in children with insulin-dependent diabetes mellitus. *J Pediat* 1981; **98**: 1011–13
56. Hauenstein EJ, Marvin RS, Snyder AL, Clarke WL. Stress in parents of children with diabetes mellitus. *Diabet Care* 1989; **12**: 18–23
57. Kovacs M, Kass RE, Schnell TM, Goldston D, Marsh J. Family functioning and metabolic control of school-aged children with IDDM. *Diabet Care* 1989;**12**: 409–14
58. Jacobson AM, Hauser ST, Lavori P, Wolfsdorf JI, Herskowitz RD, Milley JE, Bliss R, Gelfand E, Wertlieb D, Stein J. Adherence among children and adolescents with insulin-dependent diabetes mellitus over four-year longitudinal follow-up. I. The influence of patient coping and adjustment. *J Pediat Psychol* 1990;**15**: 511–26
59. Parker H, Swift PGF, Botha JL. Early onset diabetes: parents' views. *Diabet Med* 1994; **11**: 593–6
60. Burns KL, Green P, Chase HP. Psychosocial correlates of glycemic control as a function of age in youth with IDDM. *J Adolesc Health Care* 1986; **7**: 311–19
61. Ingersoll GM, Orr DP, Herrold AJ, Golden MP. Cognitive maturity and self-management among adolescents with insulin-dependent diabetes mellitus. *J Pediat* 1986; **108**: 620–23
62. Anderson BJ, Auslander WF, Jung KC, Miller JP, Santiago JV. Assessing family sharing of diabetes responsibilities. *J Pediat Psychol* 1990; **15**: 477–92
63. Weissberg-Benchell J, Glasgow AM, Tynan WD, Wirtz P, Turek J, Ward J. Adolescent diabetes management and mismanagement. *Diabet Care* 1995; **18**: 77–82
64. Wysocki T, Taylor A, Hough BS, Linsheid TR, Yeates KO, Naglieri JA. Deviation for developmentally appropriate self-care autonomy. Association with diabetes outcomes. *Diabetes Care* 1996; **19**: 119–25
65. Anderson B, Ho J, Brackett J, Finkelstein D, Laffel L. Parental involvement in diabetes management tasks: relationships to blood glucose monitoring adherence and metabolic control in young adolescents with insulin-dependent diabetes mellitus. *J Pediat* 1997; **130**: 257–65
66. Allen DA, Tennen H, McGrade BJ, Affleck G, Ratzan S. Parent and child perceptions of the management of juvenile diabetes. *J Pediat Psychol* 1983; **8**: 129–41
67. Rubin R, Young-Hyman D, Peyrot M. Parent–child responsibility and conflict in diabetes care. *Diabetes* 1989; **38** (suppl 2), 28
68. LaGreca AM. Children with diabetes and their families: coping and disease management. In Field T, McCabe P, Schneiderman N (eds) *Stress and Coping across Development*. Hillsdale, NJ: Erlbaum, 1988; 139–59
69. Follansbee DS. Assuming responsibility for diabetes management: What age? What price? *Diabet Educ* 1989; **15**: 347–52
70. Jacobson AM, Hauser ST, Wolfsdorf JI , Houlihan J, Milley JE, Herskowitz RD, Wertlieb D, Watt BA. Psychologic predictors of compliance in children with recent onset of diabetes mellitus. *J Pediat* 1987; **110**: 805–11
71. Kovacs M, Iyengar S, Goldston D. Stewart J, Obrosky DS, Marsh J. Psychological functioning of children with insulin-dependent diabetes mellitus: a longitudinal study. *J Pediat Psychol* 1990a; **15**: 619–32

72. Kovacs M, Iyengar S, Goldston D. Obrosky DS, Marsh J. Psychological functioning among mothers of children with insulin-dependent diabetes mellitus: a longitudinal study. *J Consult Clin Psychol* 1990b; **58**: 189–95
73. Kovacs M, Goldston D, Obrosky DS, Iyengar S. Prevalence and predictors of pervasive noncompliance with medical treatment among youths with insulin-dependent diabetes mellitus. *J Am Acad Child Adolesc Psychiat* 1992; **31**: 1112–19
74. Grey M, Cameron ME, Lipman TH, Thurber FW. Psychosocial status of children with diabetes in the first 2 years after diagnosis. *Diabet Care* 1995; **18**: 1330–36
75. Kovacs M, Feinberg TL, Paulauskas S, Finkelstein R, Pollock M, Crouse-Novak M. Initial coping responses and psychosocial characteristics of children with insulin-dependent diabetes mellitus. *J Pediat* 1985; **106**: 827–34
76. Kovacs M, Finkelstein R, Feinberg TL, Crouse-Novak M, Paulauskas S, Pollock M. Initial psychologic responses of parents to the diagnosis of insulin-dependent diabetes mellitus in their children. *Diabet Care* 1985; **8**: 568–75
77. Jacobson AM, Hauser ST, Willet J, Wolfsdorf JI, Herman L. Consequences of irregular vs. continuous medical follow-up in children and adolescents with insulin-dependent diabetes mellitus. *J Pediat* 1997; **131**: 727–33
78. Auslander WF, Anderson BJ, Bubb J, Jung KC, Santiago JV. Risk factors to health in diabetic children: a prosective study from diagnosis. *Health Soc Work* 1990; **15**: 133–42
79. Auslander WF, Thompson S, Dreitzer D, White NH, Santiago JV. Disparity in glycemic control and adherence between African–American and Caucasian youths with diabetes. Family and community contexts. *Diabet Care* 1997; **20**: 1569–75
80. Overstreet S, Goins J, Chen RS, Holmes CS, Greer T, Dunlap WP, Frentz J. Family environment and the interrelation of family structure, child behavior, and metabolic control for children with diabetes. *J Pediat Psychol* 1995; **20**: 435–47
81. Charron-Prochownik D, Kovacs M, Obrosky DS, Ho V. Illness characteristics and psychosocial and demographic correlates of illness severity at onset of insulin-dependent diabetes mellitus among school-age children. *J Pediat Nurs* 1995; **10**: 354–9
82. Kovacs M, Charron-Prochownik D, Obrosky DS. A longitudinal study of biomedical and psychosocial predictors of multiple hospitalizations among young people with insulin-dependent diabetes mellitus. *Diabet Med* 1995; **12**: 142–8
83. Wolfsdorf JI, Laffel LMB. Diabetes in childhood: predicting the future. *Pediat Ann* 1994; **23**: 306–12
84. Hamburg BA, Inoff GE. Predictable crises of diabetes. *Diabet Care* 1983; **6**: 409–16

2

Diabetes During Adolescence

T. CHAS SKINNER[a], SUE CHANNON[b], LESLEY HOWELLS[c] and ADELE McEVILLY[d]

[a] University Hospital Lewisham, London, UK; [b] Heath Hospital, Cardiff, UK; [c] Ninewells Hospital Medical School, Dundee, UK; [d] Children's Hospital, Birmingham, UK

INTRODUCTION

There is no widely accepted precise definition of what adolescence is, but it is commonly referred to as the transitional period between childhood and adulthood. As this not the place to discuss the social, cultural, historical or political construction of adolescence, for the purposes of this chapter adolescence is taken as referring to young people between 12 and 20 years old, thereby mapping fairly closely the teenage years.

Whatever definition you use, the adolescent years are clearly a period of rapid change and development. Children progress through the education system to compete with adults for resources and jobs. This is accompanied by continued cognitive development, enabling young people to think in increasingly abstract ways and to become less receptive to authority figures. As they compete for jobs or higher education places, teenagers are attempting to establish their identity and lifestyle, and quite early on have to make choices that will affect their long-term career aspirations. Adolescents spend increasing amounts of time away from home, and their leisure activities become less structured, with ever-diminishing adult supervision or involvement. It is during this period that we learn how to form and maintain friendships and close intimate relationship with our peers. With puberty comes the adjustment to a changing body and interest in sexual relationships. The timing of puberty can also have a substantial impact on adolescent development, with

Psychology in Diabetes Care. Edited by Frank J. Snoek and T. Chas Skinner.

early or late onset of puberty having markedly different effects on boys' and girls' psychosocial development. With all these changes occurring in a relatively short period, probably ending with the adoption of lifestyles that will endure through adulthood, it would seem reasonable to suggest that adolescence provides us with the opportunity of having a lasting and significant impact on the health and well-being of individuals.

Adolescence is a particularly critical time for young people with diabetes. Whether diagnosed in childhood or adolescence, it is during the adolescent years that the individual learns to take increasing responsibility for the management of his/her diabetes[1–3]. As they start to integrate their diabetes management tasks into their emerging lifestyles, teenagers directly experience the relationship between their actions and blood glucose tests, if they do any. This will in turn influence their beliefs about diabetes, its treatment and how they will manage it. Therefore, these will be formative years in the development of such beliefs, which, once fully integrated and accepted by the young person, may prove difficult to change.

Adolescence is also frequently seen as a time to change and intensify insulin regimens. Whether this is in response to trying to make diabetes management more flexible to fit with the young person's lifestyle, or in an attempt to improve diabetes control, intensifying regimens adds to the demands of diabetes. The additional pressures to test blood glucose and adjust insulin can mean that intensification will result in increasing intrusiveness making the social life of young people even more difficult.

Research consistently demonstrates that during adolescent there is a marked decline in metabolic control[4–6]. Although this decline is partly attributable to the physiological changes occurring at this time[7,8], the decline in self-care seen during adolescence is of equal if not greater importance[9–11]. This deterioration is particularly marked and of concern in the area of insulin administration. Although self-report data suggested that missed insulin injections were common, the pharmacy record data from the DARTS database demonstrates that about 28% of young adults do not even obtain sufficient insulin to meet their prescribed regimen[11].

In addition to insufficient insulin resulting in hyperglycaemia, repeated failure to inject insulin can result in diabetic ketoacidosis (DKA). Post-diagnoses and recurrent DKA, in the absence of other medical complications, is commonly caused by low levels of insulin administration[12], with the incidence of recurrent DKA peaking during adolescence[22].

As if these diabetes burdens were not enough, for many young people, especially those diagnosed early in life, their annual review will begin to include screening for the complications of diabetes, adding to their anxieties and emotional burden. It is not surprising, then, that young people are more likely to drop out of the system and not attend outpatient clinics[47,48]. Furthermore, with the emphasis on monitoring diet and weight, young people, particularly young females, are at a greater risk of developing disordered eating patterns[74,75], which may lead to clinical eating disorders.

This brief summary makes it clear that adolescents with diabetes are in the unenviable position of facing the same developmental tasks and demands as other young people, in addition to learning to manage and live with their diabetes. This poses healthcare professionals and parents with numerous challenges as they seek to maintain or improve diabetes control through this transitional phase, without depriving young people of the appropriate age-related experiences to enable development and growth.

This complex array of diabetes and general developmental issues has generated a wealth of literature on the psychological aspects of paediatric chronic illness, and diabetes in particular. In order to review this literature and consider the implications for diabetes care, the determinants of three outcomes will be considered: the mental health of individuals (commonly referred to as adjustment, adaptation, well-being); the health behaviour of the person with diabetes (incorporating compliance, adherence, self-care and self-management); and the health status or metabolic control of diabetes. Quality of life will not be considered in this review, as it is a relatively new construct to be incorporated into paediatric health psychology, and there is little research using validated measures upon which to draw.

To provide this chapter with a relatively coherent structure, it will move progressively from more individual psychological constructs, such as personality and beliefs, to increasingly social constructs, such as stress, and coping, before considering the role of the familial, peer and professional support the adolescent receives. Throughout, the practical implications of the research will be highlighted and areas for future research considered, with these practical implications being summarized again at conclusion of the chapter.

KNOWLEDGE AND SKILLS

It would seem natural to assume that knowledge of diabetes and its management, and competence in the accompanying injection, glucose monitoring and problem-solving skills are important determinants of patients' self-management behaviour and control of their diabetes. A series of meta-analyses and reviews consistently demonstrate that knowledge is predictive of better self-care and control[13–16], but the strength of the association is relatively modest, with standardized β coefficients ranging from 0.14 to 0.41. However, it should be noted that the association between knowledge skills and adherence is notably higher for adolescents than for adults, ($r = 0.41$ and $r = 0.15$ respectively[16]). Why this should be the case is unclear, with several conflicting explanations possible, which warrant further investigation.

Regardless of this finding, despite the abundance of education at diagnoses, it should be remembered that the emotional upheaval experienced at this time may also serve to prevent retention of knowledge. Furthermore, for those diagnosed in childhood, the vast majority of education is targeted at the parents, with a formal programme of education for adolescents being the rare exception rather than the rule. We also cannot assume that parental knowledge, skills and experience will automatically be transferred to the growing child, or that parents always have the depth of knowledge and understanding necessary for them to educate their child.

That education and skills training may well succeed in making the individual more skilled and knowledgeable is not disputed, but this does not in itself guarantee changes in the individual's behaviour and control of his/her diabetes, an issue that is frequently not considered. For example some researchers have assumed that poor self-care may be the result of adolescents lacking the skills necessary to deal with the social consequences of managing their diabetes appropriately. This resulted in interventions geared at improving adolescents' social/stress management skills[17–20]. However, in only one of these studies[19] did the intervention have a significant impact on diabetes control. Although the lack of significant results in these studies may be attributable to a number of methodological factors, it may well be that a lack of social skills is not the issue.

Thomas and colleagues[21] assessed the problem-solving skills in social situations of adolescents with diabetes. Despite the fact that the young people could generate a range of solutions to the dilemmas posed, they deliberately chose less regimen-adherent and more peer-acceptable actions. This suggests that the adolescents did not lack the social/stress management skills necessary to manage their diabetes appropriately, they consciously chose not to use them. This is further supported by data indicating that young people with the greatest social skills actually had the poorest control of their diabetes[19]. This suggests that although diabetes knowledge and skills are necessary for good diabetes management, there are no guarantees that this knowledge and skill will be utilized by the adolescent. However, it should never be assumed that adolescents have the requisite skills and knowledge for successful diabetes management. As a result, ensuring adolescents have adequate knowledge and problem-solving skills should be a fundamental first step in any programme of adolescent diabetes care or intervention for adolescents[23,24].

PERSONALITY

Since it was established that there is no such thing as a 'diabetic personality', researchers have to a large extent abandoned the examination of causal relations between personality and diabetes self-care, metabolic control and adjustment. Although a few studies have examined personality or temperament as predictors of diabetes outcomes, they have provided equivocal results[25–28,78,85,97,102]. The confusing nature of these results may well be a result of the fact that personality is still undergoing development throughout adolescence[29,30]. In addition, it is only within the last decade that personality researchers have begun to form a consensus about the core personality traits, namely the 'big five', extroversion, agreeableness, emotional stability, openness to experience/intellect and conscientiousness[31–33]. Furthermore, broad personality types in adolescents, based on the related dimensions of ego resiliency, ego control and the 'big five' personality constructs, are stable across populations and related to a range of adjustment measures in adolescents[34].

This also highlights the relatively consistent results of research that has looked at the ego development of children and adolescents with diabetes. Several studies have found that more mature ego development (impulse control, moral development, quality of interpersonal relations) is associated with better control of diabetes, both cross-sectionally[35,36], and in a 4 year prospective longitudinal study[37]. Furthermore, mature ego development has also been associated with better metabolic control and higher self-esteem[38]. With recent research indicating that ego strength (dependability, trust, lack of impulsivity) is associated with longevity and protective health behaviours[39] this is clearly an area worth further investigating.

Potentially, interventions may be able to enhance ego development, particularly impulse control, and provide long-term benefits for young people with diabetes that may also generalize to other aspects of their lives. Knowledge of an adolescent's personality may enable educators to fit their programmes, both in terms of style and content, more closely to the individual's needs. For instance, more extraverted young people may gain more from group sessions, whereas more introverted adolescents may have a greater need for social skills training.

BELIEFS, COGNITIONS AND ATTITUDES

Much of what we do and say is determined by the way we conceptualize and perceive our environment. It would therefore be rather surprising if our internal representations of ourselves and environment did not play a profound role in influencing our behaviour and our emotions. As a result, psychology has generated a plethora of theories (e.g. Health Belief Model, Theory of Reasoned Action, Protection Motivation Theory, Self-efficacy

Theory, etc.) in an attempt to provide a coherent means by which to conceptualize our cognitions and their interaction.

However, the research on adolescent diabetes has rarely set out to test any of these social cognition models, with some notable exceptions[40–43]. Instead, researchers have tended to include a diverse range of constructs in their study protocols. Therefore, rather than evaluate the theories used by researchers, conceptually similar constructs will be considered here, to evaluate their utility in predicting health outcomes in adolescent diabetes. Constructs in three key areas will be considered: (a) *illness representations*, which are constructs that refer to the individual's beliefs about his/her diabetes; (b) *self-beliefs*, which refer to the beliefs individuals hold about themselves and their abilities; and (c) *strategy or outcome beliefs*, which refer to beliefs about strategies and obstacles to managing diabetes and the consequences of these strategies and outcomes.

ILLNESS REPRESENTATIONS

Different conceptualizations or theories have been utilized to structure the way people think about their illness episodes. However, these are largely theoretically driven models, developed within a Westernized biomedical view of health and illness. An alternative approach to illness representations is to look for consistencies in the lay person's conceptualizations of illness episodes, and use these lay models as a guide. Stemming from work in medical anthropology, personal models of illness are derived from this line of reasoning. From a relatively atheoretical standpoint, researchers using a range of different methodologies have come to agree on five basic dimensions to the way we think about illness. These are: the illness's identity and associated symptoms; its cause; the consequences of the illness; how long it will last; and treatment efficacy[44–46]. Using the personal models approach has the additional benefit that the constructs used by researchers not using this paradigm can be readily transferred and interpreted within these five broad domains.

Although not explicitly measuring illness identity, some studies note that those adolescents who report more symptoms have poorer control of their diabetes[35,49]. The problem here is the direction of causality, as it would be expected that those in poor control of their diabetes, with its extremes of blood glucose levels, are more likely to experience the symptoms that are associated with diabetes, compared to those who control their blood glucose within or close to the normal range. The other aspects of an illness's identity, such as what is wrong with the patient, what is insulin, etc., are very much a part of diabetes education and, as such, would be subsumed into the area of diabetes knowledge.

Causal beliefs or attributions have received little research attention, but a couple of studies have examined the individual's attributional style. Brown and colleagues[52] found that children who tended to make more internal, stable and global attributions for negative events had better glycaemic control. The same group of researchers, looking at adjustment across three chronic illness groups, also report that a more pessimistic attributional style was associated with poorer self-rated adjustment[53].

One personal model construct that has received more attention is that of the consequences of having diabetes. These studies use measures of perceived severity of diabetes, perceived susceptibility to complications, perceived impact and a combined threat of diabetes measure, and have failed to provide any consistent results in relation to self-care or metabolic control[40–42,54–7].

A more immediate consequence of managing diabetes is the problem of severe hypoglycaemia. With the risk of coma or even death, it is not surprising that Green and colleagues[58], in a replication of adult work, found that those adolescents who were more worried about hypoglycaemia had poorer metabolic control of glycated haemoglobin. However, whether this is a function of self-management to avoid hypos, or the effects of increased anxiety has not been established. Those young people who worry excessively about hypoglycaemia, and seek to avoid it, may especially benefit from Blood Glucose Awareness Training (see Chapter 8), to have more confidence in their ability to detect the early signs of hypoglycaemia and take earlier remedial action to prevent it[97].

Although perceptions about the consequences of diabetes have been inconsistently related to self-care or metabolic control, these perceptions are consistently associated with psychological adjustment[54,55,57,59–61]. This suggests that using fear of complications to motivate young people is not an approach that should be used lightly, and that it is critical that, when discussing the complications of diabetes, young people should at the same time discuss how they can work to avoid these complications. Fear should not be used in isolation: if it is, it is frequently counter-productive, increasing anxiety and depression, which may then in turn adversely affect self-care and metabolic control.

SELF-BELIEFS

Beliefs individuals hold about themselves and their abilities can be categorized into three broad domains; value, capacity and control beliefs. Self-value beliefs, such as self-esteem and self-concept, reflect the way individuals describe or perceive themselves. These beliefs are typically measured using value judgements, self-descriptions or self-discrepancy models. However, these are primarily considered in the literature as indicators of adjustment or emotional well-being, and as such are seen to influence self-care and metabolic control in the same way as these more generic indices.

Self-capacity beliefs refer to individuals' beliefs in their ability to perform a task, and are similar to the concept of confidence. The construct widely used here is self-efficacy, which has been consistently related to adolescents' health behaviour[42,62–64], with further studies reporting an association between self-efficacy and measures of metabolic control[57,65,66]. A further study[67] found that adolescents who perceived themselves to have the energy and will power needed to manage their diabetes were in better control. Furthermore, Grey and colleagues[68] found that higher self-efficacy was associated with better quality of life, less depression and higher self-esteem.

These studies are all cross-sectional and do not resolve the issue about the direction of causality. Theoretically, with skilled support and education utilizing the principles underlying Bandura's work on enhancing self-efficacy[69], and Vygotsky's work on supporting cognitive development[70], health care professionals and parents should be able to enhance adolescents' sense of competence and confidence in managing their diabetes.

However, one major barrier to achieving this, especially in adolescents, with the unpredictable effects of growth hormones to be considered, is the apparent lack of immediate response of their blood glucose tests to their self-management efforts. If self-efficacy is to be enhanced, it is essential that health care professionals focus on young people's behaviour, not their blood glucose records or metabolic control. This involves a huge change in habit, as it requires that the consultation is focused on an adolescent's actual behaviour, which means that the adolescent has to be comfortable with being honest and feel that he/she is respected and valued unconditionally[71]. Added to this change of focus to behaviour rather than physiology, it is equally imperative that health care professionals change their emphasis from the negative, and what has not been done, to the positive, and seek out success in young people, even if 'success' only means that they actually *told* you they did not do any glucose tests.

Control beliefs refer to individuals' perceptions of the control they have over their life and environment, and can be seen to reflect their beliefs in self-determination, karma or fate. The most commonly used construct in this area is locus of control, which was initially thought of as a continuum, with an internal locus at one end (self-determining) and an external locus at the other end (luck, fate, no control). Using a general measure of locus of control, several studies reported that it was not associated with metabolic control[18,65,72,73,76–79]. However, more recent developments in this area now consider locus of control along three distinct dimensions, with the external dimension split into the roles of 'powerful others' and 'chance factors', and also highlight the need to measure control perceptions specific to the domain under investigation. In the light of these theoretical developments, researchers have used health and diabetes-specific locus of control questionnaires, but unfortunately, these studies have similarly failed to generate consistent results[7,18,81,82,84], although two studies have suggested that greater perceptions of control are related to psychological adjustment[86,87].

The failure to find a consistent relationship between perceived control and health outcomes is surprising, considering the results using this construct in adults[88,89]. However, it should be remembered that adolescence is a developmental period in which young people are being given increasing amounts of responsibility and independence. Their own behavioural responses, therefore, are at times limited by adults, and this may be reflected in their control beliefs. More pragmatically, though, the research in this area has almost exclusively relied on blood glucose control as its dependent variable, where behavioural measures are more relevant. Furthermore, this research has examined only linear associations, when it may be that more realistic beliefs are adaptive for promoting diabetes self-care and control. Believing that everything is under our control, or that everything is due to chance are self-evidently maladaptive beliefs.

STRATEGY BELIEFS

Strategy beliefs, which incorporate outcome expectancies, relate to individuals' beliefs about the strategies they may adopt to manage their diabetes, their efficacy, consequences and outcomes. Traditionally, the research in this area has used two key constructs; benefits of and barriers to (or costs of) diabetes self-management. Although results with these constructs in relation to metabolic control have been contradictory[40,41], they are consistent predictors of self-care behaviour. The more barriers to adherence reported, the poorer adolescents' self-care[41,42,90,91], and the greater the ratio of benefits to barriers/costs, the better their self-care[40,90].

Although derived from lay representations of illness, treatment efficacy is also closely related to these constructs, particularly the benefits of adherence. Where adolescents' perception of the efficacy of the diabetes management regimen has been assessed, it has been consistently related to self-care behaviour. The more efficacious they think their treatment regimen is to manage their diabetes, the better their self-care[42,55,59,92,93]. However, more recently researchers have made a distinction between efficacy of the regimen to control diabetes and efficacy of treatment to prevent complications. Although both constructs were associated with self-care, it was the short-term beliefs about controlling diabetes that were consistently the better predictors of self-care behaviour, both cross-sectionally and prospectively[50,51,55,59].

Although the research on adolescents' beliefs has covered a broad spectrum of constructs, very few have attempted to test particular social cognition models. On top of this lack of theoretical coherence, these studies are subject to a wealth of criticism. In essence, these studies are attempting to predict behaviour from cross-sectional assessment of beliefs. However, as Weinstein and colleagues recently pointed out[94], these studies are actually conducting analyses that reflect individuals' accuracy of perceptions or cognitions, rather than testing any causal hypotheses. Furthermore, almost exclusively the research reviewed here failed to control for past behaviour, when this has been shown to be the most important predictor of current and future behaviour[94]. So, although this research has identified several key constructs, it provides no clues as to which of these are determining behaviour and which are determined by behaviour. Prospective and intervention studies are clearly indicated if the role of cognitions, beliefs and attitudes are to be considered as key determinants of self-care behaviour, metabolic control or well-being in adolescents.

STRESS AND COPING

It has been postulated that stress may affect diabetes control either directly, through the stress hormones affecting blood glucose levels and insulin metabolism, or indirectly, through stress leading to changes in self-care behaviour. A number of studies have found an association between stress and glycaemic control[35,95,96,98–105], although some studies have not replicated these results[82,107–110,112,113], possibly due to relatively smaller sample sizes or the use of unvalidated measures. However, together with the adult literature, this data has led to the widely accepted conclusion that diabetic control is affected by stress in a young person's life, although these studies do not resolve the mechanisms of influence. Although several studies report no association between stress and adherence[100,101,105,110] in their 6 year longitudinal analysis of 52 children and adolescents with diabetes, Goldston and colleagues[99] found that the psychiatric diagnosis of non-compliance with medical treatment (based on DSM III criteria) was associated with life event scores, and both stress and non-compliance were associated with poor metabolic control. The substantial difference in results between this and other studies linking adherence and stress is the use of the number of days that an individual would meet a psychiatric diagnosis of non-compliance. This is at the extreme end of the self-care spectrum and dichotomizes the self-care behaviour of individuals. The strength of the association in this data suggests that there may be a floor effect in the relationship between stress and self-care, which would not be highlighted with the linear analysis used in the other studies in this area.

In contrast, when using structural equation modelling with a sample of 127 young people with diabetes, Hanson and colleagues[101] found that stress was indirectly associated with adherence via its effect on family relations. However, the effect size of this pathway was much weaker than for the direct effect of stress on metabolic control. Further support for direct physiological effects comes from a study using an exercise stress test. Yasar and colleagues found that this task induced an increase in blood sugar levels in only about a third of their sample of children and adolescents with IDDM[111]; for this subgroup only, this change in blood sugar levels correlated with changes in the blood norepinephrine and epinephrine levels, which are known to increase when experiencing psychological stress.

Although it is not possible to experimentally manipulate the life stress experienced by young people with diabetes, an alternative approach is to try and change their stress-management behaviours. Two studies have attempted to improve the stress-management behaviours of adolescents[17,20]. Both studies showed a significant improvement in daily hassles, especially those related to diabetes management, but the interventions failed to impact significantly on either self-care or glycaemic control of participants. These negative results could well be a function of a number of confounding factors, especially with the small sample sizes involved. They could be a consequence of individual differences in stress reactivity[111,116–119], which would mean that these programmes would only have a significant impact on blood glucose regulation for those young people who are highly stress-reactive. This is an issue which clearly needs resolving if the role of stress in diabetes control is to be illuminated. In addition to individual differences in reactivity, some evidence suggests that there may be substantial variation in the types of stresses people respond to[117,118]. These results, which replicate work with adults, suggest that for a stress-reactive subgroup of individuals, stress mainly affects blood glucose control through direct physiological mechanisms, although there may be also be a small indirect effect on control via health behaviour. Therefore, it would seem reasonable to conclude that offering stress-management training interventions to all young people would not be cost-effective. These approaches should be targeted at a stress-reactive minority. DuTour and colleagues'[119] data from an adult study suggests that individuals can tell how reactive to stress they are, and are possibly capable of self-selecting for this kind of intervention. However, adolescents may lack the experience and/or insight to determine whether they are stress-reactive, and some assessment may be needed.

In relation to psychological adjustment, experiencing fewer life events has been found to be consistently associated with better psychological adjustment[48,102,105,109]. However, the number of studies in this area is limited, and this work needs replication before an association can be considered definitive.

Considering the lay perspectives of people eating, drinking or smoking in times of stress, the weak relationship between stress and self-care is surprising[120]. One factor that may explain these results is consideration of individual differences, such as coping style or personality type as a mediator or moderator of the impact of stress in the adolescent's life.

Several studies have documented a move from more problem-focused or primary coping in childhood to more emotion-focused coping in adolescents[121], with young people with diabetes being no dif-ferent[72,84,87,110,122]. This raises the question whether the decline in self-care seen in many adolescents is a function of their uptake of more emotion-focused coping strategies. However, the research to date has generated conflicting results for blood glucose control, two studies reporting an association between coping style and blood glucose control[84,102], whilst two further studies report no such association[107,110]. The conflicting nature of these results is not surprising, as again association between coping and control would be expected to be indirect via their self-management behaviour. A couple of studies have reported on associations between coping and self-care, both of which supported the suggestion that more emotion-focused coping or avoidance was associated with poorer health behaviour[87,122].

However, it is the interaction between stress and coping that is probably most important, and was examined in a more detailed Japanese study by Nakumara and Kanematsu[103]. They found that more stressed adolescents were more likely to cope by using more ventilation, eating, avoiding home and praying. When looking at their self-care behaviour, it was these coping strategies in combination with high stress that were associated with poorer self-care. Similarly, when predicting diabetes control, it was those young people who had low stress and higher coping scores that had better control.

Similar results have been found for the relationship between coping strategies and psychological adjustment, with more emotion-focused coping associated with worse adaptation[72,102,110]. Research to date suggests that coping styles could play an important role in explaining the decline in self-care and metabolic control in adolescents. This is clearly an area requiring further work, but at present the data would suggest that trying to encourage young people to use a greater range of more problem-focused coping strategies may be a useful means by which to help them live with and manage their diabetes. Indeed, using coping skills training as an adjunct to intensifying adolescents' insulin regimens, had a significant impact on adolescents' metabolic control, quality of life and ability to cope with diabetes, compared with only intensifying the injection regimen[60].

SOCIAL ENVIRONMENT

The vast majority of research on young people's social environment has been focused on the family. This can be considered to consist of two broad aspects, its objective composition (such as number, age and gender of siblings, including birth order) and its subjective experience of social interactions. With the changing nature of our society, parent–child relations can take on increasingly varied forms, and although the traditional family, a child living with their two biological parents, is probably still the norm, there are increasing numbers of children in one-parent and reconstituted families.

Some studies have reported that young people in non-traditional families have poorer diabetes control than children in traditional families[123,124]. In a more detailed analysis of family composition, Marteau and colleagues[125] found that it was only children not living with a biological parent (always the mother in this study) that were in significantly worse metabolic control. However, neither of these studies made attempts to match their comparison group. With changes in family composition arising from separation, divorce, bereavement and remarriage, all of which are accompanied by changes in finances, personal resources and the family environment, it is important to at least to control for some of these factors.

This was highlighted by Hanson and colleagues[126] who compared 30 traditional families with 30 matched father-absent families. Their analysis indicated that, although there were no differences between groups on metabolic control of diabetes, the father-absent adolescents with diabetes were more adherent to their treatment than adolescents from the traditional families. Although not conclusive, this more methodologically rigorous study would suggest that it is probably not the actual family composition *per se* that is important, but the subjective elements of the family environment that is important when considering health in adolescents.

The role of the family environment in supporting the young person with diabetes is probably the most extensively researched area on adolescent and childhood diabetes. To provide a means of integrating the very disparate operationalizations used in the research, two dimensions that family researchers, reviewers and theorists have consistently identified will be used. The labels more usually used for these dimensions are *family support* and *family control*. Family support comprises behaviours which foster in an individual feelings of comfort and belonging, and that he/she is basically accepted and approved of as a person by the parents and family. Family control reflects an environment which directs the behaviour of an individual in a manner desirable to the parents, to the power base in the family[127].

A number of studies report significant associations between family support and psychological adjustment[124,128–131], with two smaller studies reporting no significant association between family support and adjustment[132,133]. In a review of the general paediatric literature, Drotar[134] concluded, that, although most studies found an association between support and adjustment, with better adjustment associated with more supportive families, this finding is by no means universal.

Although several studies report significant associations between family support and glycated haemoglobin, with greater support associated with better control[49,82,101,123,125,131,135,140], there are an equally impressive number of studies failing to support this association[73,81,84,91,121,124,128,141,143,144], with longitudinal studies also producing mixed results[121,123,136,142,143]. However, family support would appear to be relatively consistently related to self-care behaviour[42,63,82,91,101,128,139,146–148], with no identified studies failing to find an association between some aspect of family support and self-care behaviour. Furthermore, Liss and colleagues[137] found that adolescents who had been admitted for DKA subsequent to diagnosis came from less supportive family environments. The importance of family support for diabetes self-care is highlighted in the structural equation modelling of Hanson and colleagues[101]. Although family stress was directly associated with metabolic control, family relations affected diabetes control indirectly through its association with adherence. Furthermore, no one subscale of support shows consistent relations with self-care across studies. This suggests that family support is important in promoting self-care, but exactly which aspects are important remains to be resolved.

Conflict in the family is frequently cited as the key aspect in determining the level of family support, but the literature fails to provide consistent support for this[84,123]. For instance, even when using the same measures and protocol, Miller-Johnson and colleagues[139] found substantial differences in the role of conflict between adolescents receiving their diabetes care in private compared to public practices. Furthermore, although Hauser and colleagues[146] found that initial levels of adherence were associated with conflict, changes in conflict were not associated with changes in adherence over the 4 years of their prospective longitudinal study. This may be a result of conflict over minor issues being common and even normative in adolescence, with some commentators arguing that conflict in the family is essential for the development of young people's interpersonal skills[149–151]. However, it is important to remember that extreme levels of conflict, and/or conflicts that remains continuously unresolved, are likely to disrupt the family and impact on poor control. Therefore, communication and conflict resolution may be a more critical issue, as highlighted by Bobrow and colleagues[93], who examined the interaction between mothers and adolescent daughters with diabetes. They concluded that adolescent girls who had adherence problems had interactions with their mothers that were 'not conducive to opening up about deeper concerns' and that 'good adherers and their mothers were judged to be lower on seemingly unresolved conflict'. Alternatively, conflict within the family may act as a normative stress (i.e. one that is experienced by most adolescents as part of their negotiating independence from parents), or non-normative stress (in the context of family break-up), which acts to increase stress. As highlighted by Hanson and colleagues[101], family stress would seem to have both a direct effect on diabetes control and an indirect influence on adherence by affecting family relations. This also highlights the need for greater refinement in the operationalization of constructs, with minor conflict, conflict resolution, and family stress clearly overlapping and influencing one another. However, if conflict resolution is the key problem, then interventions designed to provide families with the skills and strategies to resolve conflicts, with resulting benefits for the family as a whole and for the management of diabetes, would be helpful, and this is an approach being developed in some centres[115,154].

Moving on to consider the dimension of family control, the results fail to support a strong association between measures of family control and adjustment, metabolic control or self-care, some studies reporting a significant association[73,81,84,91,122,128,130,131,133,138,140,142,144], whilst others do not support an association[49,81,82,91,95,105,121,123,124,128,136,137,139,141,143,146,152,153].

Although linear associations are not consistently evident in these studies, this may be a result of the failure to consider the possibility of non linear associations. Gustafsson and colleagues[142] split their samples into those whose family were in the balanced range and those in the disturbed range of family functioning (either above or below the balanced area). They found that participants from balanced families were in significantly better control of their diabetes than those in the disturbed range. This conception of balanced vs. disturbed family functioning clearly needs further consideration. It is more likely that the extreme ends of family functioning cause the problem, rather than looking for a continuum of family functioning that the parents and child need to move up in order to improve diabetes self-care and control.

Alternatively, the lack of consistency in results may be a consequence of the lack of specificity in the measures of family control measures. Research that has looked at the degree of parental involvement in diabetes care has produced noticeably consistent results. The greater responsibility taken by the adolescent with diabetes, and the less parental involvement, the worse their control[5,106,109,140,141,144,156]. More detailed examination of parent and child perceptions of responsibility indicated that where no-one was taking responsibility, the young person with diabetes was in worse diabetes control[155]. This handing over of responsibility needs to be not only negotiated and managed but also to match the maturity of the individual and his/her ability to take responsibility[7,156].

Adding weight to the critical role of continued parental involvement in diabetes management is research on the problem of recurrent diabetic ketoacidosis. White and colleagues[157] identified lack of parental involvement in diabetes care as a common problem in their sample of poorly controlled and recurrently re-admitted young patients. Furthermore, intervention studies[158–162] that have had a significant impact on metabolic control included a focus on strategies for negotiating appropriate levels of parental involvement and adolescent responsibility for diabetes care. Addressing this issue is also something that could be readily integrated into normal diabetes care and consultations without increasing diabetes-related conflict[158,159].

The results of these studies replicates the data on general adolescent development, which also implicates parental involvement as the single most important predictor of positive adolescent outcomes[186]. The key to understanding this approach is to acknowledge that the major developmental task of adolescence is movement away from dependence on the family, not toward complete independence but rather toward interdependence. Interdependence does not require the adolescents to distance themselves emotionally from parents, but requires a reorganization in which the family members renegotiate and redistribute responsibilities and obligations[158].

PEERS

In a recent review of research on paediatric chronic illness, Glasgow and Anderson[163] called for a number of conceptual issues to be addressed in future research. With the vast majority of research being conducted on the family, they 'recommend that greater attention be paid to the social context' in which the adolescent lives. In particular, La Greca[164,165] noted the paucity of research on the role and influence of the adolescent's peer group at a time when friendships develop and peer influence becomes increasing important. Studies have shown that peers and friends are an important source of emotional support for adolescents with diabetes[55,59,148,166]. However, it is not just the supportive behaviour of adolescents that is important. Kyngas and colleagues[147] report that some adolescents have friends who seem to dominate their lives, sometimes tempting them to break their treatment regimens and make self-management difficult. Friends can be both supportive and unsupportive, and may serve to help with some aspects of the regimen and yet hinder others[167].

Dunning[168] reported on a range of adolescents' self-management behaviours, and found that 66% reported skipping insulin injections to fit in socially. Jacobson and colleagues[86] found that 55% of adolescent newly-diagnosed diabetics did not talk about their diabetes with their friends, and 35% thought that their friends would like them better if they did not have diabetes. Simonds and colleagues[78] and Bobrow and colleagues[93] also found that adolescent diabetics were sensitive to being different, and felt that they were treated differently because of their diabetes. Meldman[166] reports that many adolescent diabetics found that having diabetes made it difficult to be spontaneous and socially acceptable, expressing fears that at parties or restaurants, having to go and take an insulin injection may result in others thinking they were drug addicts. As well as having to deal with the social pressures associated with being part of a peer group, adolescent diabetics may be more sensitive to feeling different from their peers. Additionally, Meldman found that young people were afraid of being identified as 'freaks' or 'weird' by their peers. The adolescent diabetic is aware of these pressures and states that peer support is important, 'those who did not have it wanted it, and those who had it appreciated it'[166].

Despite these descriptive studies, only a few studies have explored the relationship between the adolescents' peer support and their diabetes management or psychological adjustment. La Greca and colleagues[148] reported that peer support was associated with self-care, but this relationship did not remain after controlling for family support. However, this study did not consider the negative aspects of peer relationships, which is a key component of the social relationships, particularly in adolescence[169]. However, including the negative aspects of peer relations may not be the key to understanding the importance of peers for young people with diabetes[55,59]. Rather, as postulated by Wallander and Varni[170], adolescents need both supportive family and supportive friends if they are going to integrate diabetes management into their daily lives. This is supported by a 6 month prospective study of adolescents, where neither family or friend support alone predicted self-care behaviour, but the combination of the two did[55].

In addition to providing support for self-management, the emotional support provided by friends is likely to be associated with well-being in adolescents with a chronic illness[164]. Two studies of adolescents with diabetes[55,132] found that lower peer support was associated with poorer psychological adjustment. However, the data from a prospective study again supports the need for both supportive family and friends for optimal adjustment[58]. In addition, in a study looking at adjustment across several chronic conditions, it was the presence of both family and friend support that was predictive of better psychological outcomes[170]. From the limited research to date, it would seem that the social aspects of diabetes are important for adolescents, and that they are highly likely to put their social worlds before their diabetes management[21]. This conflict between social and diabetes pressures may also be important determinants of their emotional well-being, and therefore, diabetes care teams should strive to work alongside young people so that they can enable them to manage their diabetes but not at cost of their social life.

HEALTH CARE PROFESSIONALS

Repeated literature searching has succeeded in identifying only a few studies that focused on the role of the paediatric diabetes care team in supporting the young person with diabetes. Hanson and colleagues[128] asked 96 adolescents and their parents to complete a questionnaire assessing their attitudes towards physicians and their care team across three areas; the personal qualities of the physician; the professional competence of the physician; and the cost and convenience of health care.

They found that there was little intra-family agreement. Although paternal and maternal ratings were significantly correlated, the adolescents were more satisfied with the personal qualities of the physician than their parents, and the fathers were less satisfied with the cost and convenience of health care than mothers or adolescents. Following on from these differences, it was the adolescents' perception of their physician's personal qualities that were related to their adherence behaviour. In contrast, parental perceptions of the physician's professional competence were associated with adherence. In relation to metabolic control and hospitalization rates, only the youths' perceptions seemed relevant, with greater professional competence associated with worse control, but fewer hospitalizations. Auslander and colleagues[83] also examined mothers' satisfaction with their child's medical care. Again, parental satisfaction was associated with the adolescents' reports of self-care, but not maternal reports of adolescent self-care.

Although not the primary focus of the studies, a few other studies have considered patient–doctor relations. Burns and colleagues[81] found that adolescents who reported worse relations with their medical caregivers had worse glycated haemoglobin, but there was no association between control and the parents' reports of relations with medical caregivers. However, Bobrow and colleagues[93] found no associations between how much adolescent girls liked their doctor, whether the doctor gave them enough time, or whether they thought the doctor encouraged questions and their adherence. Similarly, McCaul and colleagues[63] found no association between adolescents' satisfaction with medical care and self-care.

The research that has been done has not contributed significantly to the field, as it has primarily relied on satisfaction measures. As Golin and colleagues[171] pointed out, satisfaction is a measure that is a combination of two constructs, expectations or demands the individual has of their care team, and their perceptions of what care they actually receive. Before collecting data on this issue, researchers should take a step back and examine the content of diabetes care. Once the differing components, such as provision of knowledge, transfer of complex skills, provision of emotional support and supporting decision making of the care teams' work are established, the quality and quantity of these facets can be assessed.

Confounding patient expectations and perceptions of care received will only serve to distort the assessment of the care teams' work. With clinicians striving to optimize their effectiveness in the wake of the DCCT results, this is clearly an area that would benefit from a wealth of theoretical and empirical development.

However, the recent work of Kyngas[147] points to a potential way forward, through asking adolescents about their perceptions of their physicians and nurses. Those adolescents who described their physicians and nurses as being more motivating in their actions were more likely to have optimal self-care. In comparison, those adolescents who described their nurses and physicians as more routine and negligent were more likely to have poor self-care. Although we can make no inferences about the direction of causality in this study, it would seem to replicate the work on adults with diabetes. This work indicates that health care professionals who give patients more autonomy and encourage more autonomous motivational beliefs are more likely to have patients with better self-care[172,173]. This clearly points to a potentially fruitful area of research, but it is essential that researchers include nurses and dieticians as well doctors, as there is a plethora of work on doctor–patient communication, but comparatively little on other health care professionals.

THEORETICAL ISSUES

Despite the wealth of research into adolescents with diabetes, the theoretical input into this research has been extremely limited. Although researchers have focused predominantly on the role of the family environment, 'few theoretical models have been offered that describe how family interactions support or interfere with the child's adaptation to the demands of diabetes treatment'[163]. This lack of theoretical input goes beyond the family context. If the research on adolescent health beliefs, cognitions or attitudes is considered, there has been no attempt to consider any developmental issues in this work. For a belief to influence behaviour, the individual needs to be taking responsibility for that behaviour, and with adolescents diabetes management this cannot be assumed. Further, as adolescents are learning to take responsibility for their own diabetes management this period may be a time of development and change in their beliefs, again a consideration that is frequently overlooked.

In addition, with the possible exception of personality/ego development, research to date has almost exclusively ignored general theories of adolescent development, such as Focal Theory[80] or Identity Development[174]. These may prove insightful in understanding the decline in metabolic control seen in adolescence, especially if these theories were tied together with the key developmental changes seen in adolescence, such as the timing of puberty, cognitive development, changes in moral reasoning, group affiliation, formation of romantic attachments, end of compulsory schooling, unemployment and employment. These changes and their possible impact on the young person's management of, and adjustment to, his/her diabetes has rarely been considered. Although some studies have included measures of Tanner stage development, in an attempt to control for the hormonal effects of puberty, studies have yet to consider the effect of timing of puberty, particularly early development in girls and late development in boys, which have been frequently associated with poorer health outcomes in the general population[51].

This lack of theoretical cohesion has resulted in largely separate domains of research that focus on the social cognition-based models and those on the family environment. Where researchers have combined constructs across domains, this has not been matched with concurrent merging and integrating of theory. Those models that are present in the paediatric literature[175,176] have rarely been utilized in diabetes research. However, there is a certain degree of overlap amongst these models, particularly within the hypotheses of stress processing and coping, and integrating them may prove to be the most expedient way forward. One problem with testing these models, though, is the vast array of constructs that need to be incorporated, and so these models need to be broken down into their constituent processes, to enable researchers to test systematically, and to develop a coherent model.

Reviewing this literature has also highlighted a number of questions that researchers have as yet to consider. The first of these is the timing of diabetes onset. When considering the population of adolescents with diabetes, there is huge variability in the duration of diabetes, with some having never known anything but diabetes as part of their life, whilst others are diagnosed in their middle to late teens. Some limited research suggest that earlier diagnosis of diabetes may be a risk factor for recurrent readmissions to hospital during adolescence[177,178]. However, little research has explored this issue or the differential impact of timing of diabetes onset on outcomes in later life. Studies frequently control for disease duration in their analysis, but do not explore the mechanism by which disease duration may be influencing these outcomes.

A further point that should be considered here is the age range of samples. Although some studies do limit their sample to adolescents, it is more common for samples to range from 6 or 8 up to 16 or 18. When analysing the data in these studies, researchers rarely report different analysis for different age groups, proceeding to analyse the sample as a whole, possibly controlling for age, along with other demographic factors. As for disease duration, age would also not be expected to have a linear association with the variables of interest. Rather, different patterns of association could be expected at different stages of development. This undoubtedly poses questions over the validity of the conclusions drawn from any studies using wide age ranges, as their results may reflect an amalgamated pattern of associations, that does not represent the real situation for either children or adolescents.

Further consideration of demographic issues poses additional obstacles to generalizing from these results. In particular, two issues are very evident, the socio-economic status and ethnicity of participants. As Glasgow and Anderson[163] have already noted, few researchers in this field publish data on recruitment rates and subsequent bias, but it seems reasonable to conclude that there is a bias towards white middle-class families. Furthermore, the vast majority of studies have been conducted in North America, further limiting the generalizability of studies. Finally, there is the issue of comorbidity, especially with concurrent additional chronic illness. Nearly every study reported here excluded individuals with concurrent chronic illness, or did not even raise the question. A significant number of individuals with diabetes also suffer from a range of other chronic illnesses (e.g. asthma, coeliac disease, cystic fibrosis). There is a good argument for excluding these individuals from analysis predicting metabolic control, due to possible impact of medication and illness effecting glucose metabolism. The argument for excluding them from analysis attempting to predict self-care or emotional health is less clear, and this exclusion severely limits the applicability of research to clinical populations.

However, this failure to utilize theory to drive forward research does have some advantages. Instead of progress being driven by armchair theorizing, there is now an abundance of data that needs to be assimilated to guide theoretical development. This review has only considered the relations between predictor constructs and diabetes outcome. This is a reflection of most of the research to date, and the analysis undertaken. This does not help with the building of theoretical models, as the interrelation between constructs needs to be explored if appropriate models and interventions are to be built. In summary, although little theory has guided a systematic building of knowledge in this field to date, the growth in adolescent developmental research and theorizing, the mass of knowledge already gained in this field to date should provide paediatric psychologists with an ideal opportunity to take this field forward.

Finally, there has been little research exploring the initial period of adaptation to diabetes in the first few months after diagnosis. This is clearly an important area, as the initial adaptation may well set the ground-work for, and may predict, long-term outcomes[114]. However, because there are rapid changes in emotional and cognitive adjustment, in conjunction with residual insulin secretion, which facilitates metabolic control over this initial 'honeymoon period', this is an extremely difficult time in which to conduct research. As a result, the first year post-diagnosis is frequently excluded from studies in the psychosocial literature, and where it is included, this is usually because of the researchers' interest in the early stages of adaptation.

PRACTICAL IMPLICATIONS FOR DIABETES CARE

Despite the limitations of the psychosocial research on adolescents with diabetes, there are still a number of important practical implications of this research. First, clinicians must maintain contact with the young people they care for. This can be difficult with the pressures that fill both the health care professionals' and the adolescents's schedules. However, if you cannot see the young people, use whatever tools you can to maintain contact, whether that be by phone or even e-mail. Without this contact it is difficult to maintain an honest, open and trusting relationship with young people, which must be the foundation on which diabetes care is built.

When you do make contact, don't make diabetes the be-all and end-all of the exchange. Adolescents, as do adults, have a life outside of their diabetes, and in some cases diabetes may be temporarily dropped from their list of life concerns. Be prepared to let go of the diabetes agenda, and focus on whatever issue is of greatest concern to the adolescents. Although this may not improve their blood glucose control directly, helping them deal with the problems in their lives, in addition to maintaining a trusting relationship, can also help them learn problem-solving skills which may be transferred into their diabetes management. Furthermore, if a problem is causing anxiety or stress, supporting a young person as he/she seeks a way through a dilemma may help to reduce these levels of anxiety and stress, and for some this may have a direct physiological effect on their blood glucose control.

Adolescents will undoubtedly feel the extra stress that is inherent in living with diabetes, and the resultant feelings of guilt, sadness, anxiety, frustration and anger. It is important that we help young people to make the distinction between their emotional responses to their diabetes and those that are part of being an adolescent. Separating negative feelings about diabetes from other issues, helps put the young person and his/her family on the same side of the fence, enabling everyone to work towards finding a way for the young person to live successfully with diabetes.

Feeling bad, sad or mad in response to the burden of living with diabetes is natural, normal and inevitable. Many parents and other adults find it hard to talk to young people with diabetes, possibly because they want to be able to help, but do not see how. As far as helping the young person deal with these emotions, parents should be reminded that they do not need to, and probably cannot, solve the problems the young person faces. However, just by talking and especially by listening to young people, by attempting to empathize and understand what the young person is going through, is a powerful aid for young people, and will in itself invariably help the young person with the dilemmas he/she faces.

It is important, during this time of change, growth and development, that blood glucose goals are kept realistic and achievable. Only 20% of the participants in the DCCT, which was a selected group of highly motivated individuals with diabetes who received intensive support from health care professionals (who in turn received a wealth of support), ever achieved a normal average blood glucose level (HbAic 6.05%), and only 5% maintained that level of control throughout the trial. In addition, these achievements were obtained in a predominantly adult population who do not have to contend with the vagaries of the physiological effects of puberty. Therefore, it is important to keep the goals that are set for young people as realistic as possible, and to remember that switching onto more intensive regimens does not guarantee better control. Insulin regimens, their benefits in terms of control and flexibility, and costs in terms of increased intrusiveness and cognitive demands must be discussed openly with young people. If their social world and/or personality do not fit a regimen, there is little point in trying to force it upon them.

There may well be times when diabetes can become overwhelming and almost too much for the young person to handle, alone or with your help. Be ready to admit that you do not have the skills or resources to help some young people and try to direct the adolescent, and/or his family, to the help they need. When referring an individual to psychological services, wherever possible try to develop contact with professionals who take an interest in diabetes. If you do not have anyone with a specialist interest, take the time to discuss diabetes with the mental professional concerned, so that he/she can distinguish between diabetes-related issues and more general issues.

One area in which it is essential to offer help as soon as possible is if you have concerns over young people's eating patterns and/or insulin manipulation, particularly in girls aged between 15 and 20 years. The problem of weight gain during puberty, with optimal blood glucose control, is a cause of concern for many teenage girls. Add to this the focus on diet restrictions inherent in diabetes management, it is not surprising that eating patterns are an issue of concern to many parents and professionals alike. Most prevalent (subclinical) eating disorders are binge eating and bulimia nervosa. Early warning signs to be alert to include: recurrent DKA, growth failure, recurrent (severe) hypoglycaemia, dieting, extreme low or high HbA1c. In addition to the strategies already discussed, a couple of other issues are important to consider with young people, if disordered eating patterns are to be prevented. Body dissatisfaction is common, if not the norm in adolescent girls, and increasingly so in boys. Given these concerns, try not to emphasize weight or weight goals. Where there was substantial weight loss at diagnosis, help the young person regain weight slowly, so that he/she has time to adjust to his/her changing body shape. Discuss weight and body image openly with the young person, including issues such as unrealistic media portrayals, genetic determinants of body shape and other methods of weight maintenance, particularly exercise. Finally, if you are concerned about a young person's eating habits, it is never too early to get advice or help; eating disorders are more intractable and a greater risk to the person with diabetes than to a non-diabetic.

Moving back to the more basic issues, it cannot be assumed that adolescents have all the requisite knowledge, skills and problem-solving ability to successfully manage their diabetes. Although having this knowledge and skills does not guarantee that the young person will use them, they are essential. Similarly it should not be assumed that parental knowledge and skills will be transferred to the adolescent, no matter how long they have had diabetes. Therefore, diabetes knowledge and skills should be reviewed at least annually, and any misconceptions or deficits can then be addressed. However, knowledge should not just be factual, as much as possible encourage and support young people to solve diabetes management problems as a way to enhance their self-efficacy and competence. In consultation with young people, resist the temptation to tell them how to achieve better control. Rather, try and help them solve the problems for themselves, so that they can learn to work through problems for themselves.

Another fundamental practical implication of the research reviewed here is in the area of adolescent responsibility. Whether it is conscious or not, much paediatric diabetes care, from professionals and parents alike, encourages young people to take responsibility for their own diabetes management. However, the research, whether descriptive or interventionist in nature, provides strong evidence to temper this push for adolescent responsibility, with many studies implying that lack of parental input and responsibility for diabetes is predictive of poorer metabolic control and DKA. Responsibility should not be forced onto young people, and should be negotiated with the young person, possibly only when the adolescent requests more responsibility. Frequently, when management tasks are handed over to young people, they are not taken on board and are simply not done. Discussions about appropriate levels of responsibility and negotiating this with parents and adolescents should form the basis of much psychosocial care for adolescents.

For those young people who have persistently poor control of their diabetes, it is essential to consider that there are many possible causes for this poor control. Obviously poor control will result from missing insulin injections, whether deliberate or not. This issue should be discussed openly with adolescents and parents alike. It is essential that young people feel able to talk about these aspects of diabetes management, so that the health care professional can explore the reasoning behind the behaviour and support the adolescent appropriately. The young woman who is skipping insulin to control weight needs vastly different care from the young woman who feels unable to take her insulin when she goes out. Alternatively, raised blood glucose levels may be the young person's way of avoiding socially embarrassing hypoglycaemia or severe hypoglycaemia in the presence of peers who have not been told about diabetes or how to respond. This aetiology of poor control requires markedly different management, possibly combining social skills training, blood glucose awareness training and revised insulin regimens to assuage the young person's fear.

For a subgroup of stress-reactive young people, high and persistent levels of stress, such as in highly conflictual families, may be the factor precipitating poor control. These young people may benefit from stress-management programmes, or approaches designed to help the family resolve conflicts, which may also help with young people's emotional well-being. This just highlights some of the possible cause of poor control, and possible approaches to the situation. However, it should be remembered that psychosocial approaches are not the only way to address these issues. Relaxing the goals of management to be more realistic within an adolescent lifestyle, pursuing less intensive insulin regimens and encouraging exercise as an alternative means of managing weight are examples of non-psychological approaches that are an equally important part of the clinician's armoury.

Many of these issues have been highlighted and received much greater practical attention by other authors, and for help in how to implement the issues raised by this chapter, we can recommend two valuable resources: *Practical Psychology for Diabetes Clinicians*[179], edited by Barbara Anderson and Richard Rubin, and *The Ten Keys to Helping Your Child Grow Up with Diabetes* by Tim Wysocki[180]. We hope this chapter has posed new questions for you, and that in conjunction with the above resources we hope that you may find one or two new answers to some of the questions you face each day.

REFERENCES

1. Wysocki T, Clarke WL, Meinhold PA, Bellando BJ, Abrams EC, Bourgeois MJ, Barnard MU. Parental and professional estimates of self-care independence of children and adolescents with IDDM. *Diabet Care* 1992; **15**(1): 43–52
2. Ingersoll GM, Orr DP, Herrold AJ, Golden MP. Cognitive maturity and self-management among adolescents with insulin-dependent diabetes mellitus. *J Pediat* 1986; **108**: 620–23
3. Allen DA, Tennen H, McGrade BJ, Affleck G, Ratzan S. Parent and child

perceptions of the management of juvenile diabetes. *J Pediat Psychol* 1983; **8**(2): 129–41

4. Mortensen HB, Villumsen J, Volund A, Petersen KE, Nerup J. The Danish Study Group of Diabetes in Childhood. Relationship between insulin injections regimen and metabolic control in young Danish type 1 diabetic patients. *Diabet Med* 1992; **9**: 834–9
5. Jacobson AM, Hauser ST, Lavori P, Willett JB, Cole CF, Wolfsdorf JI, Dumont RH, Wertileb D. Family environment and glycemic control: a four-year prospective study of children and adolescents with insulin-dependent diabetes mellitus. *Psychosom Med* 1994; **56**: 401–9
6. Hoey H, Mortensen H, McGee H, Fitzgeralt M (Hvidøre Group). Is metabolic control related to quality of life? A study of 2103 children and adolescents with IDDM from 17 countries. *Diabet Res Clin Pract* 1999; **44**(suppl): S3
7. Amiel SA, Sherwin RS, Simonson DC, Lauritano AA, Tamborland WV. Impaired insulin action in puberty: a contributing factor to poor glycemic control in adolescents with diabetes. *N Engl J Med* 1986; **315**: 215–19
8. Hindmarsh PC, Matthews SG, Silvio LDI. Relations between height velocity and fasting insulin concentrations. *Arch Dis Child* 1988; **63**: 666
9. Johnson SB, Kelly M, Henretta JC, Cunningham WR, Tomer A, Silverstein JH. A longitudinal analysis of adherence and health status in childhood diabetes. *J Pediat Psychol* 1992; **17**(5): 537–53
10. Johnson SB, Silverstein J, Rosenbloom A, Carter R, Cunningham W. Assessing daily management of childhood diabetes. *Health Psychol* 1986; **9**: 545–64
11. Morris AD, Boyle DIR, McMahon AD, Greene SA, MacDonald TM, Newton RW. Adherence to insulin treatment, glycemic control and ketoacidosis in insulin-dependent diabetes mellitus. *Lancet* 1997; **350**: 1505–10
12. Thompson CJ, Greene SA. Diabetes in the older teenager and young adult. In Court S, Lamb B (eds) *Childhood and Adolescent Diabetes*. London: Wiley, 1997
13. Brown SA. Effects of educational interventions in diabetes care: a meta-analysis of findings. *Nurs Res* 1988; **37**(4): 223–9
14. Brown SA, Hedges LV. Predicting metabolic control in diabetes: a pilot study using meta-analysis to estimate a linear model. *Nurs Res* 1994; **43**(6): 362–8
15. Brown SA. Studies of educational interventions and outcomes in diabetic adults: a meta-analysis revisited. *Patient Educ Counsel* 1990; **16**: 189–215
16. Nagasawa M, Smith MC, Barnes JH, Fincham JE. Meta-analysis of correlates of diabetes patients' compliance with prescribed medications. *Diabet Educ* 1990; **16**(3): 192–200
17. Boardway RH, Delamater AM, Tomakowsky J, Gutai JP. Stress management training for adolescents with diabetes. *J Pediat Psychol* 1993; **18**(1): 29–45
18. Gross AM, Heiman L, Shapiro R, Schultz RM. Children with diabetes: social skills training and hemoglobin A1c levels. *Behav Modif* 1983; **7**(2): 151–64
19. Kaplan RM, Chadwick MW, Schimmel BA. Social learning intervention to promote metabolic control in type 1 diabetes mellitus: pilot experiment results. *Diabet Care* 1985; **8**(2): 152–5
20. Mendez FJ, Belendez M. Effects of a behavioral intervention on treatment adherence and stress management in adolescents with IDDM. *Diabet Care* 1997; **20**: 1370–75
21. Thomas AM, Peterson L, Goldstein D. Problem solving and diabetes regimen adherence by children and adolescents with IDDM in social pressure situations: a reflection of normal development. *J Pediat Psychol* 1997; **22**: 541–62
22. Elleman K, Soerensen JN, Pedesen L, Edsberg B, Andersen OO. Epidemiology

and treatment of diabetic ketoacidosis in a community population. *Diabet Care* 1984; **7**: 528–32

23. Elamin A, Eltayeb B, Hasan M, Hofvander Y, Tuveno T. Effect of dietary education on metabolic control in children and adolescents with type 1 diabetes mellitus. *Diabet Nutr Metab* 1993; **6**(4): 223–9
24. Misuraca A, Di Gennaro M, Lionello M, Duval M, Aloi G. Summer camps for diabetic children: an experience in Campania, Italy. *Diabet Res Clinic Pract* 1996; **32**: 91–6
25. Weissberg-Benchel J, Glasgow A. The role of temperament in children with insulin-dependent diabetes mellitus. *J Pediat Psychol* 1997; **22**: 795–810
26. Rovet JF, Ehrlich RM. Effect of temperament on metabolic control in children with diabetes mellitus. *Diabet Care* 1988; **11**: 77–82
27. Steinhausen H-C. Chronically ill and handicapped children and adolescents: personality studies in relation to disease. *J Abnorm Child Psychol* 1981; **9**(2): 291–297
28. Stabler B, Lane JD, Ross SL, Morris MA, Litton J, Surwit RS. Type A behavior pattern and chronic glycemic control in individuals with IDDM. *Diabet Care* 1988; **11**: 361–2
29. John OP, Caspi A, Robins RW, Moffit TE, Stouthamer-Loeber M. The 'Little Five': exploring the nomological network of the five-factor model of the personality in adolescents. *Child Dev* 1994; **65**: 160–78
30. Robins RW, John OP, Caspi A, *et al.* The developing structure of temperament and personality from infancy to adulthood. In: Halverson CF (ed) *Major Dimensions of Personality in Early Adolescence: The Big Five and Beyond*. Hove: Erlbaum, 1994
31. Digman JM. Personality structure: emergence of the five-factor model. In Rosenzweigh MR, Porter IW (eds) *Annual Review of Psychology, 1990*, vol 41. Palo Alto, CA: Annual Reviews, pp. 417–446
32. Goldberg LR. The structure of phenotypic personality traits. *Am Psychol* 1993; **48**: 26–34
33. McCrae RR, Cost PT. Personality trait structure as a human universal. *Am Psychol* 1987; **52**: 509–16
34. Robins RW, John OP. Resilient, overcontrolled and undercontrolled boys; three replicable personality types. *J Personality Soc Psychol* 1996; **70**: 157–71
35. Barglow P, Edidin DV, Budlong-Springer AS, Berndt D, Phillips R, Dubow E. Diabetic control in children and adolescents: psychosocial factors and therapeutic efficacy. *J Youth Adolesc* 1983; **12**(2): 77–94
36. Ryden O, Nevander L, Johnsson P, Westbom L, Sjoblad S. Diabetic children and their parents: personality correlates of metabolic control. *Acta Paediat Scand* 1990; **79**: 1202–12
37. Jacobson AM, Hauser ST, Lavori P, Wolfsdorf JI, Herskowitz RD, Milley JE, Bliss R, Gelfand E, Wertileb D, Stein J. Adherence among children and adolescents with insulin-dependent diabetes mellitus over a four year longitudinal follow-up: 1. The influence of patient coping and adjustment. *J Pediat Psychol* 1990; **15**(4): 511–26
38. Jacobson AM, Hauser ST, Powers S, Noam G. The influences of chronic illness and ego development on self-esteem in diabetic and psychiatric adolescent patients. *J Youth Adolesc* 1984; **13**(6): 489–507
39. Friedman HS, Tucker JS, Schwartz JE, Martin LR, Tomlinson-Keasey C, Wingard DL, Criqui MH. Childhood conscientiousness and longevity: health behaviors and cause of death. *J Personality Soc Psychol* 1995; **68**: 696–703

40. Bond GG, Aiken LS, Somerville SC. The health belief model and adolescents with insulin-dependent diabetes mellitus. *Health Psychol* 1992; **11**(3): 190–98
41. Brownlee-Duffeck M, Peterson L, Simonds JF, Goldstein D, Kilo C, Hoette S. The role of health beliefs in the regimen adherence and metabolic control of adolescents with diabetes mellitus. *J Consult Clin Psychol* 1987; **55**(2): 139–44
42. Palardy N, Greening L, Ott J, Holderby A, Atchison J. Adolescents' health attitudes and adherence to treatment for insulin-dependent diabetes mellitus. *Dev Behav Pediat* 1998; **19**(1): 31–7
43. de Weerdt I, Visser AP, Kok G, van der Veen EA. Determinants of active self-care behaviour of insulin treated patients with diabetes: implications for diabetes education. *Soc Sci Med* 1990; **30**(5): 605–15
44. Leventhal H, Nerenz DR, Steele DJ, *et al.* Illness representation and coping with health threats. In Baum A (ed) *Handbook of Psychology and Health*. Hillsdale, NJ: Erlbaum, 1984; pp. 219–252
45. Meyer D, Leventhal H, Gutmann M. Common-sense models of illness: the example of hypertension. *Health Psychol* 1985; **4**: 115–35
46. Lau RR, Bernard TM, Hartman KA. Further explorations of commonsense representations of common illnesses. *Health Psychol* 1989; **8**(2): 195–219
47. Olsen R, Sutton J. More hassle, more alone: adolescents with diabetes and the role of formal and informal support. *Child Care, Health Dev* 1998; **24**(1): 31–9
48. Holmes CS, Yu Z, Frentz J. Chronic and discrete stress as predictors of children's adjustment. *J Consult Clin Psychol* 1999; **67**(3): 411–19
49. Anderson BJ, Miller JP, Auslander WF, Santiago JV. Family characteristics of diabetic adolescents: relationship to metabolic control. *Diabet Care* 1981; **4**(6): 586–94
50. Skinner TC, Hampson SE. Personality, personal models and self-care in type 1 diabetes. *Diabetes* 1999; **48**(suppl 1): A317
51. Skinner TC, Hampson SE. Personal models of diabetes in adolescents: a longitudinal study. *Diabet Med* 1999; **16**(suppl 1): P82
52. Brown RT, Kaslow ND, Sansbury L, Meacham L, Culler FL. Internalizing and externalizing symptoms and attributional style in youth with diabetes. *J Am Acad Child Adolesc Psychiat* 1991; **30**: 921–5
53. Schoenherr SJ, Brown RT, Baldwin K, Kaslow NJ. Attributional styles and psychopathology in pediatric chronic-illness groups. *J Clin Child Psychol* 1992; **21**(4): 380–87
54. Leung SS, Steinbeck KS, Morris SL, Kohn MR, Towns SJ, Bennett DL. Chronic illness perception in adolescence: implications for the doctor–patient relationship. *J Paediat Child Health* 1997; **33**: 107–12
55. Skinner TC, John M, Hampson SE. Social support and personal models of diabetes as predictors of self-care and well-being: a longitudinal study of adolescents with diabetes. *J Pediat Psychol* (in press)
56. Guttmann-Bauman I, Strgugger M, Flaherty BP, McEvoy RC. Metabolic control and quality-of-life self-assessment in adolescents with IDDM. *Diabet Care* 1998; **21**(6): 915–19
57. Grey M, Sullivan-Bolyai S, Boland EA, Tamborlane WV, Yu C. Personal and family factors associated with quality of life in adolescents with diabetes. *Diabet Care* 1998; **21**(6): 909–14
58. Green LB, Wysocki T, Reineck BM. Fear of hypoglycaemia in children and adolescents with diabetes. *J Pediat Psychol* 1990; **15**(5): 633–41
59. Skinner TC, Hampson SE. Social support and personal models of diabetes in

relation to self-care and well-being in adolescents with type 1 diabetes mellitus. *J Adolesc* 1998; **21**(6): 3–15
60. Grey M, Boland EA, Davidson M, Yu C, Sullivan-Bolyai S, Tamborland WV. Short-term effects of coping skills training as adjunct to intensive therapy in adolescents. *Diabet Care* 1998; **21**(6): 902–7
61. Kovacs M, Iyengar S, Goldston D, Stewart J, Obrosky S, Marsh J. Psychological functioning of children with insulin-dependent diabetes mellitus: a longitudinal study. *J Pediat Psychol* 1990; **15**(5): 619–32
62. Littlefield CH, Daneman D, Craven JL, Murray MA, Rodin GM, Rydall AC. Relationship of self-efficacy and binging to adherence to diabetes regimen among adolescents. *Diabet Care* 1992; **15**(1): 90–94
63. McCaul KD, Glasgow RE, Schafer LC. Diabetes regimen behaviour: predicting adherence. *Med Care* 1987; **25**(9): 868–81
64. Schlundt DG, Rea MR, Hodge M, Flannery ME, Kline SS, Meek J, Kinzer C, Pichert JW. Assessing and overcoming situational obstacles to dietary adherence in adolescents with IDDM. *J Adolesc Health* 1996; **19**: 282–8
65. Grossman HY, Brink S, Hauser ST. Self-efficacy in adolescent girls and boys with insulin-dependent diabetes mellitus. *Diabet Care* 1987; **10**(3): 324–9
66. Howells LAL, Wilson AC, Johnston M, Newton RW, Greene SA. Self-efficacy, knowledge and glycaemic control in young people with insulin-dependent diabetes mellitus: does perceived competence improve control? *Diabet Med* 1997; **20**: 50
67. Hentinen M, Kyngas H. Diabetic adolescents' compliance with health regimens and associated factors. *Int J Adv Nurs* 1996; **33**(3): 325–37
68. Grey M, Sullivan-Bolyai S, Boland EA, Tamborlane WV, Yu C. Personal and family factors associated with quality of life in adolescents with diabetes. *Diabet Care* 1998; **21**(6): 909–14
69. Bandura A. Health promotion from the perspective of social cognitive theory. *Psychol Health* 1988; **13**(4): 623–51
70. Vyogtsky LS. In Cole M, John-Steiner V, Scribner S, Souberman E. (eds) *Mind in Society*. Cambridge, MA: Harvard University Press, 1979
71. Rogers CR. *On Becoming a Person* Boston, MA: Houghton Mifflin
72. Band EB. Children's coping with diabetes: understanding the role of cognitive development. *J Pediat Psychol* 1990; **15**(1): 27–41
73. Evans CL, Hughes IA. The relationship between diabetic control and individual and family characteristics. *J Psychosom Res* 1987; **31**(3): 367–74
74. Steel JM, Young RJ, Lloyd GG *et al.* Abnormal eating attitudes in young insulin dependent diabetics. *Br J Psychiat* 1989; **155**; 515–21
75. Neumark-Sztainer D, Story M, Toporoff E, Himes JH, Resnick MD, Blum RWM. Co-variations of eating behaviors with other health-related behaviors among adolescents.*J Adolesc Health* 1997; **20**: 450–58
76. Lernmark B, Dahlquist G, Fransson P, Hagglof B, Ivarsson SA, Ludvigsson J, Sjoblad S, Thernlund G. Relations between age, metabolic control, disease adjustment and psychological aspects in insulin-dependent diabetes mellitus. *Acta Paediat Scand* 1996; **85**: 818–24
77. Liakopoulou M, Korvessi M, Dacou-Voutetakis C. Personality characteristics, environmental factors and glycaemic control in adolescents with diabetes. *Eur Child Adolesc Psychiat* 1992; **1**(2): 82–8
78. Simonds J, Goldstein D, Walker B, Rawlings S. The relationship between psychological factors and blood glucose regulation in insulin-dependent diabetic adolescents. *Diabet Care* 1981; **4**(6): 610–15

79. Jacobson AM, Hauser ST, Wolfsdorf JI, Houlihan J, Milley JE, Herskowitz RD, Wertileb D, Watt E. Psychologic predictors of compliance in children with recent onset of diabetes. *J Pediat* 1987; **110**: 805–11
80. Coleman J, Hendry L. *The Nature of Adolescence*. London: Routledge, 1990
81. Burns KL, Green P, Chase HP. Psychosocial correlates of glycemic control as a function of age in youth with insulin-dependent diabetes. *J Adolesc Health* 1986; **7**: 311–19
82. Burroughs TE, Pontious SL, Santiago JV. The relationship among six psychosocial domains, age, health care adherence, and metabolic control in adolescents with IDDM. *Diabet Educ* 1993; **19**(5): 396–402
83. Auslander WF, Thompson SJ, Dreitzer D, Santiago JV. Mothers' satisfaction with medical care: perceptions of racism, family stress and medical outcomes in children with diabetes. *Health Soc Work* 1997; **22**(3): 190–99
84. Weist MD, Finney JW, Barnard MU, Davis CD, Ollendick TH. Empirical selection of psychosocial treatment targets for children and adolescents with diabetes. *J Pediat Psychol* 1993; **18**(1): 11–28
85. Lane JD, Stabler B, Ross SL, Morris MA, Litton JC, Surwit RS. Psychological predictors of glucose control in patients with IDDM. *Diabet Care* 1988; **11**(10): 798–800
86. Jacobson AM, Hauser ST, Wertileb D, Wolfsdorf JI, Orleans J, Vieyra M. Psychological adjustment of children with recently diagnosed diabetes mellitus. *Diabet Care* 1986; **9**(4): 323–9
87. Band EB, Weisz JR. Developmental differences in primary and secondary control of coping and adjustment to juvenile diabetes. *J Clin Child Psychol* 1990; **19**(2): 150–58
88. Peyrot MF, McMurry JF. Psychosocial factors in diabetes control: adjustment of insulin-treated adults. *Psychosom Med* 1985; **47**(6): 542–57
89. Peyrot MF, Rubin RR. Structure and correlates of diabetes-specific locus of control. *Diabet Care* 1994; **17**(9): 994–1001
90. McCaul KD, Glasgow RE, Schafer LC. Diabetes regimen behaviour: predicting adherence. *Med Care* 1987; **25**(9): 868–81
91. Schafer LC, Glasgow RE, McCaul KD, Dreher M. Adherence to IDDM regimens: relationship to psychosocial variables and metabolic control. *Diabet Care* 1983; **6**(5): 493–8
92. Wing RR, Lamparski DM, Zaslow S, Betschart J, Siminerio L, Becker D. Frequency and accuracy of self-monitoring of blood glucose in children: relationship to glycemic control. *Diabet Care* 1985; **8**(3): 214–18
93. Bobrow ES, Avruskin TW, Siller J. Mother–daughter interaction and adherence to diabetes regimens. *Diabet Care* 1985; **8**(2): 146–51
94. Weinstein ND, Rothman AJ, Nicolich M. Use of correlational data to examine the effects of risk perceptions on precautionary behavior. *Psychol Health* 1998; **13**: 479–501
95. Auslander WF, Bubb J, Rogge M, Santiago JV. Family stress and resources: potential areas of intervention in children recently diagnosed with diabetes. *Health Soc Work* 1993; **18**(2): 101–13
96. Balfour L, White DR, Schiffrin A, Dougherty G, Dufresne J. Dietary disinhibition, perceived stress, and glucose control in young, type 1 diabetic women. *Health Psychol* 1993; **12**(1): 33–8
97. Nurick MA, Johnson SB. Enhancing blood glucose awareness in adolescents and young adults with IDDM. *Diabet Care* 1991; **14**(1): 1–7
98. Chase HP, Jackson GG. Stress and sugar control in children with insulin-dependent diabetes mellitus. *J Pediat* 1981; **98**: 1011–13

99. Goldston DB, Kovacs M, Obrosky DS, Iyengar S. A longitudinal study of life events and metabolic control among youths with insulin-dependent diabetes mellitus. *Health Psychol* 1995; **14**(5): 409–41
100. Hanson CL, Henggeler SW, Burghen GA. Model of associations between psychosocial variables and health-outcome measures of adolescents with IDDM. *Diabet Care* 1987; **10**(6): 752–8
101. Hanson CL, Schinkel AM, De Guire MJ, Kolterman OG. Empirical validation for a family-centered model of care. *Diabet Care* 1995; **18**(10): 1347–56
102. Kager VA, Holden EW. Preliminary investigation of the direct and moderating effects of family and individual variables on the adjustment of children and adolescents with diabetes. *J Pediat Psychol* 1992; **17**(4): 491–502
103. Nakumura N, Kanematsu Y. Coping in relation to self-care behaviours and control of blood glucose levels in Japanese teenagers with insulin-dependent diabetes mellitus. *J Pediat Nurs* 1994; **9**(6): 427–32
104. Viner R, McGrath M, Trudinger P. Family stress and metabolic control in diabetes. *Arch Dis Child* 1996; **74**: 418–21
105. Wysocki T. Associations among teen–parent relationships, metabolic control, and adjustment to diabetes in adolescents. *J Pediat Psychol* 1993; **18**(4): 441–52
106. Stevenson K, Sensky T, Petty R. Glycaemic control in adolescents with type I diabetes and parental expressed emotion. *Psychother Psychosom* 1997; **55**: 170–75
107. Delamater AM, Kurtz SM, Bubb J, White NH, Santiago JV. Stress and coping in relation to metabolic control of adolescents with type 1 diabetes. *Dev Behav Pediat* 1987; **8**(3): 136–40
108. Lawler MK, Volk R, Viviani N, Mengel MB. Individual and family factors impacting diabetic control in the adolescent: a preliminary study. *Matern–Child Nurs J* 1991; **19**(4): 331–45
109. Smith MS, Mauseth R, Palmer JP, Pecoraro R, Wenet G. Glycosylated hemoglobin and psychological adjustment in adolescents with diabetes. *Adolescence* 1991; **26**: 31–40
110. Grey M, Cameron ME, Thurber FW. Coping and adaptation in children with diabetes. *Nurs Res* 1991; **40**(3): 144–9
111. Yasar SA, Tulassay T, Korner A, Szucs L, Nagy I, Szabo A, Miltenyi M. Sympathetic-adrenergic activity and acid–base regulation under acute physical stress in type I (insulin-dependent) diabetic children. *Hormone Res* 1994; **42**: 110–15
112. Niemcryk SJ, Speers MA, Travis LB, Gary HE. Psychosocial correlates of hemoglobin AIc in young adults with type I diabetes. *J Psychosom Res* 1990; **34**(6): 617–627
113. Brand AH, Johnson JH, Johnson SB. Life stress and diabetic control in children and adolescents with insulin-dependent diabetes. *J Pediat Psychol* 1986; **11**(4): 481–95
114. Grey M, Lipman TM, Cameron ME, Thurber FW. Coping behaviour at diagnosis and in adjustment one year later in children with diabetes. *Nursing Res* 1997; **46**(6): 312–17
115. Wysocki T, Harris MA, Greco P, Harvey LM, McDonell K, Danda CLE, Bubb J, White NH. Social validity of support group and behavior therapy interventions for families of adolescents with insulin-dependent diabetes mellitus. *J Pediat Psychol* 1997; **22**; 635–50
116. Carter WR, Gonder-Frederick L, Cox D, Clarke WL, Scott D. Effects of stress on blood glucose in IDDM. *Diabet Care* 1985; **8**(4): 411–12
117. Aiken LS, Wallander JL, Bell DSH, McNorton A. A nomothetic–idiographic

study of daily psychological stress and blood glucose in women with type 1 diabetes mellitus. *J Behav Med* 1994; **17**(6): 535–48
118. Hanson SL, Pichert JW. Perceived stress and diabetes control in adolescents. *Health Psychol* 1986; **5**(5): 439–5
119. Dutour A, Boiteau V, Dadoun F, Feissle A, Atlan C, Oliver C. Hormonal response to stress in brittle diabetes. *Psychoneuroendocrinology* 1996; **21**(6): 525–43
120. Wdowik MJ, Kendall PA, Harris MA. College students with diabetes: using focus groups and interviews to determine psychosocial issues and barriers to control. *Diabet Educ* 1997; **23**(5): 558–62
121. Seiffe-Krenke, I. The highly structured climate in families of adolescents with diabetes; functional or dysfunctional for metabolic control. *J Pediat Psychol* 1998; **23**(5): 313–22
122. Hanson CL, Henggeler SW, Harris MA, Burghen GA, Moore M. Family systems variables and the health status of adolescents with insulin-dependent diabetes mellitus. *Health Psychol* 1989; **8**(2): 239–53
123. Auslander WF, Anderson BA, Bubb J, Jung KC, Santiago JV. Risk factors to health in diabetic children: a prospective study from diagnosis. *Health Soc Work* 1990; **15**(2): 133–42
124. Overstreet S, Goins J, Chen RS, Holmes CS, Greer T, Dunlap WP, Frentz J. Family environment and the inter-reaction of family structure, child behavior and metabolic control for children with diabetes. *J Pediat Psychol* 1995; **20**(4): 435–47
125. Marteau TM, Bloch S, Baum JD. Family life and diabetic control. *J Clin Psychol Psychiat* 1987; **28**(6): 823–33
126. Hanson CL, Henggeler SW, Rodrigue JR, Burghen GA, Murphy WD. Father-absent adolescents with insulin-dependent diabetes mellitus: a population at risk? *J Appl Dev Psychol* 1988; **9**: 243–52
127. Maccoby E, Martin J. Socialization in the context of the family: parent–child interaction. In Mussen PH (ed) *Handbook of Child Psychology*, New York: Wiley, 1983
128. Hanson CL, Henggeler SW, Harris MA, Mitchell KA, Carle DL, Burghen GA. Associations between family members' perceptions of the health care system and the health of youths with insulin-dependent diabetes mellitus. *J Pediat Psychol* 1988; **13**(4): 543–54
129. Safyer AW, Hauser ST, Jacobson AM, Bliss R, Herskowitz RD, Wolfsdorf JI, Wertileb D. The impact of the family on diabetes adjustment: a developmental perspective. *Child Adolesc Soc Work J* 1993; **10**(2): 123–40
130. Wertileb D, Hauser ST, Jacobson AM. Adaptation to diabetes: behavior symptoms and family context. *J Pediat Psychol* 1986; **11**(4): 463–79
131. Wysocki T. Associations among teen–parent relationships, metabolic control, and adjustment to diabetes in adolescents. *J Pediat Psychol* 1993; **18**(4): 441–52
132. Varni JW, Babani L, Wallander JL, Roe TF, Fraiser SD. Social support and self-esteem effects on psychological adjustment in children and adolescents with insulin-dependent diabetes mellitus. *Child Family Behav Ther* 1989; **11**(1): 1–17
133. Hauser SM, Jacobson AM, Wertileb D, Brink S, Wentworth S. The contribution of family environment to perceived competence and illness adjustment in diabetic and acutely ill adolescents. *Family Relations* 1985; **34**: 99–108
134. Drotar D. Relating parent and family functioning to the psychological adjustment of children with chronic health conditions: what have we learned? What do we need to know? *J Pediat Psychol* 1997; **22**(2): 149–66

135. Hansson K, Ryden O, Johnsson P. Parent-rated family climate: a concomitant to metabolic control in juvenile IDDM? *Family Syst Med* 1994; **12**(4): 405–13
136. Jacobson AM, Hauser ST, Lavori P, Willett JB, Cole CF, Wolfsdorf JI, Dumont RH, Wertileb D. Family environment and glycemic control: a four-year prospective study of children and adolescents with insulin-dependent diabetes mellitus. *Psychosom Med* 1994; **56**: 401–9
137. Liss DS, Waller DA, Kennard BD, McIntire D, Capra P, Stephens J. Psychiatric illness and family support in children and adolescents with diabetic ketoacidosis: a controlled study. *J Am Acad Child Adolesc Psychiat* 1998; **37**(5): 536–44
138. McKelvey J, Waller DA, Stewart SM, Kennard BD, North AJ, Chipman JJ. Family support for diabetes: a pilot study for measuring disease-specific behaviours. *Child Health Care* 1989; **18**(1): 37–41
139. Miller-Johnson S, Emery RE, Marvin RS, Clarke W, Lovinger R, Martin M. Parent–child relationships and the management of insulin-dependent diabetes mellitus. *J Consult Clin Psychol* 1994; **62**(3): 603–10
140. Waller DA, Chipman JJ, Hardy BW, Hightower MS, North AJ, Williams SB, Babick AJ. Measuring diabetes-specific family support and its relation to metabolic control: a preliminary report. *J Am Acad Child Psychiat* 1986; **25**: 415–18
141. Gowers SG, Jones JC, Kiana S, North CD, Price DA. Family functioning: a correlate of diabetic control? *J Child Psychol Psychiat* 1995; **36**(6): 993–1001
142. Gustafsson PA, Cederblad M, Ludvigsson J, Lundin B. Family interaction and metabolic balance in juvenile diabetes mellitus: a prospective study. *Diabet Res Clin Pract* 1987; **4**: 7–14
143. Kovacs M, Kass RE, Schnell TM, Goldston D, Marsh J. Family functioning and metabolic control of school-aged children with IDDM. *Diabet Care* 1989; **12**(6): 409–14
144. McKelvey J, Waller DA, North AJ, Marks JF, Schreiner B, Travis LB, Murphy JN. Reliability and validity of the Diabetes Family Behavior Scale (DFBS). *Diabet Educ* 1993; **19**(2): 125–32
145. Burroughs TE, Harris MA, Pontious SL, Santiago JV. Research on social support in adolescents with IDDM: a critical review. *Diabet Educ* 1997; **23**(4): 438–48
146. Hauser SM, Jacobson AM, Lavori P, Wolfsdorf JI, Herskowitz RD, Milley JE, Bliss R. Adherence among children and adolescents with insulin-dependent diabetes mellitus over a four-year longitudinal follow-up: II. Immediate and long-term linkages with family milieu. *J Pediat Psychol* 1990; **15**(4): 527–42
147. Kyngas H, Hentinen M, Barlow JH. Adolescents' perceptions of physicians, nurses, parents and friends: help or hindrance in compliance with diabetes self-care? *J Adv Nursing* 1998; **27**: 760–69
148. La Greca AM, Auslander WF, Greco P, Spetter D, Fisher EB, Santiago JV. I get by with a little help from my family and friends: adolescents' support for diabetes care. *J Pediat Psychol* 1995; **20**(4): 449–76
149. Noller P, Callan V. *The Adolescent in the Family*. London: Routledge, 1991
150. Grotevant HD, Copper CR. Individuality and connectedness in adolescent development: review and prospects for research on identity, relationships and context. In Skoe E, von der Lippe A (eds) *Personality Development in Adolescence*. London: Routledge, 1998
151. von der Lippe A. Are conflict and challenge sources of personality development? *Ego Development and Family Communications*. In Skoe E, von der Lippe A (eds) *Personality Development in Adolescence*. London: Routledge, 1998
152. Hauser SM, Jacobson AM, Lavori P, Wilfsdorf JI, Herskowitz RD, Milley JE, Bliss

R. Adherence among children and adolescents with insulin-dependent diabetes mellitus over a four-year longitudinal follow-up: II. Immediate and long-term linkages with family milieu. *J Pediat Psychol* 1990; **15**(4): 527–42
153. Bennett Murphy LM, Thompson RJ, Morris MA. Adherence behavior among adolescents with type I insulin-dependent diabetes mellitus: the role of cognitive appraisal processes. *J Pediat Psychol* 1997; **22**: 811–25
154. La Greca AM, Follansbee D, Skyler JS. Developmental and behavioral aspects of diabetes management in youngsters. *Child Health Care* 1990; **19**(3): 132–9
155. Anderson BJ, Auslander WF, Jung KC, Miller JP, Santiago JV, Abraham C, Hampson SE. Assessing family sharing of diabetes responsibilities. *J Pediat Psychol* 1990; **15**(4): 477–92
156. Wysocki T, Linscheid TR, Taylor AT, Yeates KO, Hough BS, Naglieri JA. Deviation from developmentally appropriate self-care autonomy. *Diabet Care* 1996; **19**(2): 119–25
157. White K, Kolman ML, Wexler P, Polin G, Winter RJ. Unstable diabetes and unstable families: a psychosocial evaluation of diabetic children with recurrent ketoacidosis. *Pediatrics* 1984; **73**(6): 749–55
158. Anderson BJ, Joyce H, Brackeyy J., Laffel LMB. An office-based intervention to maintain parent–adolescent teamwork in diabetes management. *Diabet Care* 1999; **22**(5): 713–21
159. Anderson BJ, Wolf FM, Bukhart MT, Cornell RG, Bacon GE. Effects of peer-group intervention on metabolic control of adolescents with IDDM: randomized outpatient study. *Diabet Care* 1989; **12**(3): 179–83
160. Ryden O, Nevander L, Johnsson P, Hansson K, Kronvall P, Sjoblad S, Westbom L. Family therapy in poorly controlled juvenile IDDM: effects on diabetic control, self-evaluation and behavioural symptoms. *Acta Paediat Scand* 1994; **83**: 285–91
161. Chase HP, Rose B, Hoops S, Archer PG, Cribari JM. Techniques for improving glucose control in type I diabetes. *Pediatrician* 1985; **12**: 229–35
162. Golden MP, Herrold AJ, Orr DP. An approach to prevention of recurrent diabetic ketoacidosis in the pediatric population. *J Pediatrics* 1985; **107**: 195–200
163. Glasgow RE, Anderson BJ. Future directions for research on pediatric chronic disease management: lessons from diabetes. *J Pediat Psychol* 1995; **20**(4): 389–402
164. La Greca AM. Social consequences of pediatric conditions: fertile area for future investigation and intervention? *J Pediat Psychol* 1990; **15**(3): 285–307
165. La Greca AM. Peer influences in pediatric chronic illness: an update. *J Pediat Psychol* 1992; **17**(6): 775–84
166. Meldman LS. Diabetes as experienced by adolescents. *Adolescence* 1987; **22**: 433–44
167. Schlundt DG, Pichert JW, Rea MR, Puryear W, Penha MLL, Kline SS. Situational obstacles to adherence for adolescents with diabetes. *Diabet Educ* 1994; **20**(3): 207–11
168. Dunning PL. Young-adult perspectives of insulin-dependent diabetes. *Diabet Educ* 1995; **21**(1): 58–65
169. Berndt TJ. The features and effects of friendship in early adolescence. *Child Dev* 1982; **53**: 1447–60
170. Wallander JL, Varni JW. Social support and adjustment in chronically ill and handicapped children. *Am J Commun Psychol* 1989; **17**(2): 185–201
171. Golin CE, DiMatteo MR, Gelberg L. The role of patient participation in the doctor visit. *Diabet Care* 1996; **19**(10): 1153–64

172. Williams GC, Freedman ZR, Deci EL. Supporting autonomy to motivate patients with diabetes for glucose control. *Diabet Care* 1998; **21**(3): 1644–51
173. Greenfield S, Kaplan S, Ware JE, Yano EM, Frank HJL. Patients' participation in medical care: effects on blood sugar control and quality of life in diabetes. *J Gen Intern Med* 1988; **3**(Sept/Oct): 448–57
174. Marcia JE. Identity in adolescent. In Adelson J (ed) *Handbook of Adolescent Psychology*. New York: Wiley, 1980
175. Thompson CJ, Cummings F, Chalmers J, Newton RW. Abnormal insulin treatment behaviour: a major cause of ketoacidosis in the young adult. *Diabet Med* 1995; **12**: 429–43
176. Wallander JL, Varni JW, Babani L, Banis HT, Wilcox KT. Family resources as resistance factors for psychological maladjustment in chronically ill and handicapped children. *J Pediat Psychol* 1989; **14**(2): 157–73
177. Kovacs M, Charron-Prochownik D, Obrosky DS. A longitudinal study of biomedical and psychosocial predictors of multiple hospitalizations among young people with insulin-dependent diabetes mellitus. *Diabet Med* 1995; **12**: 142–8
178. Kovacs M, Ho V, Pollock MH. Criterion and predictive validity of the diagnosis of adjustment disorder: a prospective study of youths with new-onset insulin-dependent diabetes mellitus. *Am J Psychiat* 1995; **152**: 523–8
179. Anderson BJ, Rubin RR. *Practical Psychology for Diabetes Clinicians*. Alexandria: American Diabetes Association, 1996
180. Wysocki T. *The Ten Keys to Helping Your Child Grow Up with Diabetes*. Alexandria: American Diabetes Association, 1996

3

Diabetes and Pregnancy

FRANK J. SNOEK
Vrije Universiteit, Amsterdam, The Netherlands

INTRODUCTION

Diabetes pregnancy has long been associated with a high risk of fetal malformations, spontaneous abortions, stillbirths, macrosomia and neonatal mortality and morbidity[1,2]. It was not until the introduction of glycated haemoglobin assays in the late 1970s that it became clear that the increased risk of major congenital abnormality in diabetic women was to a large extent determined by poor glycaemic control in early pregnancy[3]. Since then, several studies have demonstrated that near-normal glycaemia in early pregnancy reduces the frequency of spontaneous abortions and congenital abnormalities to a level close to that of infants of non-diabetic women[4–6]. This finding is heartening for women with established diabetes who wish to become pregnant, and underscores the need for education and pre-pregnancy counselling.

Throughout the different stages of pregnancy, from planning conception to delivery and beyond, diabetes has a significant impact and probes important psychological issues that need to be addressed in diabetes care. In the early stage, women with established diabetes may experience increased stress levels related to their worries about possible birth defects that may interfere with family planning. Diabetic women who are pregnant are faced with increasing demands and scrutiny regarding fetal development, managing their diabetes as it responds to the pregnancy, and increased medical management. In gestational diabetes, women are confronted with a serious health problem that may involve insulin therapy, and elicit anxieties

Psychology in Diabetes Care. Edited by Frank J. Snoek and T. Chas Skinner.

regarding the impact of the diabetes on the health of both the unborn child and the mother.

This chapter highlights some of the psychological issues involved in pregnancy in diabetes, with focus on women with pre-existing diabetes.

PLANNING PREGNANCY

From her work with women with diabetes in the Joslin Clinic more than 50 years ago, Priscilla White observed that: 'To many, if not all, of these women, life lacks meaning, and even may be unendurable without successful child-bearing'[7]. Fortunately, nowadays there are in principle no medical reasons for a woman with established diabetes not to become pregnant—provided she takes adequate care of her blood glucose control before conception and throughout the pregnancy. Only on rare occasions may doctors advise against pregnancy, for instance when the woman with diabetes has seriously advanced microvascular complications, and the pregnancy may accelerate these complications and cause severe physical disability or even death in the diabetic woman[8].

As it has been convincingly demonstrated that poor glycaemic control during early pregnancy greatly increases the risk of birth defects in infants of mothers with established diabetes, health care professionals have taken the attitude that women with diabetes have it in their own hands to prevent birth defects by maintaining optimal blood glucose levels before conception and throughout pregnancy. For women with established diabetes who are in poor metabolic control, the requirements of more intensive self-care and medical management can complicate decision making and give way to worries and increased stress levels. While little is known yet about the heredity of type 1 diabetes, the issue of 'passing on' the disease to the unborn child appears of increasing concern for women with diabetes who are planning a family.

Large individual differences may be observed in how diabetic women and their partners cope with the need for 'preconception watchfulness' and pregnancy planning. While some women or couples may be 'unrealistically' optimistic regarding the health risks involved, others may react over-anxiously and develop a phobia of hyperglycaemia, leading to excessive blood glucose monitoring and very frequent consultations of the diabetes health care team.

In cases where a woman does achieve near-normal glucose levels, but with *no* pregnancy occurring, the woman and her partner may perceive this as 'unjust' and difficult to accept. The woman may find it hard to keep striving for tight control, and 'give up' on her treatment adherence. While from a psychological point of view we would be inclined to advise couples struggling with infertility to take a more *laisser faire* attitude towards pregnancy, this approach may be less useful in women with diabetes, as developing a more accepting attitude may be incompatible with staying adherent to the diabetes regimen.

In contrast to what one might expect in view of the health risks involved, research suggests that most women with diabetes tend to seek medical care *after* they are pregnant, when damage to the fetus may already have occurred. In the often-cited Maine study, in which providers in a state-wide network were trained in pre-conception care and attempts were made to reach all diabetic women before pregnancy, only 34% of the diabetic pregnancies occurred in women who had received pre-conception counselling[9]. In a recent study performed by Holing *et al.*[10], it was found, in a sample of 85 women with diabetes diagnosed before the index pregnancy, that fewer than half of the pregnancies were planned. The authors conclude that most unplanned pregnancies are not contraceptive failures, but may have been consciously or subconsciously intended. Interestingly, the authors found that women who felt that their doctor discouraged pregnancy were more likely to have an unplanned pregnancy than women who had been reassured they could have a healthy baby. This finding may be biased but does seem to underscore the importance of the doctor–patient relationship[11]. Social support appears to play a significant role, as women with unplanned pregnancies are reported to be less satisfied with their partner relationship than those who have planned their pregnancies, and only eight out of 50 felt that their partners were informed about diabetes and pregnancy. Most of the women in this study with unplanned pregnancies felt that their partners did not understand the risks or the enormity of effort required to achieve good diabetes control. Unplanned pregnancies are likely to occur more often in women with low education and low income. As Janz and colleagues[12] have reported, lower income, unemployment, less education and unmarried status are all factors having a major impact on whether or not women seek preconception care. In a prospective, longitudinal study, St James *et al.*[13] made an analysis of psychosocial factors related to unplanned pregnancies, comparing women with diabetes to women with phenylketonuria (PKU). While use and type of birth control were comparable for both groups, diabetic women used condoms more often. Consistent birth control in diabetic women was associated with social support and positive attitudes towards birth control, accounting for 21% of the variance in frequency of birth control use. Having an 'internal locus of control' and higher knowledge of maternal diabetes each accounted for 6% of the variance, while sociodemographic variables were not significant factors in regression analyses. The authors conclude that the two most important factors influencing contraceptive use among diabetic women would be (a) attitudes towards contraception and (b) perception of the extent to which significant others want the woman to use contraception. Interviewing younger diabetic women revealed that fear of future complications is a major concern to them, and seems to outweigh concerns about future children. Many wondered if they would live long enough to raise their child.

In the study by Holing *et al.*[10] it was observed that most women who said their pregnancies were unplanned were using contraception less than half of the time and were happy to learn they were pregnant. The authors then conclude: 'For some women, the difficulties in fully planning and preparing for pregnancy may be outweighed by the desire to have a child; these women may subconsciously "let it happen"'.

MANAGEMENT OF PREGNANCY IN DIABETES

Diabetes has been characterized as one of the most psychologically and behaviourally demanding of the chronic illnesses[14], and in women with diabetes who are pregnant, the demands of diabetes self-management are increased further. The experience of pregnancy for a woman with diabetes is strongly influenced by the increasing demands of the diabetes treatment regimen, concerns about the health of her baby and the impact of the pregnancy on her own health. While most pregnant women with diabetes would seem intrinsically motivated to comply with the medical recommendations in order to reduce the risk of birth defects, actually performing the required self-care behaviours throughout pregnancy is a difficult task[15].

Pregnancy is in itself an emotionally stressful period, during which the woman is confronted with various psychological and physical challenges. For a woman with diabetes the 'developmental tasks' related to pregnancy are essentially the same as for any woman, i.e. developing attachment to the fetus, preparing for separation, and adopting a realistic relationship with the newborn[16,17]. Pregnancy in a woman with pre-existing diabetes is usually accompanied by a great deal of medical attention, which may lead women with diabetes to feel that their pregnancy is medicalized and being 'taken over' by health professionals, with much of the attention focused on the fetus and its growth. Already existing feelings of ambivalence and fragility in the woman may be strengthened, and complicate the process of developing attachment to the fetus and preparing emotionally for motherhood. The health risks associated with diabetic pregnancy can trigger overprotectiveness in the patient's partner and family members, thereby unintentionally contributing to her sense of vulnerability[18]. Unplanned pregnancy may cause emotional stress in women with diabetes and fears of criticism and abandonment.

Women striving for 'perfect' diabetes control may find it extremely difficult to accept any elevated blood glucose levels and become highly frustrated by the day-to-day variability in blood glucose levels that is likely to occur in insulin-dependent diabetes, regardless of pregnancy. Receiving feedback of a lowering of glycated haemoglobin can help to decrease stress levels and improve self-esteem. On the other hand, failure to improve glycaemic control can easily lead to feelings of guilt and an increase of psychological distress and, eventually, to diabetes 'burn-out'[19].

A complicating factor in diabetic pregnancy that has attracted increasing attention concerns the risk of (severe) hypoglycaemia in strictly regulated diabetic pregnancy, partly related to the suppression of counter-regulatory hormones[20]. Severe hypoglycaemia, be it as a result of pregnancy or improved metabolic control, can cause high levels of anxiety, confronting the mother-to-be with a serious dilemma. On the one hand, she strives for optimal glycaemic control to reduce the risk of birth defects; on the other hand she is fearful of hypoglycaemia, both for herself and because of the possible harm that hypoglycaemia may cause to the fetus. Impaired hypoglycaemia awareness and related worries about severe hypoglycaemia can lead the pregnant woman to accept 'safe' levels of blood glucose, thereby compromising glycaemic control. Hypoglycaemia may be one of the major reasons why women do not reach near-normal glycaemic control during pregnancy[21]. This may be particularly true for women for whom work and/or family commitments make it extremely difficult to have low blood glucose levels. In a retrospective study of 30 patients by Gold and associates[22], women who had had previous pregnancies indeed had poorer glycaemic control, particularly during the latter part of the pregnancy. An alternative explanation for their poorer control could be that these women may have experienced a previous successful pregnancy, making them overconfident, resulting in a degree of complacency in their self-management.

For every parent, delivery is a stressful event. In the case of a mother with diabetes, stress levels may be increased in view of the risk of obstetric complications related to macrosomia and pregnancy-induced hypertension (pre-eclampsia). Clinical studies indeed suggest a higher occurrence of premature labour and preterm delivery in diabetic pregnancies[23]. Little is known about how diabetic pregnancy, in both type 1 and gestational diabetes, affects the development of the maternal–infant relationship. There is some research to suggest that children from diabetic mothers are at increased risk for a variety of behavioural disturbances, partly related to the children's obesity[24].

IMPLICATIONS FOR CARE AND RESEARCH

Much progress has been made in the past decades in the medical management of diabetic pregnancy. Unfortunately, research tells us that pre-pregnancy counselling has a limited effect in changing contraceptive behaviour in women with diabetes. Unplanned pregnancies therefore remain a major problem, leading to an excessive rate of spontaneous abortions and congenital malformations among women with diabetes. Further research into possible ways of improving the efficacy of pre-pregnancy programmes are warranted. Such studies should take into account socio-economic, cultural and ethnic factors that can strongly influence a woman's acceptance, understanding and compliance with restrictions imposed by a diabetic pregnancy[25].

Health care professionals should take an active approach to pre-conception counselling. As Lorber concludes: '...any sexually active woman between menarche and menopause may become pregnant unless she has undergone surgical sterilization. Start early and counsel often'[26].

There is reason to believe that almost any patient is capable of achieving improved glycaemic control during pregnancy, if she wants to, including women with a history of persistent poor glycaemic control. In practice, however, far from all patients with diabetes achieve normoglycaemia. As we have learned from clinical practice, education is an important prerequisite for adequate diabetes self-management, but by no means a guarantee that patients will indeed adhere to the diabetes regimen. In order to help women with diabetes cope more effectively with their diabetes, we need to identify their specific psychological and behavioural barriers, e.g. low diabetes self-efficacy, fear of hypoglycaemia, and lack of social support. Only then will we be able to offer customized psychosocial interventions that can help to improve the outcome of pregnancies in diabetes and the patient's quality of life. The importance of follow-ups after delivery is emphasized by research that suggests that in many women glycaemic control quickly deteriorates after delivery, returning to suboptimal prepregnancy levels. Moreover, a high default rate for clinical appointments in the postdelivery period is not uncommon and should be anticipated[22].

The complexity of the issues involved in diabetic pregnancy clearly illustrates the need for a joint obstetric/diabetes clinic and an integrated team approach, including psychology.

REFERENCES

1. Molsted-Pedersen L. Pregnancy and diabetes. In Alberti KGMM, Krall L (eds) *Diabetes Annual 1*. Amsterdam: Elsevier 1985; 238–45
2. Greene MF. Congenital malformations. In Hare JW (ed) *Diabetes Complicating Pregnancy: the Joslin Clinic Method*. New York: Alan R Liss, 1989; 147–61
3. Leslie RDG, John PN, Pyke DA, White JM. Haemoglobin A1 in diabetic pregnancy. *Lancet* 1978; **ii**: 292–93

4. Miller E, Hare JW, Cloherty JP *et al.* Elevated maternal haemoglobin A1c in early pregnancy and major congenital anomalies in infants of diabetic mothers. *N Engl J Med* 1981; **304**: 1331–4
5. Kitzmiller JL, Gavin LA, Gin GD *et al.* Preconception care of diabetes: glycemic control prevents congenital anomalies. *J Am Med Assoc* 1991; **265**: 731–6
6. Diabetes Control and Complications Trial (DCCT) Research Group. Pregnancy outcomes in the Diabetes Control and Complications Trial. *Am J Obstet Gynaecol* 1996; **174**(4): 1343–53
7. White P. Pregnancy complicating diabetes. *Am J Med* 1949; **7**: 609–16
8. Hare JW. Complicated diabetes complicating pregnancy. *Bailliéres Clin Obstet Gynaecol* 1991; **5**: 49–67
9. Wilhoite MB, Bennert HW Jr, Palomaki GE, Zaremba MM, Herman WH, Williams JR, Spear NH. The impact of preconception counseling on pregnancy outcomes. The experience of the Maine pregnancy program. *Diabet Care* 1993; **16**: 450–55
10. Holing EV, Beyer CS, Brown ZA, Connell FA. Why don't women with diabetes plan their pregnancies? *Diabet Care* 1998; **21**: 889–95
11. Coustan DR. Pre-conception planning. The relationship's the thing (Editorial). *Diabet Care* 1998; **21**: 887–8
12. Janz NK, Herman WH, Becker MP, Charon-Prochownik D, Shaya VL, Lesnick TG, Jocaber SJ, Fachnie JD, Kruger DF, Sanfield JA, Rosenblatt SI, Lorenz KP. Diabetes and pregnancy: factors associated with seeking pre-conception care. *Diabet Care* 1995; **18**: 157–65
13. St James PJ, Younger MD, Hamilton BD, Waisbren SE. Unplanned pregnancies in young women with diabetes: an analysis of psychosocial factors. *Diabet Care* 1993; **16**: 1572–8
14. Cox DJ, Gonder-Frederick L. Major developments in behavioral diabetes research. *J Consult Clin Psychol* 1992; **4**: 628–38
15. Rosenblatt D. Adherence in pregnancy. In Myers LB, Midence K (eds) *Adherence to Treatment in Medicine*. Chur, Switzerland: Harwood Academic, 1998; 191–221
16. Caplan G. Emotional implications of pregnancy, and influences on family relationships. In Stuart HC, Prugh DG (eds) *The Healthy Child*. Cambridge, MA: Harvard University Press, 1960; 72–81
17. Kay E. Psychosocial responses to pregnant women with diabetes. In Brown FM, Hare JW (eds) *Diabetes Complicating Pregnancy: the Joslin Clinic Method*. New York: Wiley, 1995; 199–213
18. Papatheodorou NH. Diabetes and pregnancy: a psychosocial perspective. In Nuwayhid BS, Brickman CR, Lieb SM (eds) *Management of the Diabetic Pregnancy*. New York: Elsevier, 1987; 137–67
19. Polonsky WH. Understanding and treating patients with diabetes burnout. In Anderson BJ, Rubin RR (eds) *Practical Psychology for Diabetes Clinicians*. Alexandria, VA: American Diabetes Association, 1996; 183–92
20. Diamond MP *et al.* Impairment of counterregulatory hormone responses to hypoglycemia in pregnant women with insulin-dependent diabetes. *Am J Obstet Gynaecol* 1992; **166**: 70–77
21. Kimmerle R, Heinemann L, Delecki A, Berger M. Severe hypoglycemia incidence and predisposing factors in 85 pregnancies of type 1 diabetic women. *Diabet Care* 1992; **15**: 1034–7
22. Gold AE, Reilly C, Walker JD. Transient improvement in glycemic control. The impact of pregnancy in women with IDDM. *Diabet Care* 1998; **21**: 374–8

23. Oats JJN. Labour and delivery. In Dornhorst A, Hadden DR (eds) *Diabetes and Pregnancy. An International Approach to Diagnosis and Management*. Chichester: Wiley, 1996; 295–302
24. Rizzo TA, Silverman BL, Metzger BE, Cho NH. Behavioral adjustment in children of diabetic mothers. *Acta Paediatr* 1997; **86**: 969–74
25. Wootton J, Girling JC. Addressing the needs of the inner city clinics. In Dornhorst A, Hadden DR (eds) *Diabetes and Pregnancy. An International Approach to Diagnosis and Management*. Chichester: Wiley, 1996; 265–76
26. Lorber D (ed). Preconception management for the woman with diabetes. From research to practice. *Diabet Spectrum* 1995; 269–300

4

Facilitating Self-care Through Empowerment

ROBERT ANDERSON[a], MARTHA FUNNELL[b], ANITA CARLSON[c], NUHA SALEH-STATIN[c], SUE CRADOCK[d] and T. CHAS SKINNER[e]

[a] University of Michigan Medical School, Ann Arbor, MI, USA; [b] University of Michigan Diabetes Research and Training Center, Ann Arbor, MI, USA; [c] Karolinska Hospital, Stockholm, Sweden; [d] Queen Alexandria Hospital, Portsmouth, UK; [e] University Hospital Lewisham, London, UK

A NEW PARADIGM

In 1991 the education team at the University of Michigan Diabetes Research and Training Center (MDRTC) published an article that offered a new paradigm for diabetes care and education. Called 'patient empowerment, this paradigm was contrasted with the more traditional medical model approach to care and education[1]. The need for a new conceptual framework underlying diabetes care and education became apparent after the MDRTC education team spent years developing and evaluating innovative diabetes patient education programmes and materials, only to realize time and again that the intellectual, structural and financial infrastructure necessary for their implementation did not exist[2–5]. They realized that it was futile to continue to develop innovative approaches to diabetes care and hoped that they would be adopted by a health care system based on the treatment of acute illness.

The MDRTC realized that diabetes self-management was radically different from the treatment of acute illness and required a new conceptual framework to inform the behavioural, educational and clinical approaches used to treat it[6]. This realization presented a sizable challenge, because the

Psychology in Diabetes Care. Edited by Frank J. Snoek and T. Chas Skinner.

acute care system permeated health care in the USA. The US health care system had not adopted a conceptually sound approach to the treatment of chronic diseases such as diabetes. The MDRTC team felt that to be effective, a chronic disease care system had to be based on a realistic understanding of the nature of diabetes and its self-management, that would guide the subsequent development of programmes, materials and research studies. They felt that the new approach must be, first and foremost, grounded in a realistic understanding of diabetes self-management as a behavioural and educational issue.

The MDRTC team realized that patients with diabetes were fully responsible for the self-management of their illness. Furthermore, they saw that the patient's responsibility for self-management was non-negotiable, inescapable and could not be shared or assigned. They understood that the patients' responsibility for the self-management of diabetes differentiated it from the treatment of acute illnesses in such a profound way that it required a fundamental redefinition of the roles, responsibilities and relationships of patients and educators[7].

The immutable responsibility that patients have for the self-management of diabetes rests on three characteristics of the disease. First, *the most important choices affecting the health and well-being of a person with diabetes are made by the person with the disease, not by diabetes educators or physicians*. The choices that patients make about eating, physical activity, stress management, monitoring, etc. are the major determinants of their diabetes control. Each day, during the routine conduct of their lives, patients with diabetes make a series of choices that, cumulatively, have a far greater impact on their blood glucose levels, quality of life and overall health and well-being than the decisions made by the health professionals providing their care. It is not that the patient's life affects his diabetes care, it is that the patient's life *is* his diabetes care.

Second, *patients are in control of their diabetes self-management*. No matter what health professionals do or say, patients are in control of the important daily diabetes self-management decisions. Professionals may plead, persuade, cajole, threaten, or advise their patients regarding any aspect of diabetes care, but when patients leave the clinic or office they have control over their self-management choices. Patients can veto any recommendation a health professional makes, no matter how important or relevant the provider believes that recommendation to be.

Third, *the consequences of the choices patients make every day about their diabetes care accrue first and foremost to patients themselves*. Health professionals can not share directly in the risks or benefits of their patients' diabetes self-management choices. Health professionals can not share in the risk of developing retinopathy, neuropathy or cardiovascular disease, neither can they share in the cost to the patient's quality of life of making a commitment to rigorous blood glucose control. Diabetes belongs to the patient.

Most of the training of health care professionals is based on the treatment of acute illnesses in which professionals are socialized to accept responsibility to solve problems that patients cannot solve on their own. Most health professionals feel this responsibility deeply. It shapes virtually every interaction that they have with their patients. This deep-seated sense of responsibility to solve a patient's problem also influences how they define their effectiveness. *Health professionals usually feel effective when they are able to come up with solutions to their patients' health care problems and frustrated when they cannot*. When health professionals work in diabetes, an illness whose self-management is immutably the responsibility of the patient, conflict and frustration often the result for those professionals who do not engage in an examination and fundamental redefinition of their roles and responsibilities.

Health professionals, grounded in the traditional medical model, often feel that it is their responsibility to get their patients to maximize their level of glucose control in order to prevent the acute and chronic complications of diabetes. Furthermore, they usually view education as a process to accomplish this underlying goal. However, since they can not control the patient's behaviour in order to reach the goal, they are likely to feel dissatisfied with patient care and education. Much of this frustration is projected onto patients, by labelling them 'non-compliant'. The problem is that they are applying a conceptual framework derived from the provision of acute care that is incompatible with the nature of diabetes self-management.

Empowerment, on the other hand, grows out of the traditions of community psychology[8], adult education[9] and counselling psychology[10] that view the purpose of education as enabling the recipients to gain more power over their lives, increase the number of choices available to them, and enhance their ability to influence the individuals and organizations which affect their lives. Empowerment emphasizes the whole person and embraces a biopsychosocial model of disease and illness, as opposed to the more hierarchical, biological, reductionist and compliance-oriented models derived from the treatment of acute illnesses[11].

In the empowerment approach, diabetes education is viewed as a collaboration among equals designed to help patients make informed decisions about their own diabetes self-management. The knowledge necessary to make informed decisions about diabetes self-management falls into two global domains[12]. The first domain is knowledge about diabetes and its treatment, i.e. the information necessary to make cost–benefit judgements about adopting (or not adopting) various diabetes self-management options. The second domain is self-awareness about the patient's own values, needs, goals and aspirations regarding diabetes care. In education directed at this latter domain, patients are helped to examine and clarify the emotional, social, intellectual and spiritual components of their lives as they relate to the decisions they must make about their diabetes self-management. Diabetes care is fitted to the patient's life, rather than the reverse.

The patient empowerment approach to diabetes patient education seeks to maximize the self-management knowledge, skills, self-awareness and sense of personal autonomy of patients to enable them to take charge of their own diabetes self-management. Empowered patients are those that have learned enough about diabetes and themselves, so that, in consultation with health care professionals, they can select and achieve their own goals for diabetes care[1]. The evaluation of a patient education programme based on the empowerment approach should focus on patient achievement of self-selected diabetes care goals, improved psychosocial adaptation and enhanced self-efficacy. The MDRTC felt that most patients, once they have been adequately educated about diabetes, would choose appropriate health-related outcomes, such as improved glucose, blood pressure and lipid control and weight loss, as part of their diabetes care goals[1].

SWEDISH REFLECTIONS

The most important aspect of patient empowerment, as seen by the Diabetes Education and Research Centre (LUCD) at Karolinska Hospital, Stockholm, was the view of the human being and of the process of learning and change. First, every human being is seen as basically striving for health and well-being, and human behaviour is always intentional. What we might see as self-destructive behaviours—in, for instance, people with diabetes—should be seen as a result of internal or external barriers to change or to a more healthy way of living. Second, all human beings are seen as responsible adults with the capacity to learn and change and to make informed decisions about, for instance, lifestyle issues. Third, learning is seen as an internal process in the learner that changes his/her understanding and ways of coping with his/her situation, and not as solely the acquisition of new facts. Last, this learning can not take place in adults without the learner's active participation in the process by exploration, reflection and experimentation.

In the literature, a differentiation has been made between empowerment at a community level (e.g. health care organization) and at an individual or psychological level[16]. To facilitate self-empowerment can be defined as anything we do in these two areas—the consultation/educational setting (micro-empowerment) and the broader health care organization (macro-empowerment)—that enhances the possibilities for people with diabetes to participate as equal partners in the team, and to have the resources (including knowledge) needed to make informed choices and decisions regarding metabolic control, treatment and lifestyle.

Empowerment in this broad definition includes, on one hand, areas such as politics, economy, legislation, organization; and on the other hand, our personal philosophy of human beings, and our values and attitudes regarding teaching, learning and counselling. Following this, actions towards a more empowered (or less disempowered) diabetes population can be taken by health authorities, health administrators, politicians, people with diabetes, patient associations and health professionals. Furthermore, all of these groups can work at different levels—from attitudes and behaviours expressed in the consultation room to efforts at the societal level.

The personal potentials, the patient's own resources and expertise regarding his/her own situation and way of living, must be acknowledged and developed. Further, the organization of care and the organizational climate must give him/her the opportunities to develop necessary involvement, responsibility and skills in taking care of the disease. Finally, the patient and the caregiver must meet in a partnership, on equal terms, to create the most appropriate health care for the individual patient.

Empowerment in patient education is built on the notion that patient education should aim at helping the patient to be in control of the plan for treatment and self-care. Therefore, education has to involve discovery and development of the patient's own resources for change and responsibility. That is not to say that the person with diabetes does not need knowledge about his/her disease and its treatment, only that knowledge is not enough. To alter old habits, to change behaviour, sometimes to a degree that can be described as changed lifestyle, is so much more than, and something different from, learning general facts or acquiring new skills.

Thus, in the area of patient education, empowerment means the structuring of individual consultations and group meetings in a way that helps the patient to discover and develop his/her own resources for change and control. In order to 'discover and develop resources for change' one needs to have self-awareness and clarity over one's own values, needs and goals regarding diabetes care. To make cost–benefit judgements regarding diabetes care options, one needs to have knowledge about diabetes and its consequences and treatment[18]. Thus, there can be said to be one 'external'—knowledge transference and acquisition—and one 'internal'—discovery and development of resources for change—side of patient education. Most educational programmes for patients with diabetes so far have focused on the 'external' side, that is to deliver knowledge about the disease and its treatment. The models/programmes to be presented below both have as their focus the 'internal' aspect. Three basis for these programmes need special attention:

1. The patient's attitudes towards, and value and understanding of, the importance of having diabetes and taking care of it are the cornerstones

of his/her actions. However, we are often not fully aware of the sets of values behind our behaviours. Possibilities to increase awareness of self and of values and emotions regarding the disease and self-care have, therefore, to be included in patient education programmes.

2. Problems related to self-care are often found in the domain of the patient's everyday life. Thus, they are seldom strictly medical problems or problems due to lack of knowledge. Furthermore, the patient's understanding of the problem must be the basis for interventions—interventions that must be found and implemented by the patient him/herself. As educators we can help people with diabetes to explore and identify their problems in struggling with self-care and we can also support them in their search for solutions. However, in performing this task we have to take on quite a different role from our traditional one in the medical model.
3. Behaviour change needs strong commitment and careful planning. Habits are deeply rooted and rewarding behaviours which often can be performed without conscious thinking. To give up old habits and/or to develop new ones has to be a very conscious, step-by-step process with thoroughly planned actions. As educators, we can help people with diabetes to set goals and plan for action, and support them through the process of change.

THE UK STORY

In the UK, since the early 1970s, diabetes education strove to teach people the principles of how to do the 'right things' to get their diabetes 'right'. This was based on the assumption that if people performed the 'right' number of blood tests, ate the 'right' diet, took the 'right' amount of insulin and undertook the 'right' amount of exercise, that good diabetes control would ensue. Diabetes education was therefore directed towards getting people to do the right tasks, in the right amount at the right time. The job of providing this diabetes education initially formed the basis of a major component of the diabetes nurse specialist role. The role of the diabetes nurse was to teach people how to be skilled at undertaking these tasks.

Until the 1970s there was limited technology to aid the health care professionals in determining the how, what, when and where of these diabetes management tasks. This changed with the development of self-blood glucose monitoring and the recognition that people could learn to adjust their own insulin dosage. These technological advances supported this model of diabetes education, as health care professionals now saw good control as feasible and achievable by everyone. However, during the 1980s diabetes health care professionals began to experience the outcome of this approach to diabetes education. Rather than basking in the glow of unremitting success, health care professionals kept finding out what did not work. This led to increasing levels of frustration for everyone involved in diabetes care, with everyone blaming themselves and everyone else for the 'failures' of diabetes care:

Patients 'Why can't I get this right?'; 'I do everything you tell me and it's still no better'

Nurses 'What am I doing wrong?'; 'What else don't I know?'; 'This patient just can't learn this'; 'This patient has got difficult diabetes'; 'I am not a good enough teacher'

Medics 'If only they would comply?'; 'This patient isn't intelligent enough?'; 'This patient has brittle diabetes'

As a result, the training of diabetes clinicians focused on how to be a better teacher, how to be better provider of information. The fault was being squarely laid at the feet of teaching methodology, i.e. health care professionals were not enabling successful transfer of knowledge and skills to persons with diabetes. Where patients were clearly able to demonstrate expert knowledge and diabetes management skills (doing the right thing), they were then deemed to be poorly motivated and still not getting it 'right'. These lessons led to the development of innovative ways of delivering diabetes education, such as group work, development of audio-visual teaching materials and computer-based knowledge assessment tools. Diabetes specialists acknowledged that this improved educational method was successful for some individuals, but not the majority.

However, the 1990s has seen a shift to a consideration of the psychological and social aspects of diabetes. It has become increasingly acknowledged that these factors have a significant, but unclear role in determining the outcomes of diabetes education, care and management. This led to the appearance of the counselling model to diabetes care, as advocated by Shillitoe[17] and the development of the still popular Northampton Diabetes Counselling Course. Despite the obvious benefits of using counselling skills to enable health care professionals to gain insight into the perceptions of people with diabetes, a new dilemma was created for many. How could this approach be incorporated into everyday diabetes health care? A chance meeting with members of the LUCD team led to discussion of these issues, as a result of which two nurses (Sue Cradock and Jil Rodgers) sought out the funding to attend the empowerment workshops in Stockholm.

The experience of participating in the workshop taught us two key things. First, that counselling skills could be integrated into clinical care. The model advocated at this workshop made use of the counselling skills to enable patients to learn about themselves and their diabetes and potentially to enable behaviour change. Second, this model enabled the diabetes clinicians to explore the emotional aspects of diabetes management. Experience tells us that emotions are probably the biggest motivator of change, the biggest barrier to change and often the biggest reward of change. However, discussing emotional issues is often the most difficult part of the process for medically-trained health care professionals. Health care professionals have been disempowered to explore the emotional aspects of diabetes. They have been encouraged to believe that discussing emotional issues with patients would lead to 'opening a can of worms'. Once the can is open, and the patient is freely expressing his/her emotions, it has been has assumed that, as health care professionals lack the skills to 'heal or solve' these emotional issues, they may harm the patient by exploring them. This is clearly not the case—just having the opportunity to discuss issues in a safe, honest, non-judgemental environment is experienced as beneficial by the patient.

Experience of using this approach in clinical practice convinced us of two things. This approach allowed us to trust our developing belief that there was no need to blame anyone for failure. In fact that act of blaming gets in the way of helping, and the concept of failure is just another barrier to overcome. It also became apparent that this model can be incorporated into clinical care, resulting in the consultation becoming:

- A more positive experience for the patient.
- A more positive experience for the health care professional.
- More focused on active problem solving.
- More likely to result in meaningful and lasting behaviour change.
- More likely to result in improved emotional well-being for the patient.
- Reductions in the level of frustration experienced by the health care professional.

TRAINING HEALTH CARE PROFESSIONALS

Diabetes education designed to empower patients requires appropriate attitudes, knowledge, educational and counselling skills on the part of diabetes educators. This is especially true when diabetes patient education is directed at helping patients increase their self-awareness of their own values, needs and goals regarding diabetes care.

The MDRTC developed and evaluated a professional education programme for diabetes educators designed to enable them to apply the empowerment approach in their own settings. The programme was an intensive 3-day workshop, limited to 12 participants, each of whom was videotaped practising empowerment-based patient education and counselling skills each day. Each of the participants reviewed his/her videotapes each day as well. The programme was designed to provide participants with both the theoretical framework and the hands-on counselling skills necessary to apply the empowerment approach with a variety of patients. The evaluation of the programme demonstrated its efficacy in terms of changing attitudes, simulated and actual counselling skills, determined by blind ratings of audio-tapes with real patients[13].

At LUCD, Stockholm, we have organized workshops for health professionals, lasting 2.5 days, with the content, methods and structure of the workshops based on the work at MDRTC. A four-step model of patient education is presented and trained. The four steps aim at supporting the patient in: (a) identifying and exploring his/her problem; (b) exploring feelings and values regarding diabetes, self-care behaviour or other problems; (c) identifying goals and behaviours leading to these goals; and (d) committing to and planning for action. The main task and responsibility of the educator in this model is to help the person with diabetes to explore and reflect upon his/her thoughts, feelings and actions; and further, to make sure that decisions about goals and behaviour changes are made by the patient him/herself and are based on a genuine wish for change.

Some structural issues and rules in these workshops are important for the participants to get a safe environment where they can experiment with new behaviours, and a deeper learning experience:

- The small format—no more than 12 participants.
- Video-recording and viewing in groups of four.
- 'Real play', as opposed to role play—when in the role of a patient, the participant brings up a problem of his/her own.
- A facilitator in each small group who is not allowed to criticize or give any 'right' answer, but should help participants reflect on their own behaviour and the motives behind it.

Workshops were evaluated using the Diabetes Attitude Scale (DAS)[20], administered before the workshop, immediately afterwards and at follow-up. At the same points in time participants gave their responses to six statements made by people with diabetes—'What would be your first response to a patient who says: ...?'. At each stage these were currently analysed according to whether they included words or statements which were judgemental or prescribing (minus) and/or whether they encouraged the patient to explore problems or feelings (plus).

Results from these evaluations indicated that participants felt patients should have more autonomy with regard to making their own choices regarding diabetes treatment and self-care (Table 4.1). The answers to the statements from patients showed a strong move from judgemental, prescribing or neutral statements towards statements that encouraged the patient to explore and reflect upon his/her problems or feelings. Responses that

Table 4.1. Change in patient autonomy beliefs as assessed by the Diabetes Attitude Scale

Item	Agreement pre-workshop (%)	Agreement post-workshop (%)	Significance
Individuals with diabetes should be taught to choose their own management options (e.g. type of meal planning, type of glucose monitoring, type of insulin regimen)	87	93	Non-significant
Decisions about managing diabetes should be made by the physician	56	68	Non-significant
People with diabetes have the right to decide how aggressively they will work to control their blood glucose	81	93	0.035
The important decisions regarding daily diabetes care should be made by the individual with diabetes	76	91	0.011
People with diabetes should choose their own goals for diabetes treatment	70	91	0.008
Factor mean	3.46 ± 0.7	4.3 ± 0.6	0.002

encourage the patient to explore the issue and/or express understanding and empathy were given +1 point. Responses that were irrelevant to the patient's statement or missing were given a zero. If more than two of the six statements were not responded to, the whole case was coded as missing. Finally, responses expressing information or advice not asked for, blame or praise, or efforts to hand the patient over to someone else, were given the value −1. The coding was done by the author and a co-worker not involved in the project, independently and blind regarding whether before or after workshop. Disagreements (a few) were discussed until consensus was reached. Before the workshop the mean sum of points was 0.6 ± 3.2 ($M \pm SD$). Immediately afterwards this sum had increased to 3.0 ± 2.9 ($M \pm SD$), $p = 0.001$. Table 4.2 shows some examples of responses from participants in the workshop and how they were coded.

In the last hour of the workshop, the participants are asked to give their comments on what they have experienced during the workshop. At a reunion after about 3 months they are asked to comment on experiences from having tried to apply the model in everyday work. A number of challenging and rewarding experiences have been reported which are fully in line with what has earlier been reported from the MDRTC:

Table 4.2. Examples of responses to patient statements and how they were coded

Positive response (+1)	Neutral response (0)	Negative response (−1)
'I will never start taking insulin'		
'What is stopping you?' 'Can you tell me why?'	'Many patients do' 'For how long did you have diabetes?'	'Why not, you would feel much better and it would be easier to control your blood sugar'
'I hardly eat anything, and I still don't lose weight'		
'What do you think is the reason for that?'	'What time of the day do you eat most?'	'Sounds strange, perhaps you should document everything you eat for a week?'
'I do hate my diabetes'		
'Tell me how you feel'	'I'm sure there are others who feel like you do'	'I don't like to hear that'

- Difficulties in exploring patients' *feelings and values*: the educator does not feel comfortable in asking questions in this area and/or is afraid to 'open Pandora's box' ('What if I initiate something that I'm not competent to take care of?').
- Difficulties in holding back one's urge to *give advice*. In the traditional role as patient educator, much of the work has focused on finding solutions *for* the patient. Many participants feel that by 'just' helping the patient to find his/her own solutions, they have not done a good job. Also, when the patient's choice is not what the educator think is the 'best one', an internal conflict can be experienced which, if too strong, threatens the new behaviour.
- Patients prefer a *passive role*. Traditionally, the educator has been the active, giving, partner and the patient the passive, receiving, part in the encounter. Even if this has not been fruitful, resistance to change can be strong.
- Reported rewarding aspects of using the model are a greater capacity to see what is one's own responsibility and what is the responsibility of the patient; a greater capacity to hold back one's own ideas and wait for the patient to find his own solutions; and also less time spent on motivating or persuading patients.

In the UK, empowerment workshops for health care professionals—predominantly nurses based in primary and secondary care—have been run by a group of nurses (Sue Cradock, Jil Rodgers, Florence Brown and Rosie Walker), for 2 years and supported by a colleague from the MDRTC and LUCD. Based on the model already described, the workshops have two components. First, before actually attending the workshops, participants are asked to mimic having diabetes for a week. Then they attend a 2 day workshop, involving a brief lecture, group discussions and 'real play' rehearsal of an empowerment consultation, which was videotaped and discussed in the small groups. These workshops have been evaluated using the dame approach as in the USA and Sweden. Participants were asked to complete the Diabetes Attitude Scale before mimicking diabetes, immediately before the workshop and at the end of the workshop. In addition, at the start and at the end of the workshop, participants were asked to indicate their response to hypothetical patient statements (e.g. see Table 4.2).

One of the most emotional and challenging experiences of the workshop, as perceived by the facilitators, is the mimicking of diabetes. Participants were asked to follow a prescribed diabetic of lifestyle, a fixed diet, two injections a day, four blood glucose test a day and an exercise programme. At the beginning of the workshop participants are encouraged to share their experiences of living with diabetes for a week. At these workshops we have been constantly struck by the powerful emotions this experience generates:

- 'I felt really guilty, like I could not stick to this for a week, let alone a lifetime'.
- 'I felt angry at the programme organizers for putting me through this'.
- 'It got in the way of everything, and my husband wanted to know when it would be over'.
- 'It was not what I tell my patients to do, so I followed my own regimen'.
- 'I was embarrassed to tell people what I was doing'.
- 'I did not need to do it, I know about diabetes and I inject myself all the time to show patients how to do it'.

These responses highlight just some of the emotions and responses brought out by this discussion. They confirmed in our minds, and those of participants, the mass of emotions generated by living with diabetes, if only for a week. The value of this experience for any health care professional, in recognizing the power of the emotional experience of diabetes care, cannot be understated.

These experiences of life with diabetes, and the group work undertaken in the workshops, led to a number of changes in participants' attitudes. Using repeated measures analysis of variance, compared to their initial responses on the Diabetes Attitude Scale, at the end of the workshop participants reported a greater need for specialist training for health care professionals caring for people with diabetes ($F=4.32$; $df=2$; $p < 0.02$). Similarly, participants reported a stronger belief in the need for patients to have more autonomy ($F=5.40$; $df=2$; $p < 0.007$). Both of these effects appear to a result of the combination of mimicking diabetes and the workshop, see Figures 4.1 and 4.2. Participants also reported a more positive attitude to poor self-care at the end of the workshop ($F=9.08$; $df=2$; $p < 0.001$) than before mimicking diabetes. However, this effect appeared to be influenced largely by the workshop ($t = -3.65$; $df=37$; $p < 0.001$) and not by mimicking diabetes (see Figure 4.3).

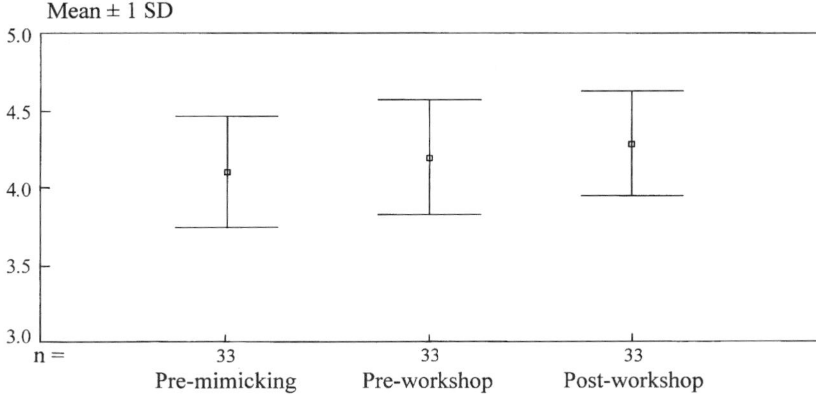

Figure 4.1. Change in need for specialist training

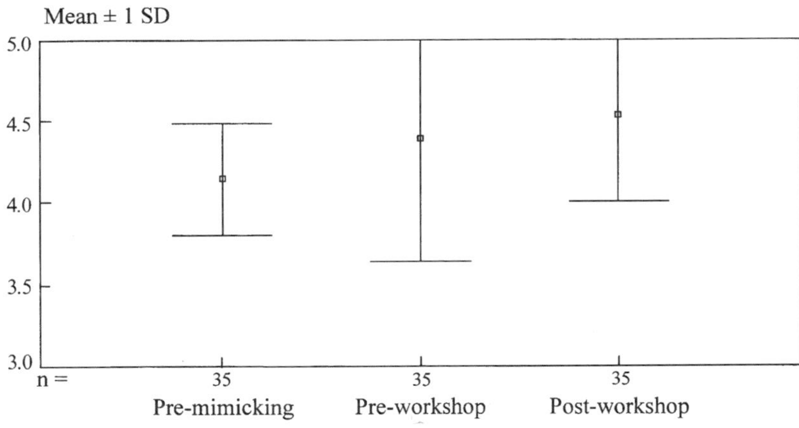

Figure 4.2. Change in patient autonomy

In light of DCCT and UKPDS results, the fourth change evident in participants' response to the DAS is of interest. Compared with the baseline measure, at the end of the workshop participants were less likely to support the belief that tight blood glucose control will prevent complications ($F = 3.96$; $df = 2$; $p < 0.03$: see Figure 4.4). This does not mean that participants did not believe that tight control would prevent complications, no participant disagreeing with this statement. However, it does suggest that participants were more likely to acknowledge the fact that there are

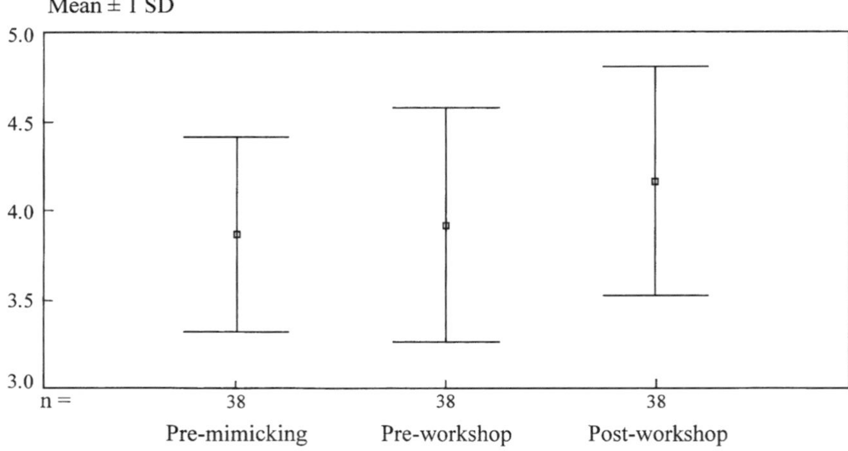

Figure 4.3. Change in attitude to poor self-care

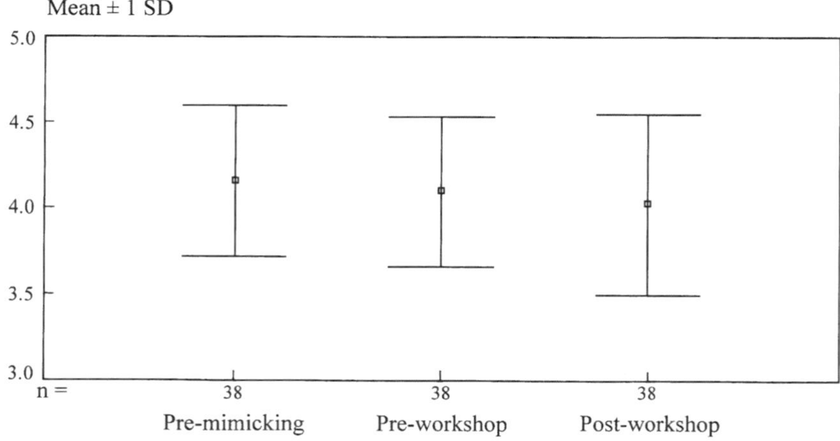

Figure 4.4. Change in control prevents complications

individuals with a history of tight control who do get complications, and vice versa. In the light of the workshop discussions around what motivates self-care behaviour, this result may reflect a more realistic appreciation of the patients' own thoughts, rationalizations and the probabilistic nature of the relationship between blood glucose control and complications.

EMPOWERMENT EDUCATION FOR PATIENTS

After determining that they could train educators, the MDRTC next designed a study to determine whether participation in a patient empowerment programme would result in improved psychosocial self-efficacy and attitudes toward diabetes, as well as a reduction in blood glucose levels.

Developed by Catherine Feste, the programme comprised a series of six 2–3 hour seminars, focusing on diabetes and self-care as experienced by the participants, and with a view to assisting participants[14,21] in: (a) identifying and setting realistic goals; (b) applying a systematic problem-solving process to eliminate barriers; (c) coping with circumstances that can not be changed; (d) managing different kinds of stress; (e) identifying and obtaining appropriate social support; and (f) improving their ability to be self-motivated.

The material includes a book for the group facilitator including a presentation of the empowerment concept, the philosophy behind the structure and content of the sessions, and the role of the facilitator. Also, for each of six sessions, there is a lecture to be given and advice on how to structure the session. The material also includes a number of work sheets for the participants to use. Each session has the same structure: a mini-lecture is given on the subject of the day (a–f above); the participants work with the subject, supported by the worksheets, in groups of four to six; and a final discussion is held in plenum.

This study was conducted as a randomized, wait-list control group trial. The intervention group received a six-session empowerment programme. Six weeks after the programme, both groups provided follow-up data. The intervention group showed gains over the control group on four of the eight self-efficacy subscales[15] and two of the five diabetes attitude subscales. Also, the intervention group showed a significant reduction in glycosylated haemoglobin levels. A 6 week follow-up analysis of data from all programme participants showed sustained improvements in all of the self-efficacy areas and two of the five diabetes attitude subscales, and a continuing modest improvement in blood glucose levels[14]. This study indicated that patient empowerment education is an effective approach to developing educational interventions for addressing the psychosocial aspects of living with diabetes. Furthermore, a patient empowerment approach is conducive to improving blood glucose control.

The material and process presented above have been translated into Swedish by the team at LUCD. Preliminary versions have been piloted with four groups of patients (in total 70 participants) in four different settings (patient association, the LUCD, and two different primary health care centres). The participants in the first group were interviewed by independent interviewers (student nurses). In the last session they were also asked to comment, in writing, on their immediate feelings and thoughts about the seminars. Further, the facilitators, after each session, evaluated the session on a number of parameters. From these evaluations some points should be should be mentioned:

- Participants felt inspired and encouraged to be more active in taking care of their disease—'I got a "kick" and I eat better now, which also shows on my blood sugar'; 'It is very useful to meet others with diabetes. I have learned a lot. It has been very encouraging in a way I can not express.'
- Participants expressed increased awareness about self in relation to self-care—'I had my objectives set earlier, but now I see them more clearly'; 'I understand now that it's I who have to do it'; 'Of course, I knew earlier what is important (in self-care), but during these seminars it became more clear, more concrete sort of...'.
- Participants reported that existing knowledge about diabetes had deepened—'We learned everything on a deeper level'; 'I have taken a lot of courses over the years, but this gave me new insights'.

When asked about the specific content of the seminar and to what extent it had been useful, responses were more varied. Many participants did not explicitly express that they were better equipped to set goals, solve problems, handle stress, etc. The facilitator evaluations after each seminar also showed strong doubts about whether or not participants had had time to integrate the subject of the day. Time became short partly because of the participants' eagerness to ask about medical issues. Even though many (17–18 out of 21) had participated in a number of patient education programmes before, the demands in these seminars to put the knowledge into action, or to apply it in everyday self-care, showed that the knowledge acquired was not properly integrated. Also, the language used in mini-lectures and worksheets might have been too sophisticated for many of the participants. A finding in the students' interviews showed that participants with a high 'sense of coherence' more often reported that they found the content of the seminars useful, than participants with low 'sense of coherence'[22]. Based on these and other findings, the material and the format will be revised and a final version will be finished in autumn 1999. A 2 day workshop is planned for the training of diabetes educators to provide the programme.

INTERNAL REASONING, DIABETES EXPERIENCES AND EMPOWERMENT IN A MULTI-CULTURAL SOCIETY

Culture can be appraised as one way in which people interpret, make sense of, and order their experiences and then communicate them to others[23]. Helman[24] defined culture as a set of guidelines (both implicit and explicit) that an individual inherits and which defines ways to view and experience the world emotionally and behave in relation to other people. The author states that culture has an important influence on the person's many aspects of life, his/her beliefs, behaviours, religion, family, clues, language and attitudes to illness and health. All this has its effect on health and health care. Linguistic barriers, different ways of interpreting happenings and different attributes of the meaning of the illness experience and treatment value can cause problems in communication and understanding when the patient and staff have different cultural backgrounds.

The patient, when faced with the challenge of daily dealing with his/her diabetes, tries to make sense of that within the frame of his/her knowledge, skills and the consequences of actions taken. The actions taken in order to manage his/her diabetes are governed by this understanding. Thus, achieving a good metabolic control and reducing the risk of late complications is controlled by the patient's understanding. As diabetes care mostly falls within the patient's own domain, it is essential for the health care staff to focus their treatment plan at promoting the patient's competence to accomplish his/her task. In doing this, the basis must be the patient's pre-understanding of what has happened to him/her. Therefore, competence in managing diabetes cannot be achieved by providing the patient with lists of routines to be done nor the mere supply of facts.

Fitzgerald and colleagues[25] studied the impact of dietary restrictions on African–Americans and Caucasians with non-insulin-dependent diabetes mellitus (NIDDM). Results showed that social support among Caucasians was an important factor in whether or not the patients follow the dietary recommendations, while for African–American patients the most important factor was the patient's attitude to diabetes. The authors recommended that health educators need to assess the psychosocial effects of diabetes on the patient's personal and social life. Furthermore, they concluded that interventions should aim at assisting the patients in recognizing their feelings about diabetes, and how these feelings influence their behaviour in the management of their illness or in following the self-care recommendations.

Rankin[26] studied the quality of life and social environment as reported by Chinese immigrants with NIDDM in a descriptive cross-sectional study. The purpose of the study was to ascertain factors related to the management of diabetes in the selected sample. He used Klienman's questions concerning the meaning of diabetes and could describe a non-medical model of causality of diabetes. The implications of this study for practice were to emphasize assessment of the specific educational, psychosocial and quality-of-life issues. In planning educational interventions, one must be culturally sensitive to the different emotional, educational, social and vocational needs in this group.

Even with the general knowledge acquired about certain cultures, one cannot generalize all patients from that culture. Dimou[27] proposed that one should not infer from the cultural or ethnic generalizations, but instead try to assess the conceptions and understanding of each individual.

Andersson and colleagues[28] explored the factors that influence the management of a chronic disease in two groups, Chinese–Canadian and Euro–Canadian women with diabetes. The authors proceeded with a hypothesis that women's patterns of self-management would be related to (a) ethnicity and/or (b) fluency in English. Their findings suggested that the way in which a woman managed her diabetes was not reducible to her ethnicity. Instead, the contextual features of her life, along with her ability to access resources, seemed to organize the way in which she managed her diabetes.

In our study[29] the experiences of Arabic-speaking immigrant patients on how they live with diabetes and manage their illness in daily life was examined. The initial assumption was that problems in the encounter between this group of patients and their Swedish health care providers were due to cultural and linguistic differences. The study then developed through three phases. During the first phase we described problems as perceived by Arabic-speaking patients and their health care providers. This was carried out by first interviewing both patients and health care providers. The result was a list of problems identified by both, but there was a discrepancy as to what was seen as the problem. In the next step, we arranged a workshop where patients, interpreters and health care providers were invited to discuss these problems. The results indicated that even though culture is a factor in the problems occurring in the encounter, it is but just a small part.

The next step was to elicit the patients' own experience and understanding of living and managing their diabetes, through semi-structured in-depth interviews. A conceptual model was developed describing patients' understanding of diabetes and its management (Figure 4.5). The model was made up of the following concepts and their meanings in the understanding of diabetes. The concept of the *meaning of having diabetes* is described as the impact of developing diabetes, not only from the physical but also from the emotional and social viewpoints. The *onset of diabetes* is the period when the patient was first discovered to have diabetes, describing the reasons to which the patient ascribed his/her diabetes. *Care for myself* is the strategy that the patient developed to manage his/her diabetes as he/she judged to fit best. This included not only the medical but also the social and psychological aspects. The 'care for myself' is often regarded by most health care providers as negative behaviour. This is not necessarily true, at least not as conceived by the patient. *Self-care* is what the patient was told to do to take care of his/her diabetes, i.e. usually a treatment regime described as a set of routines which the health care providers believed would best serve the patient. 'Care for myself' is the patient's modification of self-care, or even the alternative to

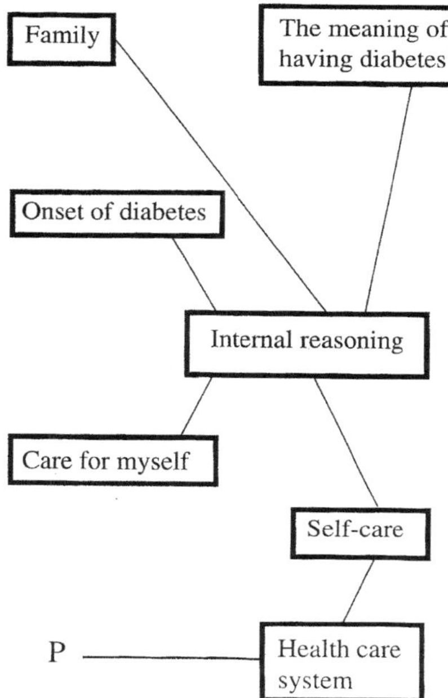

Figure 4.5. The conceptual model that describes how patients can understand diabetes and how it' affects their lives. P is the patient

the self-care recommended by the health care providers. As long as this 'care for myself' is not acknowledged by the health care providers, it will always compete with self-care. The *health care system* is usually constituted of the treating doctor, the diabetes nurse educator and sometimes other members of the team. Sometimes the family, neighbours and friends give advice and help the patient to manage his/her diabetes. The concept of the *family* involves the meaning and the function of family members in the patient's life, including his/her diabetes.

The patient's understanding of diabetes and the different ways of reasoning were summarized in a process called *'internal reasoning'*. This is the process that the patient uses to explain to him/herself the phenomenon of having diabetes and its consequences on his/her daily life. Through internal reasoning the patient can put the different aspects of the phenomenon together to make a whole meaning and to explain the relationship between the different parts of diabetes. All these concepts are interlaced and affect each other, with the process of internal reasoning governing this relationship.

The third and last phase of the study was an intervention where the above group of patients were followed up during a period of 6–33 months. Two kinds of interventions were observed. The first was teacher-centred, where the patient was passive. The second type of intervention was patient-centred, where the patient was active, reflective and experimenting until he/she found the ways to manage his/her diabetes according to his/her understanding. During this kind of intervention, the role of the health provider was supporting the patient and helping him/her reach his/her objectives. It was during this kind of intervention that behavioural changes occurred and learning took place[30].

Silverman[31] has indicated that human actions are based on making sense of reality and argued that human action has an internal logic. Thus, the main concept in the model that we named 'internal reasoning' could be compared to Silverman's 'internal logic'.

Kleinman[32] has introduced the Explanatory model, which was defined as the 'the notions about an episode of sickness and its treatment that are employed by all those engaged in the clinical process'. Both patients and health care providers have explanatory models in which explanations and alternatives to therapy are provided.

Strandford and colleagues[33] studied the personal illness models of diabetes among pre-adolescents and adolescents using Klienman's questions. Their results indicate that personal models are important tools and that they can help health care providers in planning education and implementing interventions.

The health care providers' model, on the other hand, is often based on medical facts and scientific causes, while the patients' model is based on personal experience, social, intellectual and cultural meanings of the illness[31]. In the encounter between the health care provider and the patient, where each has a different explanatory model of the disease or illness, there are bound to be difficulties.

The empowerment approach stems from humanistic education and community psychology. The philosophy behind it is that the patient and the health care providers are equals. The patients are seen as having both the ability and responsibility to make choices and take decisions. Empowerment is defined as the process where patients gain control and mastery over their life[34,35] Thus, patient education in which empowerment is the goal aims at improving the patients' quality of life by enabling them to make informed choices regarding their illness management. In this respect, these choices made are based on the patients' change in understanding regarding his situation.

The proposed model could be used as an aid to illustrate areas of patients' understanding which should be brought to the surface. It could be an asset in order to overcome the cultural barriers and have access to the individual's own understanding in relation to his/her cultural background, as well as social and personal experiences in relation to the illness. It also shows the different movements that the patient makes during different phases of life. Learning and changing one's understanding is a continuous process.

Price[36] proposed another model of learning diabetes self-management based on interviews with 20 IDDM patients in order to explore their learning experiences. Her model is composed of sequential phases that evolve over time, and is influenced by four factors: personal considerations, monitoring activities, specific cognitive skills for diabetes problem solving and definitions of control. While this model recognizes the importance of personal experiences and perceptions of what 'works for me', it can take a long time for the patient to reach an understanding and change his/her behaviour, since it depends a lot on trial and error.

Culture and ethnic background is but a small part of patients' understanding of diabetes. For health providers to be able to plan effective interventions leading to changes in patients' behaviour, they need to strive to understand how patients think and feel about their diabetes and help them accomplish the task of managing their diabetes and their daily lives. The internal reasoning model could be used as a helping tool to access patients' understanding of their experiences of the illness. This will facilitate the planning of more effective interventions.

Patients with diabetes, regardless of their cultural background, learn how to manage their diabetes and maintain acceptable HbA1c levels through a qualitative change of their understanding and the meaning of having and managing diabetes. In practice, this starts with the patients learning to test their blood glucose levels and learning to interpret these results in relation to their activities of their daily life. These activities include the relationship between blood glucose variations in association with food intake, exercise, stress, family life and social activities. This route provides a holistic perspective of patients managing their diabetes.

Supporting a patient in changing the conception of his/her diabetes and its management was a more effective educational strategy than the traditional ones. The use of both the interview and the model will increase the quality of the consultation and lead to a relatively rapid improvement of the patients' metabolic control.

Our follow-up of the interventions and the subsequent analysis using the model indicated that a patient changed his/her illness management only when an intervention was focused on supporting the patient in his/her change of understanding. The model is to help staff to plan how to best support the patient and to plan this together with the patient. Meaningful learning occurs when the patient's life experiences are used as a source of knowledge; the patient is encouraged to reflect on this knowledge and expert knowledge is to be supplied on the patient's demand. This type of learning will affect the patient's understanding of diabetes, which will result in a change of actions and better metabolic control and thus decrease the risk of developing late complications.

ADDITIONAL EVIDENCE FROM DIABETES RESEARCH

In addition to the work described here, there are two lines of research in the diabetes literature to suggest that an evidence base for this approach is emerging in the peer-reviewed literature, the descriptive research, followed by the intervention research.

Kyngas and Hentinen[37] interviewed a number of adolescents about their perceptions of their health care professionals, specifically their physicians and nurses. The adolescents' descriptions of their carers' behaviour were put into three or four categories. Two of these categories were common to both nurses and physicians; 'motivating'—asks, listens and takes notice of adolescent's opinion, decisions concerning care are made together, action of professionals is influenced by adolescents; and 'routine'—professionals act according to their goals, ask the same questions every visit, and answers are ignored. For physicians, the other two categories were 'authoritarian' and 'negligent'. For nurses, the other category was 'behaving according to physician's instruction'. What is important to note is that those adolescents whose health care professionals were described as motivating (which is closely related to the description of empowerment), were substantially more likely to have been rated as having 'good compliance', which in turn was related to better control of diabetes.

Along similar lines, Street and colleagues[19] studied the consultations of nurses with patients with type 2 diabetes attending a $3\frac{1}{2}$ day diabetes education course. The recorded consultations were coded by assistants blind to the purpose of the research. After controlling for baseline HbA1, follow-up HbA1, taken 2–3 months after the consultations, was predicted by features of the nurse–patient interactions. Specifically, after interacting with nurses who were more controlling and directive in their communication, patients experienced poorer metabolic control.

Another important descriptive study was recently published by Williams and colleagues[38]. They conducted a prospective study of 128 adults with diabetes. Their data indicated that when the health care climate was experienced as being rich with provision of choice, information about the problem, acknowledgement of the patient's emotions and minimal pressure to behave in particular ways, patients display improved physiological outcomes, in this case glycosylated haemoglobin. Furthermore, Williams demonstrated the process by which an empowering consultation may lead to improved patient outcomes. Their prospective data indicated that patients who experienced a more autonomy-supportive health care climate reported more autonomous motivation (experienced a sense of volition, self-initiation and personal endorsement of the behaviour), rather than controlled motivation (people felt pressured to behave by some interpersonal or intrapsychic pressure). This sense of autonomous motivation mediated the association between an autonomous health care climate and blood glucose regulation.

In a review of research on the role of patient participation in a visit to a doctor, Golin and colleagues[39] concluded that patient participation was associated with self-care. They hypothesized that increased patient participation in the consultation would influence subsequent self-care, through improving the fit between the treatment regimen and patients' lifestyle. This would clearly make it more likely that the individual would enact the treatment recommendations. In addition, by permitting patients to communicate their concerns and priorities to the provider they are more likely to receive more of the information they want and need, rather than what the health care professional thinks they want, the result of which may be greater relevance of information and subsequent improved use of knowledge and skills. Therefore, it is not surprising that prospective studies have found a direct link between patient participation and expression of their views and subsequent self-care.

Furthermore, a couple of studies have shown that increased information giving, meeting of patients' expectations, and expression of empathy effect patients' satisfaction with their medical care more than do the costs of care or the technical competence of the physician[40,41] Individuals were more satisfied with interactions in which they expressed their own opinions, and also reported feeling less motivated to adhere when they were scolded by a provider. Therefore, it would seem that there is a sound theoretical rationale and increasing descriptive data to support the argument for a more empowering approach to consultations. This descriptive data cannot demonstrate a causal relationship, which can only be demonstrated through intervention studies. However, there are at least two published intervention studies that provide further support for the principles of empowerment.

Greenfield and colleagues[42] conducted a randomized controlled trial of an intervention designed to improve patients' participation in their diabetes care. In a 20 minute session just before the regular clinic visit, the participants reviewed their medical records with a clinical assistant, guided by a diabetes algorithm. Using systematic prompts, the assistant encouraged participants to use the information gained to negotiate medical decisions with the doctor. In the control group, the participants just reviewed standardized educational material. The intervention was successful in terms of changing the nature of the consultation. The experimental group were more active, asking more questions, speaking more, and obtaining more information. At follow-up the participants in the intervention group showed significant improvements in glycosylated haemoglobin and fewer functional limitations. Furthermore, there was a significant correlation between more effective information seeking and follow-up glycosylated haemoglobin. It should also be noted that the increase in patient participation did not result in a lengthening of the clinic visit time.

Building on this work, Kinmonth and colleagues[43] conducted a randomized controlled trial of training primary care professionals in more 'patient-centred' care. This was operationalized by encouraging professional carers to review the evidence for patient-centred care, and provide them with relevant skills training, such as active listening and negotiation of behaviour change. In addition, patients in the intervention group received a booklet encouraging them to ask more questions. All newly diagnosed patients with type 2 diabetes at the 41 participating practices were then followed for a year. The intervention participants subsequently reported better communication with health care professionals, greater treatment satisfaction and better emotional well-being. These benefits were achieved without adversely affecting glycaemic control. The authors concluded that the 'study shows the power of the consultation to affect patients' health and well-being'.

Neither of these interventions was overtly based on the empowerment model, and only focused on certain aspects of the model as described above. However, in conjunction with the work previously described in this chapter, the data indicates that giving patients more choice, actively listening to them and answering their questions—in effect empowering them to take care of their diabetes—will result in improved physical and emotional health. However, it must be noted that to date, the authors are not aware of any study that has fully tested the empowerment model. Studies report changes in health care professionals' attitudes towards patients having more autonomy, choice and involvement in their diabetes care, as a result of attending 'empowerment training workshops'. There is, as yet, no published data to indicate that this results in changes in health care professionals' behaviour in clinical practice, and that this will result in improvements in patients' health. Bearing this in mind, we feel that the literature briefly reviewed here suggests that patients' physical and emotional health will be enhanced if an empowerment model is adopted. Thus, there is the beginning of an evidence base for this model of diabetes care, but a full test of the model is needed.

CONCLUDING THOUGHTS

This chapter has summarized the processes that led the authors to reconceptualize diabetes education and care. We have described how we have taken our colleagues down the same path, through our training workshops. We have highlighted the research, both our own and that of our colleagues, which we feel provides evidence for the effectiveness of this approach. We as a group are convinced, on philosophical, theoretical, experiential and evidential grounds, that this approach must be comprehensively tested in the world of diabetes care.

Some readers may feel that this chapter has not touched their world of diabetes care, for example: *How does this approach affect your practice? Does this take more time and resources? Does this replace diabetes education programmes?* Therefore, we would like to end by presenting the story of one clinician's experience using this approach.

Helen is a 20 year-old single female, diagnosed by her GP, who had had type 1 diabetes for 2 years when she was admitted to intensive care for 24 hours in severe diabetic ketoacidosis, with no concurrent illness. Whilst still an inpatient, conversations revealed that Helen had, over the previous few months, reduced the number of injections she was taking. She said that this was initially because the injections were painful, but that as a consequence of weight loss following insulin skipping, she had persisted with this behaviour. Following discharge she was taught the relationship between circulating insulin levels, blood glucose levels and ketoacidosis. For the next few weeks she appeared to be managing her diabetes effectively. Subsequently, she self-referred to the diabetes nurse specialist, complaining of backache, after her GP had failed to diagnose any pathology. Her random blood glucose was 25 mmol/l, and her urine was positive (+ + +) to ketones.

STOP: *Please now take a few moments to think about your plan of action at this time.*

Using the approach advocated in this chapter, Helen was first asked what her explanation of the pain was, but she had no causal explanation. After listening to Helen describe her health over the last few days, the clinician reflected back to Helen the set of symptoms she was experiencing (polyurea, fatigue, polydypsia, kidney pain, tender and sunken eyes). Helen was then encouraged to explore what these symptoms meant to her, in relation to her experiences of living with diabetes. Discussing these symptoms led Helen to reveal the amount of insulin she had administered over the past few days, and she acknowledged the probable association between her current health and lack of insulin. The possible management options were then explored with her, including admission to hospital. Helen chose to go home, take some insulin, measure her blood sugars and contact the diabetes centre if further assistance was required. The next morning Helen rang and asked for further information about controlling high blood sugars—despite administering her usual doses of insulin, her blood sugars were still high (>20).

STOP: *Please now take a few moments to think about your usual plan of action at this time.*

In response to statements about her current insulin not working, the clinician checked Helen's level of understanding, specifically the need to use higher-than-normal dosages of insulin during period of hyperglycaemia. This enabled Helen to suggest a number of potential options, which were discussed with the diabetes nurse. As Helen was still experiencing the symptoms of hyperglycaemia, she chose to take an additional shot of insulin and increase her normal dosage for the next 24 hours. Throughout this 48 hour period, the diabetes nurse specialist gave *no advice or recommendations* to Helen; rather, she described the various options and probable outcomes for each potential solution that Helen raised. All information that was given to Helen was given only in response to her requests. Helen was informed that the diabetes nurse specialist would be happy to see her if she wanted to talk further about her insulin management. Helen dropped in to the diabetes centre the following day.

STOP: *Please now take a few moments to think about your plan of action at this time.*

After a little wait, Helen met with the diabetes nurse specialist. After asking 'Helen, why are you unhappy?', Helen revealed that she felt that people were perceiving her as fat. This made her feel angry, frustrated, she 'just could not be bothered', which resulted in missed insulin injections. Over the next few days, she managed her diabetes markedly more effectively (blood glucose levels 10–14 mmol/l). Furthermore, she acknowledged the need for further help and the possibility of psychological support was discussed.

A number of key points should be noted from this case study:

- Helen was the individual who solved her own problems (this works to increase her confidence, competence and esteem).
- Helen received detailed technological and physiological information (this information was not only received, but processed, acted upon and reinforced through experiencing the results of her decisions).
- Helen has acknowledged her emotional struggle with diabetes and is considering psychological support (interpersonal therapy requires an active acceptance and desire to work at difficulties to succeed; this is difficult to achieve through clinician-driven referrals).

- Helen remained out of hospital, improved her self-care, started to enhance her emotional well-being and successfully reduced her blood glucose levels.

REFERENCES

1. Funnell MM, Anderson RM, Arnold MS, Barr PA, Donnelly MB, Johnson PD, Taylor-Moon D, White N. Empowerment, an idea whose time has come in diabetes education. *Diabet Educ* 1991; **17**: 37–41
2. Anderson RM. The challenge of translating scientific knowledge into improved diabetes care in the 1990s. *Diabet Care* 1991, **14**: 418–21
3. Anderson RM, Fitzgerald JT, Funnell MM, Barr PA, Stepien CJ, Hiss RG, Armbruster BA. Evaluation of an activated diabetic patient education newsletter. *Diabet Educ* 1994; **20**: 29–34
4. Funnell MM, Donnelly MB, Anderson RM, Johnson PD, Oh MS. Perceived effectiveness, cost, and availability of patient education methods and materials. *Diabet Educ* 1992; **18**: 139–45
5. Arnold MS, Butler PM, Anderson RM, Funnell MM, Feste C. Guidelines for facilitating a patient empowerment program. *Diabet Educ* 1995; **21**: 308–12
6. Anderson RM. Patient empowerment and the traditional medical model: a case of irreconcilable differences? *Diabet Care* 1995; **18**: 412–15
7. Anderson RM, Funnell MM, Arnold MS. Using the empowerment approach to help patients change behavior. In Anderson B, Rubin R (eds) *Practical Lessons from Psychology for Diabetes Clinicians*. Alexandria, VA: American Diabetes Association, 1996; 163–72
8. Rapport J. Terms of empowerment exemplars of prevention: toward a theory for community psychology. *Am J Community Psychol* 1987; **15**: 12–47
9. Wallerstein N, Bernstein E. Empowerment education: Freir's ideas adapted to health education. *Health Educ Q* 1988; **15**: 379–94
10. Combs AW, Avila DL, Purkey WW. *Helping Relationships*, 2nd edn. Boston, MA: Allyn and Bacon, 1978
11. Engel GL. The need for a new medical model: a challenge for biomedicine. *Science* 1977; **196**: 129–36
12. Anderson RM, Funnell MM, Arnold MS. Beyond compliance and glucose control: educating for patient empowerment. In Rifkin H *et al*. (eds) *Diabetes*. New York: Excerpta Medica International Congress Series, 1991; 1285–9
13. Anderson RM, Funnell MM, Barr PA, Dedrick RF, Davis WK. Learning to empower patients: the results of a professional education program for diabetes educators. *Diabet Care* 1991; **14**: 584–90
14. Anderson RM, Funnell MM, Butler P, Arnold MS, Fitzgerald JT, Feste C. Patient empowerment: results of a randomized control trial. *Diabet Care* 1995; **18**: 943–9
15. Anderson RM, Fitzgerald JT, Funnell MM, Feste C. Diabetes Empowerment Scale (DES): a measure of psychosocial self-efficacy. *Diabetes* 1997; **46**: 269A
16. Brown F. Counselling for patient empowerment. *Pract Diabet Int* 1996; **12**(6): 189–90
17. Shillitoe R. *Counselling People with Diabetes*. Leicester: British Psychological Society, 1994
18. Feste C. A practical look at patient empowerment. *Diabet Care* 1992; **15**(7): 922–5

19. Street RL, Piziak VK, Herzog J, Heijl J, Skinner G, McLelan L. Provider–patient communication and metabolic control. *Diabet Care* 1993; **16**(5): 714–21
20. Anderson RM, Fitzgerald JT, Gorenflo DW, Oh MS. A comparison of the diabetes-related attitudes of health care professionals and patients. *Patient Educ Counsel* 1993; **21**: 41–50
21. Feste CC. *Empowerment: Facilitating a Path to Personal Self-care*. Elkhart, IN: Miles Diagnostic Division, 1991
22. Anotnovsky A. *Unraveling the Mystery of Health. How People Manage Stress and Stay Well*. San Francisco, CA: Jossey-Bass, 1987
23. Kleinman A, Eisenberg L, Good B. Clinical lessons from anthropologic and cross-cultural research. *Ann Intern Med* 1978; **88**: 251–8
24. Helman CG. *Culture, Health and Illness: an Introduction for Health Professionals*, 2nd edn. Oxford: Butterworth, 1990
25. Fitzgerald JT *et al.* Differences in the impact of dietary restrictions on African–Americans and Caucasians with NIDDM. *Diabet Educ* 1997; **23**(1): 41–7
26. Rankin S *et al.* Quality of life and social environment as reported by Chinese immigrants with non-insulin-dependent diabetes mellitus. *Diabet Educ* 1997; **23**(2): 171–7
27. Dimou N. Illness and culture: learning difference. *Patient Educ Counsel* 1995; **26**: 153–7
28. Andersson JM *et al.* Living with a chronic illness: Chinese–Canadian and Euro–Canadian women with diabetes—exploring factors that influence management. *Soc Sci Med* 1995; **41**(2): 181–95
29. Saleh-Statin N. Arabic-speaking patients with diabetes: how they understand and learn to manage and live with their diabetes. Doctoral dissertation, Department of Public Health and Caring Sciences, Uppsala University, 2000
30. Anderson RM. The personal meaning of having diabetes: implications for patient behaviour and education or kicking the Bucket Theory. *Diab Medic* 1986; 85–9.
31. Silverman D. *The Theory of Organization*. London: Heinemann, 1970
32. Kleinman A. *Patients and Healers in the Context of Culture*. Berkeley, CA: University of California Press 1980; 104–8
33. Strandford *et al.* Personal illness models of diabetes: preadolescents and adolescents. *Diabet Educ* 1997; **23**(2): 147–51
34. Funnell MM, Anderson RM, Arnold MS, Barr PA, Connelly M, Johnson PD, Taylor-Moon D, White NH. Empowerment: an idea whose time has come in diabetes education. *Diabet Educ* 1991; **17**: 37–41
35. Anderson RM, Funnell M, Arnald MS. Beyond compliance and glucose control: educating for patient empowerment. In Rifkins H, Colurd JA, Taylor SI (eds) *Diabetes*. Amsterdam: Elsevier Science, 1991; 1285–9
36. Price MJ. An experiential model of learning diabetes self-management. *Qual Health Res* 1993; **3**(1): 29–54
37. Kyngas H, Hentinen M, Barlow JH. Adolescents' perceptions of physicians, nurses, parents and friends: help or hindrance in compliance with diabetes self-care? *J Adv Nurs* 1998; **27**: 760–69
38. Williams GC, Freedman ZR, Deci EL. Supporting autonomy to motivate patients with diabetes for glucose control. *Diabet Care* 1998; **21**(3): 1644–51
39. Golin CE, DiMatteo MR, Gelberg L. The role of patient participation in the doctor visit. *Diabet Care* 1996; **19**(10): 1153–64
40. Hall DA, Roter D, Katz N. Meta-analysis of correlates of provider behavior in medical encounters. *Med Care* 1988; **26**: 657–75

41. Waitzkin H. Information giving in medical care. *J Health Soc Behav* 1985; **26**: 81–101
42. Greenfield S, Kaplan S, Ware JE, Yano EM, Frank HJL. Patients' participation in medical care: effects on blood sugar control and quality of life in diabetes. *J Gen Intern Med* 1988; **3**: 448–57
43. Kinmonth AL, Woodcock A, Griffin S, Spiegal N, Campbell MJ. Randomised controlled trial of patient-centred care of diabetes in general practice: impact on current well-being and future disease risk. *Br Med J* 1998; **317**: 1202–8

5

Stage of Change Counselling

YVONNE DOHERTY[a], PETER JAMES[b]
and SUSAN ROBERTS[b]
[a]Fife Primary Care NHS Trust, UK; [b]Northumbria Health Care NHS Trust, North Shields, UK

NATURE OF THE PROBLEM

THE NEED FOR SELF-MANAGEMENT

Diabetes management requires a number of deliberate and largely conscious behaviours of significant complexity. In type 1 diabetes, the individual must alter food, insulin and physical activity on an hour-by-hour, day-by-day basis. In type 2 diabetes, management of medication, food consumption and physical activity are critical to good outcomes. For all people with diabetes there is a need to monitor blood glucose levels and make predictions, using bodily indications of hyperglycaemia or hypoglycaemia and external cues, such as time of day and physical activity. The person is also required to use health care services to screen for early signs of complications, and engage in preventive activities, such as foot care. This range of behaviours needs to be maintained by an individual within the context of helpful and unhelpful peer and social pressures, domestic and economic responsibilities and distracting life events.

If self-management is inadequate and blood glucose falls too low, the individual suffers problems of hypoglycaemia—disruption to activity, loss of control, embarrassment or fear, loss of driving license, hospital admission or, on rare occasions, death. However, if blood glucose is high for too long there

Psychology in Diabetes Care. Edited by Frank J. Snoek and T. Chas Skinner.

is a risk of kidney failure, heart disease and loss of vision and limbs. The costs of poor self-management are thus enormous in terms of the impact upon quality of life, especially in the physical, emotional and social domains. Most recent studies suggest that 8–9% of NHS expenditure is spent treating the complications of diabetes alone[1,2].

THE DISCREPANCY BETWEEN IDEAL AND REAL SELF-MANAGEMENT

The ultimate aim is that people with diabetes enjoy the best possible quality of life with minimum disruption. Health care professionals have identified a set of behaviours to which an individual 'should' comply (Table 5.1), although the emphasis will vary according to the service. Patients fall significantly short of staff ideals, as illustrated in column two of Table 5.1. There are difficulties inherent in attempting to measure compliance, the main being that self-report measures overestimate actual behaviour[3]. People may also look after some aspects of their regimen, but neglect others. This has given rise to the notion of *'levels of self care'*[4] a more helpful concept than traditional categories which label individuals as those that either do or do not self-manage.

Research suggests that lower levels of compliance are associated with regimens that are complex, life-long and prophylactic[17]. This helps to explain low levels of compliance, although there is a variation across diabetic conditions and variables[18]. A greater understanding of the psychological issues involved is needed in order for staff to develop the necessary skills to

Table 5.1. Levels of compliance to recommended self-care behaviours

Behaviour	Level of compliance (%) (%)	Reference
All aspects of the regimen	7–40	5 6
Taking medication or insulin	70–80	7 8 6
Blood monitoring	57–70	9 6
Dietary recommendations	65–76	10 11 12
Physical activity	19–30	13 14
Foot care	28	15
Attendance at clinic appointments	75	16

help patients. In this way the gap between ideal and real self-management can be narrowed.

STAFF ATTITUDES

Poor levels of compliance can be difficult for staff, given both the pressure of meeting targets set by national and international bodies[19] and the relentless reminder of risk from complications demonstrated in patients with whom staff may have had long and established relationships. This can result in negative and detrimental attitudes towards 'non-compliant' patients, which can have a deleterious effect on rapport, patients' self-esteem and motivation. Staff could be in danger of assuming that poor control is directly related to inferior self-management and that good control is always achieved by *'ideal'* self-management. However, this is not necessarily the case, as there are constitutional and environmental factors that shape both diabetes control and the development of complications (Figure 5.1). Health professionals do not appear to have fully grasped the complexities of self-management[20], as there is not a unified set of commonly agreed behaviours applicable to all people with diabetes, and hence patients need to learn their own repertoire[3].

Staff beliefs about what is a 'good' outcome and their ability to encourage a greater sense of self-determination and autonomy in their patients are factors that influence improved glycaemic control[21]. Staff can also uninten-

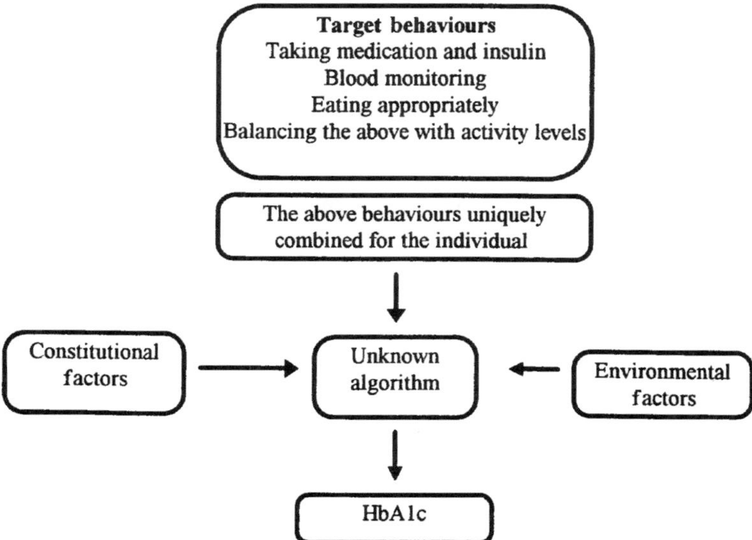

Figure 5.1. The relationship between self management behaviours and outcome

tionally enhance misconceptions about diabetes, such as the notion of 'mild' diabetes, which may impact upon the person's attitude towards his/her self-management[22]. For example, it is easy for a well-intentioned health care professional without specialist diabetes knowledge to suggest that routine blood monitoring will improve control, or that 'hypos' are completely avoidable with self-care. Therefore, staff wishing to facilitate behaviour change need to ensure that the targeted behaviour is worthwhile and the goals set are realistic. This may involve staff engaging in peer or multi-disciplinary group discussions to ensure that their beliefs and attitudes towards self-management behaviour are consistent with the evidence.

Applied psychological theory should be able to help patients and staff in the pursuit of improved self-management. There are relevant theories, but limited empirical evidence to draw upon. This chapter will cite the psychological principles that have proved valuable in health care and clinical implications will be discussed. These will, in part, be based upon the authors' experiences in a 3 year pilot project on change counselling in a routine diabetes service[23]. Ultimately, the authors hope to stimulate a number of disciplines into contributing to this crucial endeavour and highlight the scope for change.

THE TRADITIONAL APPROACH

THE ROLE OF EDUCATION

Knowledge is needed in order to self-manage diabetes. Many people with diabetes learn by trial and error. Information can come from other people with diabetes, lay sources (books, magazines and the Internet), or directly from medical experts, in which case it may be more consistent and accurate. A wide range of patient education programmes have been developed and evaluated over the last 20 years. Meta-analyses show that they increase patients' knowledge about diabetes and lead to improvement in some areas of self-management, but they do not appear to have a significant impact upon overall diabetes control[24,25]. In fact, some studies have found little relationship between level of knowledge and diabetic control[26]. The general conclusion is that patient education is a vital component of diabetes care, but is not sufficient in isolation[27].

There is a difference between knowledge and skill acquisition. The latter needs attention to modelling, practice and feedback. It is unclear how well these are incorporated into diabetes education programmes, although authors now acknowledge that simple knowledge transfer is not enough[28]. Attempts to use behavioural models from learning theory in education programmes have had some additional benefit[29] and there are guidelines from adult education theory that may enhance the effectiveness of routine education. These include the use of different learning stages and styles[30], and specific approaches for the acquisition of skills, rather than knowledge alone[31].

BEYOND COMPLIANCE AND ADHERENCE?

Compliance is the extent to which a person's behaviour coincides with medical advice[32]. Early research showed that compliance correlated with the extent to which patients understood, remembered and were satisfied with the information provided[17]. As much as 16% of the variance in 'compliance' could be explained by these factors. However, there are still discrepancies between 'ideal' and 'real' informational care and improvements need to be made[18]. Simple strategies have been shown to improve recall and are summarized in Table 5.2. Other interesting examples of effective informational care include the use of the Internet[33] and visual cards in ethnic populations[34].

Individuals often value non-health aspects of their life more highly such as social relationships and occupational status. Collaborative consultations[37] and joint decision making is needed to allow a patient to balance the desired health outcome with other aspects of his/her life. The health care professional needs to learn to facilitate behaviour change in a way that takes into account the person's overall choices and values and is not detrimental to his/her quality of life[21,35]. Consequently, a person's self-care, lack of symptoms, social functioning and emotional well-being need to be considered as separate, but relevant, domains. This is the essence of a patient-centred approach.

In health care, this is reflected in movement away from 'compliance', which implies an authoritarian 'do as I say' approach, to the use of the term 'adherence', with its evocation of greater self-determination and collaboration. In diabetes the term 'self-management', defined as the set of skilled

Table 5.2. Techniques to increase the understanding and memory of verbal communications. Based upon reference[38]

Technique	Improvement in recall (%)
Primacy: present the most important information first	↑36
Stressing importance: emphasize the most important information	↑15
Simplification: use shorter words and sentences	↑13
Repetition: restate important information	↑14–19
Use specific statements rather than general statements	↑35

behaviours engaged in to manage one's own illness[36], moves even further from the traditional stance in acknowledging that in order to achieve good control a person actually needs to be a self-motivated technician with the overall responsibility and burden of managing the disease[18].

Professionals often do not know exactly how patients achieve good control, so facilitating self-management will involve helping individuals to find their own best combination of behaviours[3]. The chronic disease management research suggests people develop a set of 'coping strategies', and there is no ideal way to manage successfully. In fact, it is most helpful to have a range of skills to use in different situations[39]. Thus, the challenge for health care professionals is to help each patient find his/her optimum way of self-managing.

THEORETICAL FOUNDATIONS TO CHANGE COUNSELLING

INTRODUCTION

Change counselling can be defined by its *philosophy*, desired *outcomes* and *methods*. The *philosophy*, based upon the counselling tradition, aims to empower people sufficiently to be able to help themselves[40,41]. The professional's objective is to be an equal partner in this process as the 'client' attempts to change. The desired *outcome* is the person achieving the best quality of life; balancing disease prevention with overall functioning and well-being. Change counselling *methods* draw upon the most relevant and applicable models from the behavioural sciences, which include: an understanding of the way emotions distort rational thinking; how cognitions (thoughts, assumptions and beliefs) ultimately determine behaviour; and how behaviour is shaped by learning processes.

In change counselling, theoretical and practical components can be assembled into a sequence of steps, according to the way people might make changes in their lives[42]. This provides the health care professional with a framework for breaking down the task of change counselling into a series of stages. It entails identifying the person's stage of change and then providing the most relevant form of help. The underlying theory and empirical support for this approach is presented first in order to describe and clarify each change counselling component and is followed by a description of the process.

COUNSELLING AND MOTIVATIONAL INTERVIEWING

Counselling

The core conditions of counselling (Table 5.3) have been found to be predictive of better outcomes in talking therapies[43]. Behaviour change counselling, therefore, incorporates these so that at the end of the consultation the patient should perceive that the health care professional was understanding, genuine, warm, non-judgemental and caring. Guidelines are available for health care staff who wish to learn and apply a counselling approach[41]. It is not necessary to train as a counsellor, but it does involve a shift in style away from a directive approach (i.e. suspending advice giving at times) in favour of eliciting the individual's thoughts and feelings[44]. The attitude of staff towards patients is seen as a prerequisite to effective working, and in diabetes services the counselling approach will be necessary for change counselling consultations to be effective. This is supported by recent research suggesting that those individuals who rated the professional to be 'patient-centred' achieved better diabetes control[45], and that adolescents' perceptions of carers were related to diabetes self-management[46]. While the approach is insufficient alone, it facilitates a trusting and collaborative relationship upon which to develop the change counselling intervention.

Essential counselling skills (Table 5.4) include the use of questions and reflections to explore patient perspectives. Summaries can also be employed to improve recall, clarify understanding and demonstrate that staff have been listening. Self-reflection and supervision are essential for health care professionals maintaining a patient-centred stance. Each and every patient is unique, and staff must attempt to understand each individual's particular needs and style of diabetes self-management. This is consistent with patient empowerment.

Table 5.3. Core conditions of counselling

Core conditions	Description
Empathic	Attempting to understand the problems from the other person's viewpoint and demonstrating it
Non-judgemental	Accepting the person's opinions and values without evaluating
Genuine	Not playing out a 'role' with the individual, i.e. open and honest communication.
Concrete	Clarifying meanings and being specific, e.g. what, when. How exactly did you feel?
Warm	Showing care, being interested and positive towards the individual

Table 5.4. Core counselling skills

Skill	Description	Function
Open question—a question that does not restrict the response to a yes or no	These questions usually start with: • How • What • When • Where e.g. 'What do you think are the most important aspects of your diabetes care?'	Encourages exploration of the issues, and elaboration of thoughts and feelings. Helps the person to talk and is patient-centred
Reflections—a re-statement of all or part of what someone has just said	• *Simple* or 'parroting', where part of the indiv dual's statement is repeated • *Paraphrase:* the restatement is changed before being fed back e.g. 'So, from what you've been saying, you have been thinking about stopping smoking'	Demonstrates the helper has been listening, improves rapport, allows clarification and encourages the person to talk
Summary—restatement of the main points of a consultation or part of a consultation	'So, today we have been discussing your concerns about smoking. On one hand, you know it would improve your health, save you money and give you a real sense of achievement. However, on the other hand, you worry about coping with the cravings and any potential weight gain and would like to think it through at home'	Improves recall, demonstrates listening, provides a formulation of the problem and possible action. It can bring part of a consultation to a close before moving on. Used at the end of a consultation

Motivational interviewing

Motivational Interviewing, is defined as a '*directive, client-centred counselling style for eliciting behaviour change by helping clients explore and resolve ambivalence*'[47]. Rollnick and Miller[47] argue that this approach is more than just a set of techniques, but encompasses a style and *spirit* which is patient-centred and facilitative. The key elements in motivational interviewing, which have developed over several years, are shown in Table 5.5.

The resolution of ambivalence is at the core of the approach. It recognizes that people often have conflicting views about making changes to their lives. An example would be people who would like to stop smoking, as it will save them money and improve their health, but they feel unable to cope with

Table 5.5. Key elements of motivational interviewing. Based upon reference 47

- Motivation to change is elicited from the person and not imposed by the health care professional
- It is the person's task, and not the health care professional's, to identify and resolve ambivalence
- Direct pressure does not resolve ambivalence
- The counselling style is generally a quiet and eliciting one
- The 'counsellor' is directive in helping the client to examine and resolve ambivalence
- Readiness to change is not a 'client' trait but fluctuates over time
- The relationship is more like a partnership than expert/recipient roles

everyday hassles and stress without cigarettes. The health care professional's task, using a motivational interviewing approach, is to highlight the ambivalence and facilitate the person's resolution of the issues, without persuasion. This reduces the likelihood that a patient will become resistant to health care staff and emphasizes the pursuit of patient-generated options.

The approach has been developed mainly in the area of alcohol dependence. Initial studies found that therapist empathy was a significant predictor of weekly alcohol consumption[48] and further research demonstrated that motivational interviewing gave better outcomes than traditional approaches[49,50]. Since ambivalence about engaging in change is common for people with diabetes, it has been argued that this approach could be employed in diabetes care[51]. In a weight reduction programme with women with type 2 diabetes, a group given an intervention using motivational interviewing principles achieved a significantly higher rate of adherence and better glycaemic control[52]. Change counselling programmes should therefore encompass these empirically supported consultation guidelines[53].

THE TRANSTHEORETICAL MODEL OF BEHAVIOUR CHANGE

Prochaska and DiClemente[54] investigated the process of change in an observational study that followed smokers who were attempting to stop independently. They observed that individuals went through a number of discernible stages in the change process, which led to the Transtheoretical Model of Change (Figure 5.2). Six stages of readiness were described: precontemplation, contemplation, determination, action, maintenance and relapse. Each stage represents an amalgamation of attitudes, intentions and behaviours[55]. This model has subsequently been used to describe the process of change in a wide variety of behaviours, such as exercise[52], smoking[56], healthy eating[57] and diabetes self-management[58].

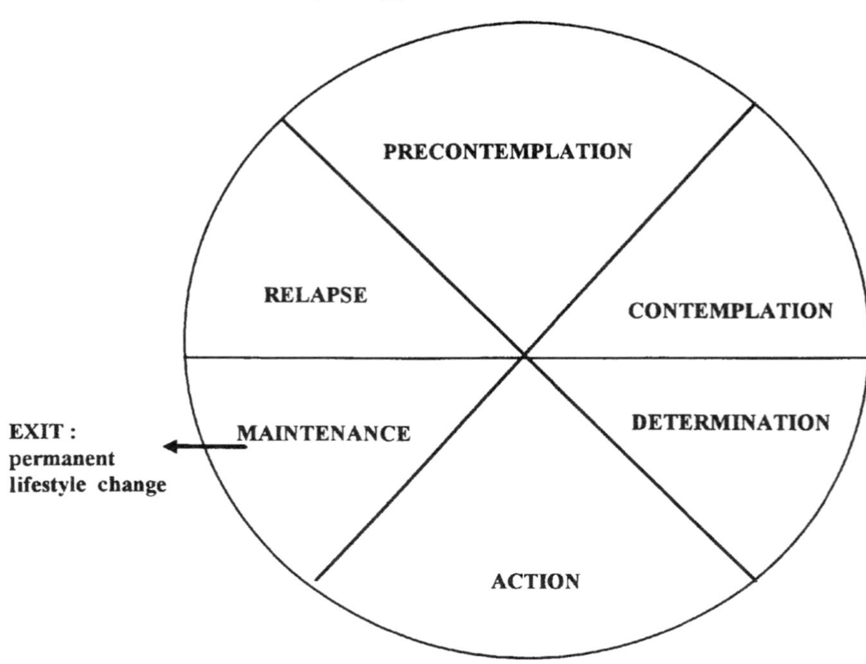

Figure 5.2. The Transtheoretical Model of Behaviour Change. Based on reference 54

Individuals in *precontemplation* are either unaware that the behaviour is a problem for them or are avoiding or unwilling to consider behaviour change. At this stage the people may display some of the characteristics of resistance[50], evidenced by avoiding discussion, minimizing or denying that the behaviour is problematical or defending their actions[59]. The people move into *contemplation* when they become able to think about and discuss their behaviour. They now acknowledge that the behaviour might be problematical or that they have something to gain from change, but have not decided whether to make the change because the advantages do not outweigh the associated barriers or losses. At the *determination* stage, the individual intends to make the change, develops action plans, reviews final blocks or barriers and considers how these might be overcome. In *action*, the individual is adopting the new behaviour whilst contending with the strength of old habits. After several months, the new repertoire has to be kept going, *maintained*, long enough for it to become the norm. At this point individuals may exit 'the cycle' into permanent lifestyle change. Alternatively they may *relapse*, having given up the intention to make or maintain the change.

The change process was initially seen as progression in a circle. Evidence now suggests there is movement forwards and backwards, with the potential for relapse to occur at any point in the process. This has led some authors to conceptualize the model as a spiral[60]. For the purposes of this chapter it will be conceptualized as shown in Figure 5.2. However, it should not be seen as just an orderly process—people do move backwards. Also, there is some reason to believe that the stages are not absolutely discrete, and sometimes movement is along a continuum[61]. Nevertheless, the model has proved to be useful in research, has been widely used in health education training[62] and has high face validity for staff and patients.

The Transtheoretical Model of Change emphasizes that individuals will normally make changes without intervention from a health care worker. For example, Prochaska[63] argued that people will move from precontemplation to contemplation as a result of a developmental event (e.g. reaching 40) or an environmental event (e.g. a comment that they smell of cigarette smoke). However, if the emotions, cognitions and behaviours associated with each stage could be identified, health care professionals, using counselling and motivational interviewing principles, could facilitate progress more effectively. Research is needed to test out these clinical assumptions, although developing the necessary methodology will be challenging[64].

PSYCHOLOGICAL MODELS TO HELP UNDERSTAND SELF-MANAGEMENT

Social cognition models

The psychological literature has investigated in considerable detail the beliefs that predict a person's intention to engage in a health-enhancing behaviour. These models can help guide the clinician in terms of the most relevant topics to explore.

The Health Belief Model (Figure 5.3), proposed by Becker[65], argues that people acquire beliefs about perceived disease severity, susceptibility and the perceived benefits over barriers for change; these combine to increase the 'likelihood of taking action'. The Health Belief Model has been extensively researched in diabetes, with the use of psychometric measures for each health belief dimension[66]. They are usually significantly associated with self-management but account for a small amount of the variance[67]. Consequently, they provide a relevant but insufficient explanation of the process, although they are widely referred to by clinical staff. However, the model does not cite the importance of intention as a mediating variable, and does not embrace other non-health beliefs that might determine behaviour change. It therefore needs to be integrated within a wider model.

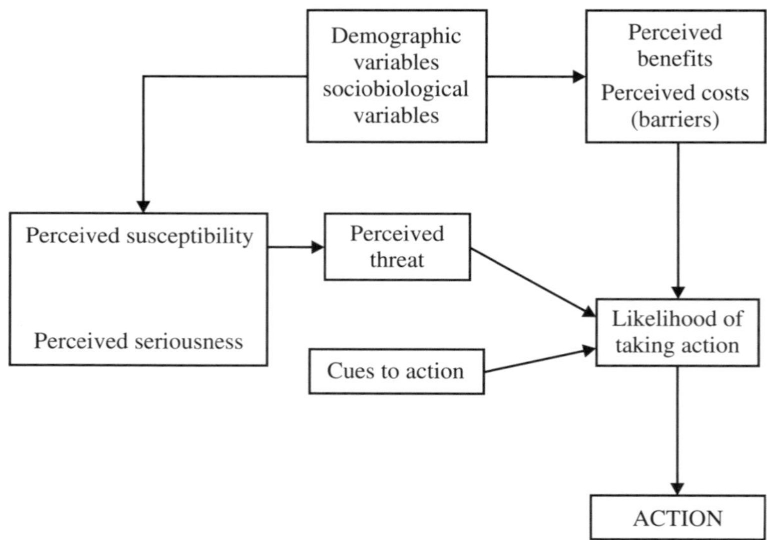

Figure 5.3. The Health Belief Model. Based on reference 65

Some psychological models assume that self-management behaviours are under volitional control, and therefore the single best determinant of future behaviour is a person's reasoned 'intention to change'[68]. The Theory of Reasoned Action[69] predicted that an intention to behave results from two variables: (a) a favourable attitude towards the behaviour, and (b) from norms that suggest that valued others would approve of the individual engaging in the behaviour. A third variable, namely self-efficacy, or the person's belief in his/her ability to carry out the behaviour was added and the model then became known as the Theory of Planned Behaviour[70].

The Health Action Process model[71] (Figure 5.4) attempts to combine research findings and serves as the best summary to date of the relevant variables. It emphasizes the importance of outcome expectancy ('What's in it for me?') and self-efficacy ('Can I do it?'). It adds an important further predictor of behaviour, namely cognitions that result in plans about initiating the behaviour, e.g. 'I will start going for a walk on Monday with my friend' (i.e. action plan) and thoughts that predict difficulties in maintaining the behaviour and develop appropriate coping strategies, such as distraction or focusing upon the gains of change (i.e. action control). The model emphasizes a set of beliefs that can in part determine and motivate towards an intention to behave, but then need to be translated into cognitive plans for action and maintenance. They provide a checklist of beliefs to explore with

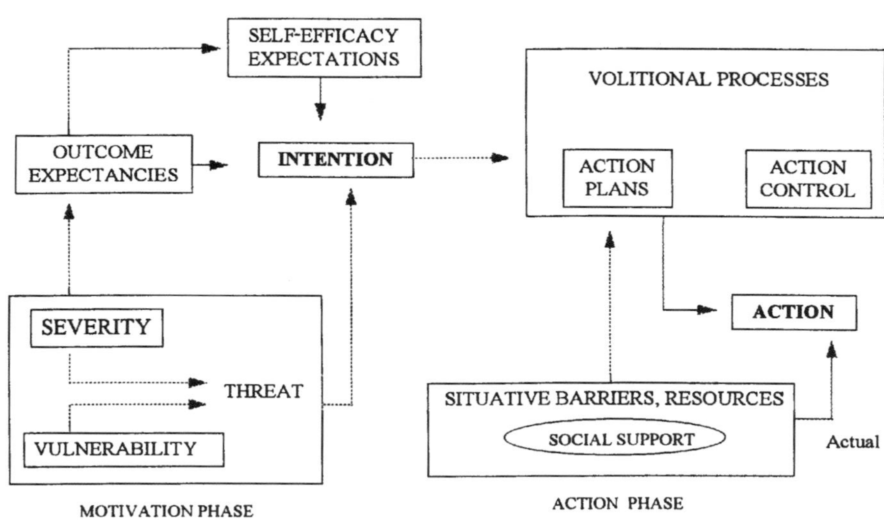

Figure 5.4. The Health Action Process Approach[71] (Schwarzer 1992)

the patient and thus influence the likelihood of self-management. These attitudes and beliefs are evident initially during the precontemplative stage of readiness, but are most important during the contemplative stage. The action plan and action control of the Health Action Process model are relevant in the determination and action stages.

Behavioural processes

Behavioural theory argues that actions are shaped by their antecedents and consequences. If a behaviour is positively reinforced, by either a pleasant sensation, praise or the cessation of something unpleasant, then individuals are more likely to engage in that behaviour again. If adverse consequences follow behaviour, then it is less likely to occur again. Crucially, it is the immediate consequences that shape behaviour, not long-term gains. In diabetes self-management this is problematic, as the immediate consequences of some elements of the regimen are not instantly reinforcing and the gains are only evident in the long term.

Reinforced behaviour that is preceded by a cue, or trigger (known as a stimulus), will then be initiated by the presentation of the 'stimulus' alone, and will seem automatic. Improving self-management may involve disrupting the cues that trigger unhelpful behaviour, or deliberately introducing new triggers that will initiate the new behaviour. Shillitoe[72] describes the use of these behavioural principles to improve self-management in diabetes care and these techniques have proved to be beneficial in obesity[29] and diet[73]. They involve manipulation of the stimuli and the inclusion of more immediate positive reinforcers.

For new behaviours to become automatic, they would need to be followed by positive reinforcers and preceded by strong triggers or cues. This is the ideal, as the new behaviour would not have to be consciously thought about in order to be maintained. Unfortunately, most lifestyle changes in diabetes self-management have no immediate reinforcers, the cues for the new behaviour are subtle, and the cues for old behaviours are very strong. If the behaviour is to be maintained, it will have to be consciously thought about each time and reinforced. For patients with diabetes, health issues may not be given highest priority when other life events or needs demand conscious attention. Behavioural principles generate strategies for increasing success during the action and maintenance stages[74].

Emotional processes

Emotions have an impact upon the way people think and behave, and strong emotions may disrupt the cognitive and behavioural processes described so far. They may arise due to problems in adjusting to the diagnosis of diabetes[75,76], diabetes related fears of complications[77,78], negative hypoglycaemic events[79], or because of external and unresolved life events. The emotional impact of an event may be amplified by individual differences in emotional lability, conditioning, coping and levels of social support[80,81].

Strong emotions lead to defence mechanisms which seem to act by distorting or denying the reality of the situation which then protects the conscious mind from further distress[82]. This may be the underlying explanation for the theoretical model forwarded by Janis[83], which predicts that high or low fear-arousing messages will not motivate healthy behaviour. Moderate levels of fear may be most useful, as they emphasize the importance of change without engaging defence mechanisms. Strong emotion may also disrupt rational thought processes, leading to more erroneous beliefs. If thinking about diabetes elicits strong negative, unpleasant emotions, behavioural principles would suggest that the individual will respond by trying to reduce the frequency of such unpleasant thoughts. The person will thus 'avoid thinking about it' and remain precontemplative.

Low or depressed mood leads to increased pessimism with respect to the perceived benefits of change and to reduced self-efficacy, which are both crucial motivating factors. Low mood may stem from the bereavement process, triggered by the diagnosis itself and the constant stream of diabetes-related losses that a person experiences[84]. There may be other reasons for low mood, such as negative life events, but whatever the aetiology it will have a major impact upon the person's capacity to self-manage. Screening to detect depressed mood may be helpful in patients who are attempting significant lifestyle change. A simple scale, such as the Hospital Anxiety and Depression Scale[85], can screen out patients who should either be excluded from behaviour change counselling, or need help for their problems as a precursor to work on self-management. It would then be important for the person to receive the appropriate treatment, either pharmacologically or with cognitive therapy.

CHANGE COUNSELLING—ASSEMBLING THE COMPONENTS

Research indicates the value of combining motivational interviewing, the change cycle and an understanding of psychological processes to influence diabetes-relevant behaviours, such as taking exercise, quitting smoking and establishing a healthier diet. The Stage of Change model has not been fully evaluated by randomized control trials, but evaluations carried out in a number of areas suggest its potential efficacy[86]. Messages specific to a person's stage of change have been shown to increase the uptake of mammography and smoking cessation[87,88]. These behaviours are highly relevant to diabetes, especially type 2, where the focus is upon healthy eating, exercise and taking medication. In type 1, insulin-dependant diabetes, successful self-management is more complex, given the greater interdependency of behaviours (e.g. monitoring, diet and insulin dose adjustment). Nevertheless, similar principles should apply to complex behaviours, provided that the action plan, action control and acquisition of skill is addressed in more detail.

A pilot study supporting the use of these methods[52] randomized individuals with type 2 diabetes into two groups that focused on weight reduction. One group included a motivational intervention ($n = 6$) and the second followed a standardized behavioural weight control programme ($n = 10$). Significant benefits in glycaemic control and in adherence to the weight reduction programme were reported in the motivational group. A 4 month follow-up showed that both groups had lost weight, with no significant differences but a trend in favour of the motivational group. The authors report the advantages of a motivational intervention, but note the need for further investigation with a longer follow-up period (the real test of weight reduction programmes), a larger sample size to improve the power of the study and a tighter experimental control.

In summary, empirically supported models for behaviour change have been widely used in medical settings. Counselling and motivational interviewing largely dictate the recommended style of empowerment, but the skills are not usually taught to health care staff[20]. These techniques aid the development of appropriate rapport in order for the individual's readiness to change to be identified using the change cycle. The prevailing psychological models can then help to formulate which emotional, cognitive or behavioural barriers might be stopping individual progress around the cycle with the employment of appropriate specific strategies to complete the process[89]. Given the current level of knowledge, this represents the most logical way to understand and facilitate self-management.

CHANGE COUNSELLING IN PRACTICE

NEGOTIATING TIME TO WORK

At each consultation patients may come with new needs, e.g. physical health problems, requests for information and for reassurance. They may want their toe nails cut, or a new insulin pen. The health care professional may have his/her own screening and surveillance agenda and, as time is strictly limited, priorities may be very different. Self-management may never be discussed. Indeed, there may be some collusion to avoid the subject; the patient avoids a sense of failure and the health care professional keeps the topic safe and supportive. Therefore, if change counselling is to facilitate self-management, it must first be on the agenda.

One approach to raising the issue is to specify subgoals within the consultation, as in general practice[90]. In a diabetic clinic, a 'road map' (Figure 5.5) has been piloted[23]. It makes the agenda negotiated and explicit by defining and agreeing the purpose of the next part of the consultation, thus empowering the patient and prompting the health care professional. It starts with the person's life beyond his/her diabetes, and then considers the person's diabetes agenda ('What would you like from today?'). It then considers the clinician's agenda (e.g. screening, treatment and education). Options for self-management follow, such as specific target behaviours, assessment of the individual's stage of change and the employment of a stage-specific strategy or intervention.

The 'road map' expects some self-management work to be covered, and thus motivates the member of staff to reach this part of the consultation. It can also provide a record that is useful within a multidisciplinary clinic across and within clinics, such as the annual review process, and allows for follow-up of self-management issues.

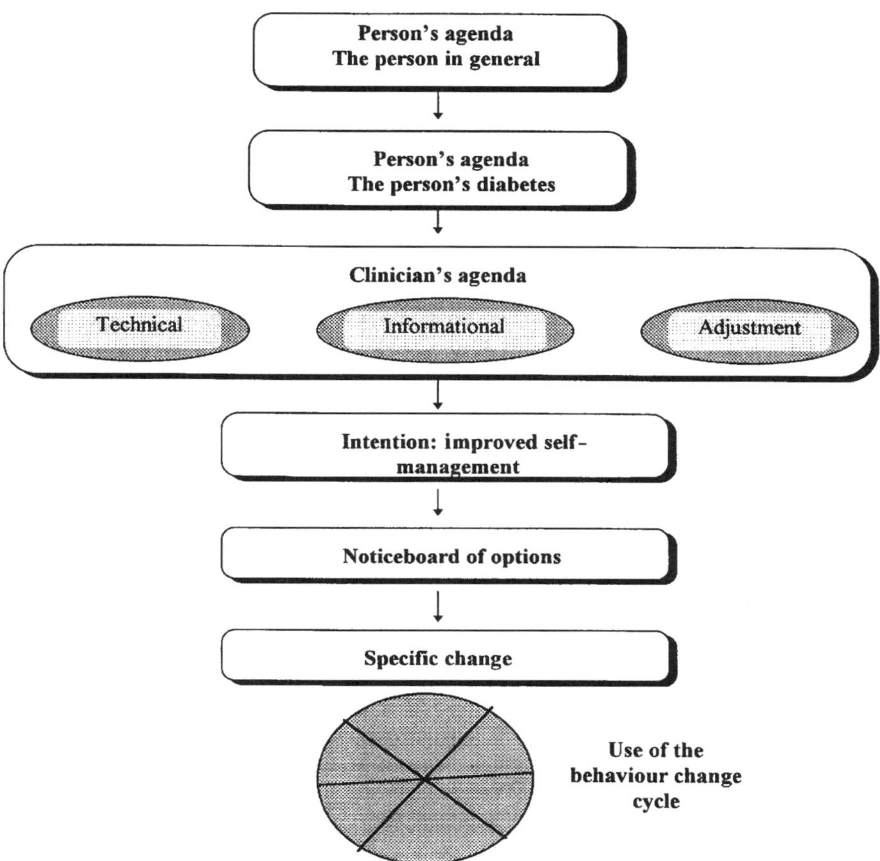

Figure 5.5. The consultation roadmap

DEFINING THE DESIRED OUTCOME

The additional challenge in diabetes is to target the most important behaviour from a potentially long list of self-management behaviours. Counselling models[41] would suggest that the individual should define the next health-enhancing change. So if, for example, the patient would like to focus on increasing the amount of fibre in his/her diet, then this should be the target behaviour in the hope that other changes will follow. Unfortunately, in diabetes more critical changes may be necessary. Patients may be missing insulin injections or medication. Negotiation and challenging may be necessary, and is more likely to be successful if good rapport has been established using counselling methods. A 'risk factor tool' can aid this process by highlighting the options and potential benefits of each behaviour. Variations on this approach have been described[51].

ASSESSING READINESS TO CHANGE

Patients can simply be asked to rate, on a scale of 0–10, how ready they are to make a change. Prochaska and DiClemente[92] suggest the use of an algorithm in order to determine the actual stage of change. They identified six stages: in *precontemplation*, individuals are not currently engaged in the behaviour change and do not intend to change in the next 6 months. In *contemplation*, the individual is considering changing in the next 6 months. When individuals are in the *determination* stage, they are planning to make a change in the next 30 days and have made at least one attempt. Those in *action* have started the change in the last 6 months, and those in *maintenance* have managed the change and have kept it going for 6 months or longer. This can be a complex system to employ.

Other methods of assessing readiness to change include the use of questionnaires which employ stage-specific statements. Heather *et al.*[93] developed a tool specifically for use with alcohol and there have been

Please look at the statements below. Which one best describes how you feel right now about improving your diabetes self management?

	Which statement fits for you Tick [√] one only
There is no need for me to think about my diabetes	☐
I don't want to think about my diabetes	☐
It's a waste of time thinking about my diabetes	☐
I am weighing up the advantages and disadvantages of improving my diabetes	☐
Sometimes I think I might benefit from improving my diabetes but haven't decided yet	☐
I have definitely decided to improve my diabetes	☐
I am planning how to improve my diabetes	☐
I am actually trying to improve my diabetes and started to do something about it	☐
I have managed to improve my diabetes, I just need to keep it going	☐
I have now improved my diabetes and I am trying to avoid slipping back into my old ways	☐
I have given up trying to improve my diabetes	☐
I have not been able to keep the change going	☐

Scoring key: The first three items would suggest the individual was precontemplative. Items four and five refer to contemplation, six and seven determination and eight suggests early action. Nine and ten would indicate attempts at maintenance with eleven and twelve indicating relapse.

Figure 5.6. A method to aid assessment of stage of change for diabetes self-management

Being more active ?

Please look at the six pictures and statements below. Which best describes how you feel **right now** about being more active?

Which picture fits for you? (Tick (✓) one only)

- ❑ ***Staying put***
- ❑ ***Wondering where to go***
- ❑ ***Planning***
- ❑ ***Taking the first steps***
- ❑ ***I've made it thus far***
- ❑ ***I'm back to where I started***

Which statement fits for you? (Tick (✓) one only)

- There is no need for me to think about being more active. ❑
- I don't want to think about being more active. ❑
- It's a waste of time thinking about being more active. ❑
- I am weighing up the advantages and disadvantages of becoming more active. ❑
- Sometimes I think I might benefit from becoming more active, but haven't decided yet. ❑
- I have definitely decided to be more active. ❑
- I am planning how to be more active. ❑
- I am actually trying to be more active. ❑
- I know that I should do more activity and have started to do something about it. ❑
- I have managed to be more active, I just need to keep it going. ❑
- I am now more active and trying to avoid slipping back into my old ways. ❑
- I have given up trying to be more active. ❑
- I have not been able to keep the change going. ❑

Figure 5.7. An assessment method using stage-specific pictures and statements for a specific behaviour

How do you feel about Smoking ?
I'M NOT BOTHERED.... SMOKING'S NOT DOING ME ANY HARM...
AVOIDING, NOT THINKING
WHAT AM I GOING TO MISS
THINKING
WHAT'S IN IT FOR ME
I HAVE A PLAN
PREPARING / PLANNING
WHY DID I BOTHER?
RELAPSED
I'VE STOPPED
STARTING
TONIGHT
NATIONAL NON-SMOKER OF THE YEAR
KEEPING IT GOING

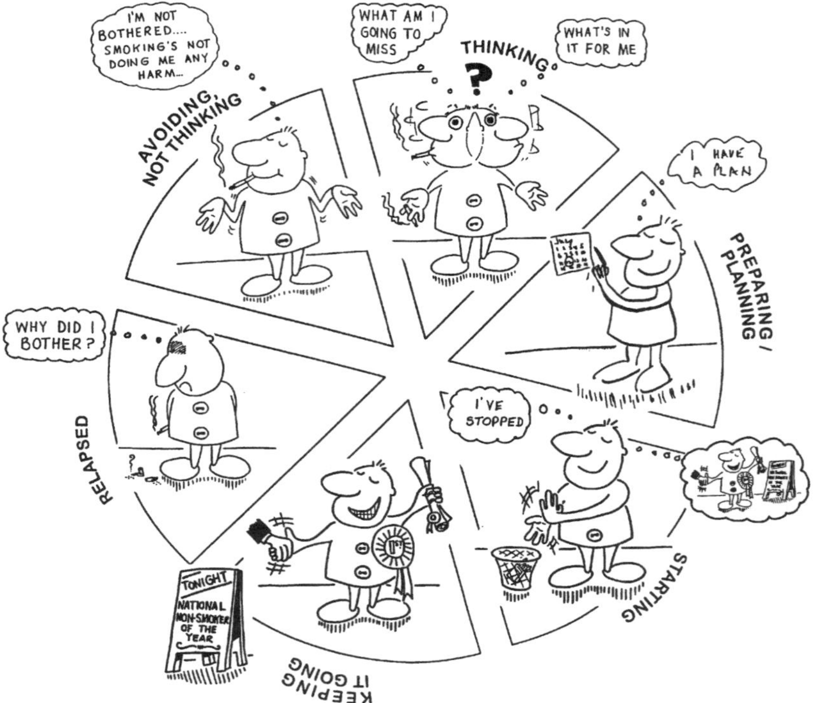

Figure 5.8. An assessment method employing behaviour change cycle with pictures

attempts to adapt these for diabetes services.[58] Diabetes-specific statements have been developed from the 'Readiness to Change' Questionnaire (Figure 5.6) but the transfer of this method into diabetes care is yet to be tested. This was viewed to be necessary before assessing the stage of change for a specific behaviour, such as physical activity or smoking. If individuals are precontemplative for their overall diabetes self-management, this would need to be addressed before moving on to specific behaviours. Similar tools can be employed to assess stage of change (Figure 5.7) for a specific behaviour, and visual images alongside stage-specific statements enable concurrent validity to be tested[94]. Alternatively, the behaviour change cycle can be described using illustrations, and the patients asked to indicate which representation applies to them (Figure 5.8). Ultimately, the practitioner can use clinical judgement. The measures illustrated are in their infancy, but an initial pilot suggests some validity to this approach[95]. Using the tool shown (Figure 5.7) in a small sample ($n = 11$), the level of reported physical activity matched closely the individual's stage of change. Furthermore, progression around the cycle was in accordance with increases in the self-reported frequency of physical activity. Much more work is needed to further test the validity and reliability of this tool.

PRECONTEMPLATION

Overcoming the emotions

In diabetes, adjustment to the condition itself is a problem[96,97]. The diagnosis implies future losses and there is a need to acknowledge the life-long adjustments needed to accommodate and manage the process from the beginning[84]. In a sample of 1159 people with diabetes, 60.4% experienced strong emotional reactions at the time of diagnosis and 23% would have liked more emotional support[75]. Poor adjustment, as with other conditions, can be related to the way the individual was informed of the diagnoisis[98], poor social support[99], rigid belief structures[100] or a poor range of coping strategies[39]. Bereavement counselling models can be used to facilitate adjustment[101]. People are encouraged to talk through the loss and the negative impact in a way that leads to emotional catharsis[41] and emotional habituation. This requires the use of open questions that direct attention to the emotional feelings associated with loss; open questions that encourage discussion and reflections that demonstrate understanding.

A second source of negative emotion is the fear of complications[77] perhaps made worse by the vicarious experience of older relatives or hospital visits. Clinicians can help by providing appropriate information and allowing individuals to question their catastrophic thinking about vulnerability, seriousness or the extent to which complications can be avoided (e.g. medical advances in screening and treatment). Maximal motivation will occur with moderate amounts of fear. If this is not achieved by informational care alone, then allowing people to talk about complications and fears in the right environment (as shown in Table 5.2) can lead to some emotional calming. Graded exposure helps individuals with diabetes-related phobias or obsessions, and needs to be conducted or supervised by an appropriately qualified practitioner.

Severe hypoglycaemia fits the diagnostic criteria for a traumatic event as it involves a threat to life in association with feelings of helplessness[102]. Following a traumatic event, strong and often distorted memories are stored which can be very emotionally distressing when recalled[103]. In order to manage this distress, individuals may avoid recalling the event and also avoid potentially similar situations. This may explain why some individuals maintain elevated blood sugar levels, although phobic fear of hypoglycaemia can develop without a traumatic event[79]. However, in the case of trauma, problems can be identified by asking the person to recall the distressing events to see whether he/she can still be upset by recalling them. Simple therapeutic interventions include encouraging people to repeatedly recall these experiences and elicit their beliefs about the experience until they became desensitized by repetition[104]. However, this must be done with caution. An individual should never be forced into this dialogue, as unresolved distress can cause further trauma. More severe cases should be referred for psychological help.

If people sense that they are being pushed into something that they do not own, they react with resistance[59]. In the diabetes clinic, this is likely to be covert and demonstrated by continued poor self-management. Resistance is a reflection of the person's experience and not a personality trait[50]. It may have accumulated from previous hospital or GP visits, especially if in the past the approach has been authoritarian, overly critical and negative. Resistance is an obstacle to increased awareness of the problem and the benefits of behavioural change. To overcome this barrier, it helps to encourage deliberate expression of resistance by asking open questions. The most valuable technique is *rolling with resistance*[50], in which the health care professional does not necessarily agree with the person's comments but nevertheless reflects them back to demonstrate listening and empathy. This approach is likely to assist the patients to move on in their thinking and explore their own needs, rather than justifying their behaviour to the staff member. A sophisticated version of rolling with resistance is the double-

Table 5.6. Rolling with resistance

Patient comment	Staff 'role'
Examples of rolling with resistance	
No I don't think that the amount I drink does me any harm	So, you really can't believe that you could be doing any harm to yourself
Smoking, that's the catch-all of the medical profession. I think my main problem is stress	All everybody seems to talk to you about is smoking when really you believe all your problems are related to stress
Well, I suppose I could if you think it would help	Perhaps you know what we want, but you're not so sure yourself
I just can't take my BMs. I'm too busy at work and I forget, and once I've finished work, by the time I've picked up the kids and got home, I don't have time	Its hard to find time to do your BMs. At work you are too busy and at home you can't find the time
Examples of double-sided rolling with resistance	
I don't think I can do anything	So you can't do much but you have been worried about your eyes
Don't tell me I should lose weight, it's how I've always been	So you get a bit cross when losing weight is suggested but you don't want to go on insulin

sided reflection, where the beliefs of the patient are fed back, highlighting the patient's ambivalence by including the positive aspects of change (Table 5.6).

Addressing misconceptions

Leventhal and colleagues[105] established that people's beliefs about physical illness are first accumulated via past life experience, media influences and the information gained from family or friends[106]. They are then ordered into personally unique illness representations which are used to make sense of subsequent information. This means that people do not passively receive the information they are given during education programmes. It is filtered through an illness representation where errors occur as information is distorted to fit with existing 'knowledge'. Misconceptions are therefore to be expected.

Each individual's illness representations has five constructs. In diabetes these would be: (a) *identity*—the symptoms associated with the patients' diabetes and the type of diabetes they have; (b) *timeline*—the individuals' perception of how long their diabetes will last; (c) *consequences*—beliefs regarding the impact the diabetes will have upon their functioning and quality of life; (d) *control/cure*—whether the diabetes can be cured or controlled; and finally (e) *cause*—whether the diabetes is caused by stress, a virus, genetics or some other factor. Inaccurate beliefs can be one of the reasons why individuals are not considering change. For example, they may believe they have 'mild diabetes' and that they do not need to try too hard to reduce their blood sugars; or that diabetes medication is addictive, or insulin has side effects, and so miss the occasional injection or tablet. They may be unable to make the connection between blood glucose levels and serious complications, perhaps believing that no symptoms means no damage.

These misconceptions can be hard to detect, as they may have been developed over time. The individuals will assume their belief is correct and does not need to be checked out. The practitioner's counselling skills can help to elicit misconceptions by using open questions, such as, 'What do you think is the most important thing to do for your diabetes control?'. It is crucial to check the individuals' beliefs before giving information, as they will tend to select the information that fits best with their own belief system. Informational care must start with the patients' models and also check subsequent understanding. If a misconception is identified, the practitioner can provide information but must also discuss the evidence the individual is using to support that belief. This is most effective when carried out within the core style using the counselling skills presented previously, as too many questions may feel like interrogation and precipitate resistance. Table 5.7 includes some strategies that can help individuals to question their beliefs.

Table 5.7. Strategies to help question misconceptions

1. Ask the person to identify and question the evidence of his/her belief
2. Ask him/her to consider his/her response if a good friend made this suggestion
3. Test out the reality of his/her belief. This process can be enhanced by asking the individual to attend to or collect information on the subject, such as all articles in the newspapers that report the benefits and risks of the target behaviour, e.g. cigar smoking. This can also prevent 'selective attention', i.e. only noting information that fits with one's own beliefs (e.g. cigar smoking prevents Alzheimer's disease)
4. Rather than seeing something as either black or white, ask the person to consider seeing it in shades of grey

Establishing salience

There are many distractions in everyday life. They cannot all be processed, so only a fraction are given our limited attention[107]. If thoughts about diabetes self-management are to be chosen, there has to be sufficient relevance or salience for the individual. Human beings are agreed to be rational processors of information calculating how they can personally achieve the most advantageous outcome[106]. Their needs include self-esteem, control, comfortable emotions, relationships, and a sense of achievement. Health issues may have low salience in comparison, especially when the advantageous outcome is the potential avoidance of complications in the distant future!

Thus, movement out of precontemplation involves 'hooking' someone into thinking about self-management, and so information needs to emphasize gains that are personally relevant. This means identifying the person's major needs and anticipating the way these would be threatened by poor self-management or enhanced by improved control. Table 5.8 provides some illustrations as to how health care professionals can tailor general information about diabetes to the person in a way that makes it relevant. For example, a person who values his/her fitness and enjoys competitive sports

Table 5.8. Examples of personally relevant information

Patient: 'Losing weight, it's so hard, I can't see how it will help anyway, it's not what I eat. The thing that bothers me the most at the minute is those pains in my knees'

Helper: 'So it would be hard for you to lose weight (reflection). Did you know that losing weight would lesson the pressure on your knees and that would help with the pain? You might even be able to get around more easily'

Patient: 'Stopping smoking and my diabetes, that's all everyone talks about. I don't want to stop smoking. It's this breathlessness that bothers me'

Helper: 'So you don't want to think about stopping smoking (reflection), but it actually might help with your breathlessness and means you could walk further without stopping'

Patient: 'I really hate blood monitoring—it hurts, it's messy and embarrassing, especially at work. I want someone to help me with these hypos I keep getting, they are really starting to get me down'

Helper: 'So, blood monitoring is really not for you (reflection) but it could help with your hypos. Getting a handle on your blood sugars really helps to determine how much insulin you need'

could be motivated by maintaining his/her performance for Sunday football by sustaining good control, whereas an individual who enjoys needlework could be motivated by the gains of preserving his/her eyesight.

CONTEMPLATION

When a person is in the contemplation stage, he/she typically has a range of ambivalent thoughts about making the change. 'Ambivalence' describes an individual who is experiencing opposing thoughts and feelings about an issue at the same time. It is important in behaviour change counselling that both sides of the argument are addressed[59]. If insufficient attention is given to the negative aspects of change, these will invariably come to the fore at a later stage and undermine any progress. The simplest way to do this is to help a patient make a thorough pros and cons list (Figure 5.9). This may include non-health issues, such as finances, reaction of relatives, models for children or grandchildren, ability to get into clothes. People are also motivated to behave in a similar way to those they perceive to be like them, or whose opinion they value, as described in the Theory of Reasoned

	Pros of change	Cons of change
consequences for me		
consequences for other people		
my reactions		
the reactions of others		

Figure 5.9. Pros and cons list (the decisional balance). Based upon reference 60.

Action[68]. This helps to explain the value of video role models or group programmes in diabetes care. When helping to construct a pros and cons list, it is often useful to consider the Health Belief Model[65]. This is a reminder of the importance of balancing perceived severity and vulnerability, combined with how avoidable the risks are, against perceived barriers to making change. It is important that health care professionals help patients to understand risk accurately, as inaccurate understanding may result in the patient feeling vulnerable and susceptible to complications he/she perceives to be unavoidable. This is particularly important, since trials suggest that people can only reduce their chance of developing complications, and cannot be guaranteed a healthy life[108]. In summary, the question for the patient is, 'what's in it for me?' It is only when he/she has considered both sides of the equation, from both a health and a non-health perspective, that he/she can be clear about their intention.

Detailed questionnaires based on the Health Belief Model exist to assess people's beliefs about complications, i.e. vulnerability, susceptibility, seriousness, barriers[109]. These methods may take too long to apply in routine clinical work. But the health care professional can employ a number of open-ended questions to identify potential gains or losses with respect to the change. These prompts might start with non-health aspects, move on to health and complications and finish with peer group issues.

Self-efficacy is the individual's belief that he/she can perform the behaviour required to achieve the desired outcome[110], e.g. 'I want to lose weight, but will I be able to pass the bakery on my way home without buying a muffin?'. Self-efficacy is usually assessed by asking people how confident they feel about achieving the changes they are planning, on a scale of 0–10 and in a variety of situations (0 = not at all confident, to 10 = completely confident). Self-efficacy can be increased by referring to examples of personal achievement in the recent past, by using normative data showing that people in similar positions have been able to make these changes, and by breaking the task down into small manageable tasks, thus increasing mastery. The behaviour change cycle can be employed to normalize the process, particularly relapse, and by emphasizing that small incremental changes, or even progression around the cycle, are indicators of success. A problem may arise when negative emotions emerge and distort thinking, resulting in self-doubt[111]. One approach is to ask patients to note when they become low or pessimistic in mood, and then identify the thoughts that were going through their heads at those times. These can then be discussed and 'restructured' if they include distortions or incorrect inferences (Table 5.7). Many guidelines are available[112], although few have applied this approach to diabetes.

The optimism and behaviour of the health care professional may also have a bearing on an individual's subsequent self-efficacy. However, this needs to be used cautiously so that the patient does not feel under pressure.

DETERMINATION

When a person is clear about the outcome he/she wants to achieve, and this is expressed in a way that can be monitored and recorded, e.g. number of blood glucose monitoring measures in a day, then he/she is more likely to achieve the change. The health care professional needs to help clarify specific but tailored plans according to the acronym SMARTS (Table 5.9). This approach has been cited in the care of diabetic adolescents[113]. In addition to this, some form of self-monitoring, such as keeping a diary, can also be motivating and will influence the development of an action plan. Motivation lists (Table 5.10) can act as reminders of 'What's in it for me?' and a relapse

Table 5.9. Elements of a SMARTs action plan. Based upon reference 62

Specific	The plan needs to be clear, so rather that 'cutting down' the person needs to specify what he/she will do, e.g. walk for half an hour, three times a week; have chips twice a week
Measurable	It should be possible to monitor or gauge the person's progress. This is easier if the aims are specific, as described above
Agreed	The plan is negotiated—the person is not forced into the decision by the health care professional
Realistic	The plan is achievable—the person is not deciding to run a marathon. Progress needs to be made in small incremental steps in order to build self-efficacy
Time-specific	There needs to be a clearly defined start point and agreement about how often, how long and when progress will be reviewed
Support	Support has been found to be an important element in the change process for the health professional, family and friends

Table 5.10. The motivation list of a woman with type 2 diabetes

Reasons why I want to lose weight:

- Legs rub, so I would lose sore legs
- Feel less self-conscious
- Wear smaller clothes
- Be healthier
- Not be so sweaty
- Be fitter, i.e. be able to do more strenuous walks and other things—aerobics, etc.
- Getting in the car better, the seat belt fitting better
- Be proud of what I have achieved
- Join in more with the kids
- Doing something for me, not for anyone else
- Get into a leather jacket size 16
- Get into a pair of size 16 jeans
- Wear shoes that fit instead of having to buy shoes one or two sizes too big
- Be confident in anything I do without being put down by people around me

prevention strategy can identify, ahead of time, actions to employ in a difficult ('high risk') situation. These strategies help transform the individual's intention to change into appropriate action.

However, there are a number of problems that can still arise to frustrate good intentions. Firstly much of an individual's behaviour is habitual or automatic, as described earlier; triggers or cues exist to initiate routine behaviours. In this way, a person does not consciously have to think about what to do next, leaving capacity for other activities. This is known as 'stimulus control', and the theory predicts that unless the person introduces a new set of stimuli to remind him/her of the new change, old cues will trigger previous behaviour. Therefore, it is useful to help people to plan in detail how they would reorganize their lives to incorporate new cues or triggers and ignore old stimuli. For example, someone intending to cut down on sweet biscuits may still need to avoid walking down the supermarket aisle, reaching for the biscuits and putting them in the trolley. He/she may need to reorganize his/her route through the supermarket, either to miss this shelf or to avoid the aisle. For some people, this sort of behavioural intervention will be paramount if they are to succeed; examples include written memos to identify permissible food[114] and verbal prompts from staff for self-monitoring charts[115]. Detailed planning (see Table 5.11 as an example for physical activity) facilities subsequent changes.

Human beings are able to rehearse mentally for events, thus making their subsequent performance a little better. People can be encouraged to anticipate the changes that they might make and imagine the change in order to predict its impact. In this way many problems can be identified in advance and coping strategies developed.

Some of the changes people plan will deny them pleasurable experiences or ways of coping, e.g. smoking or eating. It is helpful to plan an alternative. Stress management or relaxation would need to be employed for those who use cigarettes for calming. A person eating inappropriate food as a reward would need to substitute the food for equally enjoyable rewards.

Table 5.11. Example of the essential questions needed to complete an action plan for physical activity

1. What activity?
2. Where and when?
3. For how long?
4. Who with?
5. What is the target?
6. How will the person reward him/herself?
7. What will the person do if he/she 'slips'?
8. What are the potential blocks and barriers?
9. How will the person overcome these?

For some there will be final blocks or barriers to be overcome before initiating a behaviour, such as the reactions of other people to blood monitoring at work, the difficulty of eating at regular times when meetings run over, etc. At this point a problem-solving approach is needed. The health care professional may give advice, but the basic principles of counselling emphasize that people do better when they generate their own solutions[41]. A simple protocol suggests: (a) identify the problem; (b) brainstorm solutions; (c) choose a solution; (d) implement the chosen option; (e) evaluate its success. This sequence can be repeated if necessary, or the individual may decide on a number of options to implement simultaneously.

ACTION

An individual's conscious intention, directed via an action plan with a series of appropriate cues, should now lead to a change in behaviour. If the immediate consequences (within a minute or two) are pleasant, then the behaviour will be self-reinforcing and the pattern will be strengthened over subsequent days and weeks. However, many of the changes appropriate to diabetes do not have a short-term benefit, and indeed the long-term benefits over several years cannot be guaranteed. In fact, the discomfort of blood testing, the reminder of having diabetes, denying certain foods, taking more insulin, with increased risk of hypoglycaemia, all have immediate negative consequences. Behavioural processes now act to reduce the likelihood of this behaviour occurring again and it is likely to reduce in frequency if the person does not review his/her intention, action plan and set of cues for the new behaviour. These factors explain why many people are unable to maintain changes. There are a number of ways to reinforce motivation and maintain change. First, individuals can use a form of mental self-praise, e.g. 'Well done—a step in the right direction', which will act as a reinforcer. Second, they can actually give themselves some immediate reward or token of a subsequent reward. There is also little doubt that external praise can also bridge this reinforcement gap, hence someone who can provide encouragement on a daily basis can significantly assist the person. In the early days of change, a 5 minute telephone call from a specialist nurse could help to keep the behaviour going at a crucial stage. Other potential helpers include family members or friends, buddying systems to provide support, or groups of people in a similar situation.

During the initial stages of the action phase, the person is trying out in reality what he/she has previously been only thinking about theoretically. New negative emotions may emerge that disrupt thinking or behaviour. A cognitive therapy approach[111] that addresses negative automatic thoughts may be appropriate for those who become pessimistic about their ability to maintain change. In addition, the negatives for change now become more evident, and problem-solving approaches may prove helpful. The positive reasons for change may become less salient, so the motivation list may need to be revisited and rehearsed. The action plan itself may have been unrealistic or need modification, and the cues that control behaviour may need attention. Finally, other pressures or problems in life may relegate the intention to change to a lower order, even if by simple distraction. Social support or back-up from the health care services may be vital in this respect.

One way of construing the behavioural approach is to draw a gradient, which is made steeper by the lack of immediate reinforcements, by negative consequences becoming evident, by strong cues for the old behaviour and weak cues for the new, with little social support. The steeper the gradient, the more the person will need a motivation 'head of steam', (i.e. a good supply of intention and external reinforcers). It is only then that the personal intentions will be translated into behaviour change that can be maintained.

MAINTENANCE

In most cases, a behaviour will have to be continued for several months before it becomes the new norm and the individual can become less vigilant. This time period can vary according to the behaviour and individual differences. For smoking, this may take a year or two, for controlled drinking several years. In the maintenance stage, all the principles and problems identified in the action phase still apply. However, it is inevitable that people will sometimes forget to keep the change going and maybe go 'off the rails' for several days. For individuals prone to 'all-or-nothing' thinking, this may precipitate a total relapse. It is therefore essential that preparatory work is done to define the difference between a *lapse* (a temporary phenomenon) and *relapse* (in which the attempt to change is abandoned). This is known as the 'abstinence volition effect' in Marlott and Gordon's[116] Relapse Prevention Model (Figure 5.10), in which an individual interprets a slip as a relapse and in consequence is more likely to relapse fully.

The research is quite clear that people benefit from identifying and preparing for potential problems in the future, i.e. relapse prevention[116]. For example, where a break in routine is envisaged, e.g. going on a holiday, a plan can be drawn up for a slightly altered routine. The 'old' routine can then be resumed when the person returns. New habits may be disrupted by other changes, such as Christmas, illness or negative life events.

The notion of 'high-risk situations'[116] has developed from drug and alcohol work. This suggests that certain environments make it difficult to continue the new behaviour. For instance, in the pub or at a party peers may put pressure on an individual to smoke. The company of certain people who

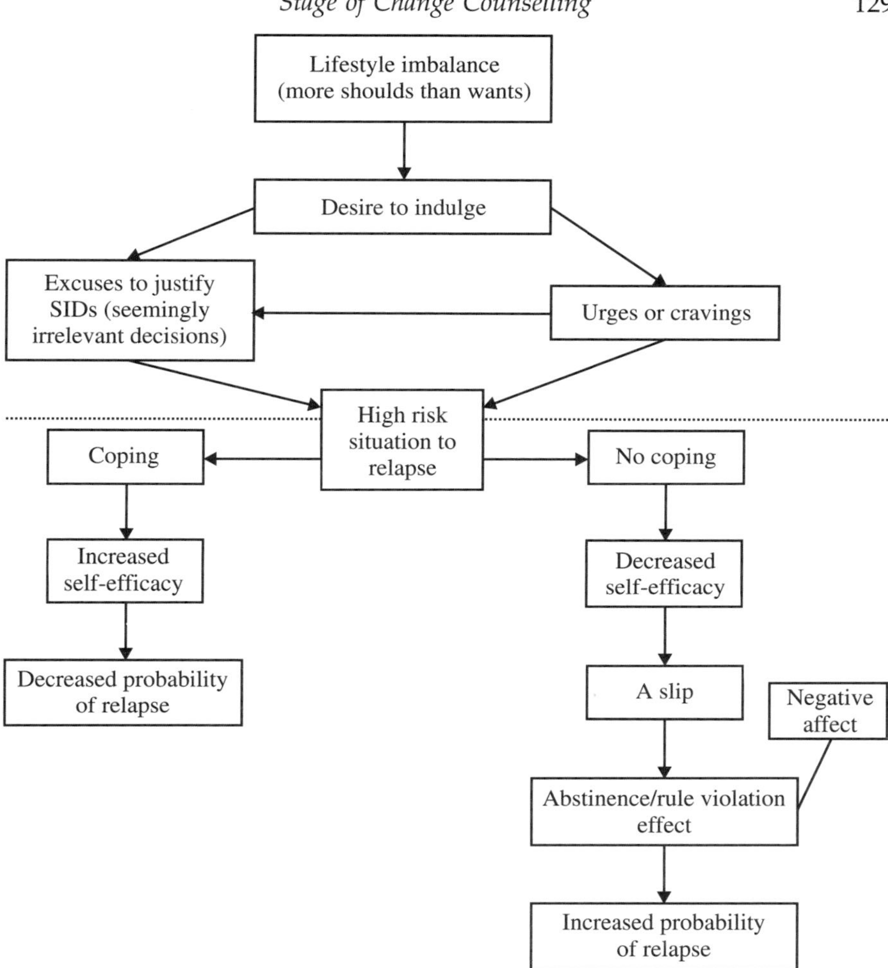

Figure 5.10. Relapse Prevention Model. Based upon reference 116.

always have alcohol in the fridge or a bowl of sweets on a coffee table can be an irresistible temptation. Before a new behaviour is established, the individual may need to avoid these situations or develop the appropriate coping strategies. According to the model, 'coping' in a high-risk situation will lead to increased self-efficacy and therefore a decreased probability of relapse in the future.

Another important idea is 'lifestyle imbalance' (Figure 5.10), which suggests that if patients feel that they spend most of their time doing what they *should* do, rather than what they *want* to do, they will have an increased desire to treat themselves, either by eating, drinking, smoking or omitting a behaviour such as blood monitoring or physical activity. For example, individuals working long hours may have a desire to reward themselves. Urges or cravings and related thought processes are activated that make it okay to 'slip' (e.g. 'one cigarette won't harm me'). The individual might make a decision which seems unimportant (a SID) (Figure 5.10), but which results in the person finding him/herself in a 'high-risk situation', such as at the pub or at the house of a friend who smokes. There may be insufficient time to explore this model with every patient, but it can provide a useful framework to help the patient to predict potential relapses and evaluate 'What went wrong?'. Some short-hand terms for relapse prevention include *uppers* (a positive event increases a desire to celebrate), *downers* (low mood or a negative life events can result in slips), *rows* (arguments, etc.) and *joining the club* (peer pressure)[116]. These situations will occur and slips might result. However, the most effective relapse prevention strategy is for the individual to view the slip as a hiccup rather than a relapse and re-establish his/her previous behaviour.

Above all else, social support or continued interest by the health care professional will be of upmost importance in maintaining change. A traditional clinic approach involving appointments every 2 months and consultations with different health care professionals does not provide the most conducive environment or relationship to facilitate change and offer support. Appropriate help might involve telephone calls (How are you? How's your diabetes? How's the change going?) or letters to demonstrate interest and support in reinforcing the change. If health issues are not discussed, other problems may take precedence. Health care professionals who encourage people to embark on change therefore need to consider the amount of support they can realistically provide.

RELAPSE

Research on smoking cessation, combined with clinical observations of a wide variety of patients, suggests that people relapse many times before then going on to ultimate success in making change. Smokers have been found to make three to four action attempts before they become maintainers[117]. The aim during the relapse stage is, first, to help people evaluate what went wrong, and to see if they can move back through precontemplation to contemplation again, having learnt new lessons about themselves and the changes they were considering. Aspects to consider in this process include reviewing negative emotions that might again distort thinking. Open-ended questions addressing these feelings are a useful way to help people 'express' their feelings. Second, a systematic approach to identifying what went wrong is required. Relapse can then be normalized, and not viewed to be predictive of future failure. Indeed, it can be argued that when people learn from these experiences they are more likely to be successful when they progress around the cycle the next time.

CHANGE COUNSELLING AND DIABETES SERVICES

EVERYDAY USE

There are potentially four different ways in which change counselling methods might be used in typical diabetes services: (a) the health care professional could employ the method within a routine clinic or home visit, spending time clarifying an individual's stage of change and employing a stage-specific strategy; (b) during a formal annual review, where self-management issues could be put on the agenda and explored more routinely; (c) change counselling methods could be used more extensively for targeted (high-risk or high-need) patients, with special clinics and more consultation time. These clinics could provide patients with continuity, allow the health professional to assume a key worker role and facilitate the development of a consistent relationship; (d) these principles could be used by a service to define the ethos (counselling/motivational), protocols (open-ended questions, reflections, patient summaries, screening for emotional/behavioural barriers), intermediate outcome measures (stage of change, self-efficacy and quality of life), and the content of locally produced information leaflets.

In reality, it is hard for staff to change their existing routines, and evidence suggests that it is hard to maintain new ways of working[23,118]. A service wishing to adopt the methods outlined in this chapter will need to manage change in a similar fashion to their patients? Do the members of the service own the changes, have they been allowed to voice their fears or resistance, have they reviewed the pros and cons, have they thought through the details of introducing the change and agreed SMARTs plans, is there praise and support for the changes, and are the cues or reminders in place to create new routines? Specially trained staff with dedicated sessions to pursue this may be more effective. However, there is a strong suggestion from a development project that change counselling skills cannot be separated from diabetes skills, as the patients' agenda demands that both are needed within one consultation[23]. Training in change counselling skills is necessary, as nurse training does not routinely address change counselling competencies.

STAFF TRAINING

A set of competencies[23] can be defined which are necessary to carry out change counselling, involving specific attitudes, knowledge and skills. Doherty *et al.*[23] trained a multidisciplinary team in a set of change counselling competencies. They found that the trainee staff very quickly acquired the essential attitude and the necessary knowledge. However, it took intensive training over several months to develop the skills, as evidenced via observation of interactions with clients, role play exercises and completion of a competency checklist. Doherty *et al.*[23] note that it was difficult to determine the extent to which competencies were applied in the clinic situation, but self-report and video evidence suggested that it did not readily generalize to routine clinics. Whilst the authors had hoped that a training manual might be an effective training method, as it could be widely disseminated, the staff reported this to have been the least useful of the training methods attempted. Personal supervision with video examples of staff's work was rated as the most useful method. This is consistent with the way staff learn other significant psychologically-based therapies, such as counselling, behaviour therapy and cognitive therapy.

Doherty *et al.*[23] also noted, based upon staff ratings of efficacy and use, that in the range of change counselling competencies some were more difficult to acquire and apply than others. The core style and counselling skills were more readily implemented, whilst the most difficult skills to acquire were those dealing specifically with emotion, such as rolling with resistance and dealing with loss and adjustment. Staff also found it difficult to replace well-rehearsed skills and strategies, such as informing people or providing solutions with new skills, i.e. eliciting thoughts and feelings and patient-generated solutions to problems.

Given the time and commitment needed for training, staff involved in diabetes care may want to develop some basic skills in change counselling, with a smaller number acquiring change counselling competencies in greater detail, thus offering a specialist role. This would be consistent with the finding that although staff are enthusiastic about change counselling methods, it probably takes more time and continued supervision than is currently conceived for the skills to be demonstrated in clinics on a routine basis[118]. It is likely that a series of increasingly complex change counselling skills will need to be defined and taught in smaller learning units, such as the 'Readiness to Change Ruler'[51]. The training methods are likely to involve manuals to provide the basic knowledge component. However, there is a need for workshops that use video- or computer-generated models to facilitate skills learning via practice and feedback.

Finally, explicit attention is needed to ensure that the competencies are then used in patient consultations by reviewing cases and observing clinics, via audio and video recordings within the context of peer or individual supervision.

FUTURE DEVELOPMENTS

The principles underlying change counselling are widely cited in the research. They have received empirical support in other applications, and have high face validity. However, they remain largely untested in diabetes care. Evaluation is now needed, especially to ascertain the health benefits and costs. One of the main difficulties remains to be maintenance of the intervention throughout the period of the study. As recent research indicates, only 19% of the staff initially trained were employing the intervention at 2 year follow-up[118]. Therefore, there is a need for us to addressing our own behaviours, attitudes and clinic structures.

It is unlikely that the underlying theory in change counselling will change considerably in the next 10 years. The challenge is to isolate and refine the most useful components, and then translate these into useful clinical procedures. Clinicians ultimately need procedures which are either largely patient-determined or can be easily acquired and administered in 'noisy clinics'.

ACKNOWLEDGEMENTS

The completion of this chapter was only made possible by a grant from the British Diabetic Association. We would also like to thank all the staff in the diabetes team who took part in the project and allowed themselves to be videoed; Nicky Asbury, Polly Ashworth and Debra Hall who provided a great deal of support and inspiration; and the Healthy Hearts team, who began this endeavour in cardiovascular disease.

REFERENCES

1. Alberti KGMM. The costs of non-insulin-dependent diabetes mellitus. *Diabet Med* 1997; **14**(1): 7–9
2. Currie CJ, Gill L, Peters JR. Cost of diabetes-related complications. *Diabet Med* 1996; **13**: S57
3. McNabb WL. Adherence in diabetes: can we define it and can we measure it? *Diabet Care* 1997; **20**(2): 215–18
4. Glasgow, RE, Wilson W, McCaul KD. Regimen adherence: a problematic construct in diabetes research. *Diabet Care* 1985; **8**: 300–301
5. Fox CH, Mahoney MC. Improving diabetes preventative care in a family

practice residency programme: a case study in continuous quality improvement. *Fam Med* 1998; **30**(6): 441–5
6. Cerkoney KA, Hart LK. The relationship between health belief model and compliance of persons with diabetes mellitus. *Diabet Care* 1980; **3**: 594–8
7. Morris AD, Boyle DI, McMahon AD, Green SA, MacDonald JM, Newton RW. Adherence to insulin treatment in diabetes mellitus. *Lancet* 1997; **350** (9090): 1305–10
8. Skaer TL, Scalar DA, Markowski DJ, Won JK. Effect of value added utilities on prescription refill compliance with diabetes mellitus. *J Clin Pharm Therapeut* 1993; **18**: 295–9
9. Hoskins PL, Alford JB, Handelsman DJ, Yue DK, Turtle JR. Comparison of different models of diabetes care on compliance and self-monitoring of blood glucose by memory glucometer. *Diabet Care* 1988; **11**: 719–24
10. Schmidt LE, Klover RV, Arfken CL, Delamater AM, Hobson D. Compliance with dietary prescriptions in children and adolescents with insulin-dependent diabetes mellitus. *J Am Dietet Assoc* 1992; **92**: 567–70
11. Christensen NK, Terry RD, Wyatt S *et al.* Quantitative assessment of dietary adherence in patients with insulin-dependent diabetes mellitus. *Diabet Care* 1983 **6**: 245–50
12. Glasgow RE, McCaul KD, Shafter LC. Self-care behaviour and glycaemic control in type 1 diabetes. *J Chron Dis* 1987; **40**: 399–41
13. Kamiya A, Ohsawa I, Fujii T, Nagai M, Yamanouchi K, Oshida Y, Sato Y. A clinical survey on the complance of exercise therapy for diabetic patients. *Diabet Res Clin Pract* 1995; **27**: 141–5
14. Kravitz RL, Hays RD, Sherbourne CD, Di Matteo MR, Rogers WH, Ordway L, Greenfield S. Recall of recommendations and adherence to advice among patients with chronic conditions. *Arch Intern Med* 1993; **1543**: 1869–78
15. Barth R, Campbell LV, Allen S, Jupp JJ, Chisholm DJ. Intensive education improves knowledge compliance and foot problems in type 2 diabetes. *Diabet Med* 1991; **8**: 111–17
16. Hammersley MS, Holland MR, Walford S, Thorn PA. What happens to defaulters from a diabetic clinic? *Br Med Clin Res Educ* 1985; **291**(6505): 1330–32
17. Ley P. *Communicating with Patients*. London: Croom Helm, 1988
18. Ruggiero L, Glasgow RE, Dryfoos JM, Rossi JS, Prochaska JO, Orleans CT, Prokhorov AV, Rossi SR, Greene GW, Reed GR, Kelly K, Chobanian L, Johnson S. Diabetes self-management: self-reported recommendations and patterns in a large population. *Diabet Care* 1997; **20**(4): 568–84
19. St Vincent Declaration Action Programme. *Diabetes Care and Research in Europe*. Geneva: World Health Organization, 1992
20. Lorenz RA, Bubb J, Davis D, Jacobson A, Jannasch K, Kramer J, Lipps J, Schlundt D. Changing behaviour: practical lessons from the diabetes control and complications trial. *Diabet Care* 1996; **19**(6): 648–52
21. Williams G, Pickup J, Keen H. Psychological factors and metabolic control: time for reappraisal? *Diabet Med* 1988; **5**: 211–15
22. Murphy E, Kinmouth AL. No symptoms, no problem? Patients' understandings for non-insulin-dependent diabetes. *Family Pract* 1995; **12**(2): 184–92
23. Doherty YA, Hall D, James PT, Roberts SH, Simpson J. Change counselling: the development of a training programme for the diabetes team. *Patient Educ Counsel* 2000 (in press)
24. Brown SA. Meta-analysis of diabetes patient education research: variations in intervention effects across studies. *Res Nurs Health* 1992; **15**: 409–19

25. Padgett P, Mumford E, Hynes M, Carter R. Meta-analysis of the effects of educational and psychological interventions on management of diabetes mellitus. *J Clin Epidemiol* 1988; **41**: 1007–30
26. Coates VE, Boore JRP. Knowledge and diabetes self-management. *Patient Educ Counsel* 1996; **29**: 99–108
27. Beeney LJ, Dunn SM. Knowledge improvement and metabolic control in diabetes education: approaching the limits? *Patient Educ Counsel* 1990; **16**: 217–29
28. Glasgow RE, Osteen VL. Evaluating diabetes education: are we measuring the most important outcomes? *Diabet Care* 1992; **15**(10): 1423–37
29. Wing RR, Venditti, E, Jakicic JM, Polley BA, Lang W. Lifestyle intervention in overweight individuals with a family history of diabetes. *Diabet Care* 1998; **21**(3): 350–59
30. Honey P, Mumford A. *A Manual of Learning Styles*, 3rd edn. Maidenhead: Honey, 1992
31. Reid MA, Barrington H. *Training Interventions: Managing Employee Development*, 4th edn. London: Institute of Personnel and Development, 1994
32. Sackett DL, Snow JC. Magnitude of compliance and non-compliance. In Haynes RB, Taylor DW, Sackett DL (ed) *Compliance in Health Care*. Baltimore, MD: Johns Hopkins University Press, 1979
33. McKay HG, Feil EG, Glasgow RE, Brown JE. Feasibility and use of an Internet support service for diabetes self-management. *Diabet Educ* 1998; **24**(2): 174–9
34. Hawthorne K, Tomlinson S. One-to-one teaching with pictures—flashcard health education for British Asians with diabetes. *Br J Gen Pract* 1997; **47**: 301–4
35. Coles C. Educating the health care team. *Patient Educ Counsel* 1995; **26**: 239–44
36. Goodall TA, Halford KW. Self-management of diabetes mellitus: a critical review. *Health Psychol* 1991; **10**(1): 1–8
37. Stott NCH, Rees M, Rollnick S., Pill RM. Innovation in clinical method: diabetes care and negotiating skills. *Family Pract* 1995; **12**(4): 413–18
38. Ley P, Llewelyn S. Improving patients' understanding, recall, satisfaction and compliance. In Broome, A, Llewelyn S (eds) *Health Psychology: Processes and Applications*, 2nd edn. London: Chapman and Hall, 1995
39. Maes S, Leventhanl H, deRidder DTD. Coping with chronic diseases. In Zeidner M, Endler N (eds) *Handbook of Coping: Theory, Research and Applications*. Chichester: Wiley, 1996
40. Rogers CR. *Client Centred Therapy: Its Current Practice. Implications Theory.* New York: Houghton Mifflin, 1951
41. Burnard P. *Counselling Skills for Health Professionals*. London: Chapman and Hall, 1989
42. Prochaska JO, DiClemente CC. Towards a comprehensive model of change. In Miller WR, Heather N (eds) *Treating Addictive Behaviours: Process of Change*. New York: Plenum, 1986; 1007–30
43. Traux C, Carkhuff R. *Toward Effective Training in Counselling and Psychotherapy.* Chicago, IL: Aldine, 1967
44. James PT. Counselling those with diabetes. *Diabet Nurs* 1995; **20**: 8–9
45. Williams GC, Freedman ZR, Deci EI. Stage theories of health behaviour: conceptual and methodological issues. *Health Psychol* 1998; **17**(3): 290–99
46. Kyngas H, Hertinen M, Barlow J. Adolescents' perceptions of physicians, nurses, parents and friends: help or hindrance in compliance with diabetes care? *J Adv Nurs* 1998; **27**(4): 760–69

47. Rollnick S, Miller WR. What is motivational interviewing? *Behav Cogn Psychother* 1995; 325–34
48. Miller WR, Baca LM. Two year follow-up of bibliotherapy and therapist-directed controlled drinking training for problem drinkers. *Behav Ther* 1983; 441–8
49. Miller WR. Motivational interviewing: research, practice and puzzles. *Addict Behav* 1996; **21**(6): 835–42
50. Miller WR, Rollnick S. *Motivational interviewing: preparing people to change additive behaviour.* New York: Guilford, 1991
51. Stott NCH, Rees M, Rollnick S, Pill RM, Hackett P. Professional responses to innovation in clinical method: diabetes care and negotiating skills. *Patient Educ Counsel* 1996; **29**: 67–73
52. Smith DE, Heckemeyer CM, Kratt PP, Mason DA. Motivational interviewing to improve adherence to a behavioural weight-control program for older obese women with NIDDM: a pilot study. *Diabet Care* 1997; **20**(1): 52–4
53. Rollnick S, Kinnersley P, Stott N. Methods of helping patients with behaviour change. *Br Med J* 1993; **307**: 188–90
54. Prochaska JO, DiClemente CC. Stages and processes of self-change in smoking toward an integrative model of change. *J Consult Clin Psychol* 1983; **5**: 390–95
55. DiClemente CC, Prochaska JO. Processes and stages of change. Coping and competence in smoking behaviour change. In Shiffmand S, Wills TA (eds) *Coping and Substance Abuse*. San Diego, CA: Academic Press, 1985.
56. Dijksta A, DeVries H, Roijackers J, Van Breukelen G. Tailored interventions to communicate stage matched information to smokers in different motivational stages. *J Consult Clin Psychol* 1998; **66**(3): 549–57
57. Glanz K, Patterson PE, Kristal A. Stages of change in adopting health diets: fats, fibre and correlations of nutrition intake. *Health Educ Qu* 1994; **21**: 499–519
58. Trigwell P, Grant PJ, House A. Motivation and glycaemic control in diabetes mellitus. *J Psychosom Res* 1997; **43**(3): 307–15
59. Miller WR. Motivational interviewing with problem drinkers. *Behav Psychother* 1983; **1**: 147–72
60. Prochaska JO, DiClemente CC, Norcross JO. In search of how people change: applications to addictive behaviours. *Am. Psychol* 1992; **47**(9)P 1102–14
61. Sutton, S. Transtheoretical model of behaviour change. In Baum A, Newman S, Weinman J, West J, McManus C (eds) *Handbook of Psychology, Health and Medicine*. Cambridge: Cambridge University Press, 1997
62. Health Education Authority. *Helping People Change: Training Course for Primary Care Professionals HEA*. Oxford: National Unit for Health Promotion in Primary Care, 1993
63. Prochaska JO. Why do we believe the way we do? *Canad J Cardiol* 1995; **11**(suppl A): 20–25A
64. Weinstein ND, Rothman AJ, Sutton SR. Stage theories of health behaviour: conceptual and methodological issues. *Health Psychol* 1998; **17**(3): 290–99
65. Becker MH. The health belief model and personal health behaviour. *Health Educ Monogr* 1974; **2**: 324–508
66. Bradley C (ed). *Handbook of Psychology and Diabetes: a Guide to Measurement in Diabetes Research and Practice*. Chur, Switzerland: Harwood Academic, 1994
67. Glasgow RE, Hampson SE, Strycker LA, Ruggiero L. Personal model beliefs and socio-environmental barriers related to diabetes self-management. *Diabet Care* 1997; **20**: 556–61

68. Ajzen I, Fishbein M. The prediction of behaviour from attitudinal and normative beliefs. *J Personality Soc Psychol* 1970; **6**: 466–87
69. Fishbein M, Ajzen I. *Belief, Attitude, Intention and Behaviour: an Introduction to Theory and Research*. Reading, MA: Addison-Wesley, 1975
70. Ajzen I. From intentions to actions: a theory of planned behaviour. In Khul J, Beckman J (eds) *Action Control: from Cognition to Behaviour*. Berlin: Springer-Verlag, 1985
71. Schwarzer R. Self-efficacy in the adoption and maintenance of health behaviours: theoretical approaches and a new model. In Schwarzer R (ed) *Self-Efficacy: Thought Control of Action*. Washington, DC: Hemisphere, 1992
72. Shillitoe RW. *Psychology and Diabetes*. London: Chapman and Hall, 1988
73. Glasgow RE, Toobert DJ, Hampson SE. Effects of a brief office-based intervention to facilitate diabetes dietary self-management. *Diabet Care* 1996; **19**(8): 835–42
74. Mendez FJ, Belendez M. Effects of a behavioural intervention on treatment adherence and stress management in adolescents with IDDM. *Diabet Care* 1997; **20**(9): 1370–75
75. Beeney LJ, Barkry AA, Stewart MD. Patient psychological and information needs when the diagnosis is diabetes. *Patient Educ Counsel* 1996; **29**: 109–16
76. Pibernik-Okanovic M, Roglic G, Prasek M, Metelko Z. Emotional adjustment and metabolic control in newly diagnosed persons. *Diabet Res Clin pract* 1999; **34**: 99–105
77. Hendricks LE, Hendricks RT. Greatest fears of type 1 and type 2 patients about having diabetes: implications for diabetes. *Diabet Educ* 1998; **24**(2): 168–73
78. Berlin I, Bisserbie JC, Eiber R, Balssa N, Sachon C, Bosquet F, Grimaldi A. Phobic symptoms, particularly the fear of blood and injury are associated with poor glycaemic control in type I diabetic adults. *Diabet Care* 1997; **20**(2): 176–81
79. Irvine A, Cox D, Gonder-Frederick L. The Fear of Hypoglycaemia Scale. In Bradley C (ed) *Handbook of Psychology and Diabetes*. Chur, Switzerland: Harwood Academic, 1994
80. Greenberg LS, Safran JD. *Emotion in Psychotherapy*. New York: Guilford, 1987
81. Guthrie E. Emotional disorder in chronic illness: psychotherapeutic interventions. *Br J Psychiat* 1996; **168**: 265–73
82. Ivinson MHL. The emotional world of the diabetic patient. *Diabet Med* 1995; **12**: 113–16
83. Janis IL. *Psychological Stress: Psychoanalytic and Behavioural Studies of Surgical Studies*. New York: Wiley, 1958
84. Lindgren CL, Burke ML, Hainsworth MA, Eahes CG. Chronic sorrow: a lifespan concept. *Scholar Inqu Nurs Pract* 1992; **6**(1): 27–42
85. Zigmond AS, Snaith RP. The hospital anxiety and depression scale. *Acta Psychiat Scand* 1983; **67**: 361–70
86. Ashworth P. Breakthrough or bandwagon? Are interventions tailored to stage of change more effective than non-staged interventions? *Health Educ J* 1997; **56**: 166–74
87. Skinner CS, Strecher VJ, Hospers H. Physicians' recommendations for mammography: do tailored interventions make a difference? *Am J Public Health* 1994; **84**(1): 43–9
88. Strecher VJ, Kreuter M, Den Boer DJ, Kobin S, Hospers HJ, Skinner CS. The effects of computer-tailored smoking cessation messages in family practice settings. *J Family Pract* 1994; **39**(3): 262–70
89. Perz CA, DiClemente CC, Carbonari JP. Doing the right thing at the right time?

The interaction of stages and processes of change in successful smoking cessation. *Health Psychol* 1996; **15**(6): 462–8

90. Pendleton D, Schofield T, Tate P, Havelock P. *The Consultation: an Approach to Learning and Teaching*. Oxford: Oxford University Press, 1984
91. Rollnick S, Heather N, Gold R, Hall W. Development of a short 'readiness to change' questionnaire for use in brief, opportunistic interventions among excessive drinkers. *Br J Addict* 1992; **87**: 743–54
92. Prochaska JO, DiClemente CC. Stages of change in the modification of problem behaviours. In Hersen M, Eisher RM, Miller PM (eds) *Progress in Behaviour Modification*. Newbury Park, CA: Sage, 1992
93. Heather N, Rollnick S, Bell A. Predictive validity of the readiness to change questionnaire. *Br J Addiction* 1993; **88**: 1667–77
94. Rollnick S, Heather N, Bell A. Negotiating behaviour change in medical settings: the development of brief motivational interviewing. *J Mental Health* 1992; **1**: 25–37
95. Stone D, Challinor R. Health Hearts: Food and exercise group. Cardiovascular Disease Prevention Conference IV, London, September, 1998
96. Goldman JB, Maclean HM. The significance of identity in the adjustment to diabetes among insulin users. *Diabet Educ* 1998; **24**(6): 741–8
97. Jacobson AM, Hauser ST, Willett JB, Wolfsdorf JI, Dvorak R, Herman L, De Bgroot M. Psychological adjustment to IDDM: 10 year follow-up of an onset cohort of child and adolescent patients. *Diabet Care* 1997; **20**(5): 811–18
98. Maguire P. Breaking bad news. In Baum A, Newman S, Weinmann J, West R, McManus C (eds) *Cambridge Handbook of Psychology, Health and Medicine*. Cambridge: Cambridge University Press, 1997
99. Sarafino E. *Health Psychology: Biopsychological Interactions*. New York: Wiley, 1990
100. Moorey S. When bad things happen to rational people. In Salkovskis P (ed) *Frontiers in Cognitive Therapy*. New York: Guilford, 1996
101. Worden JW. *Grief Counselling and Grief Therapy: a Handbook for the Mental Health Practitioner*, 2nd edn. London: Routledge, 1991
102. Reid WH, Wise MG. *DSM-IV Training Guide*. New York: Brunner/Mazel, 1995
103. Charlton PFC, Thompson JA. Ways of coping with psychological distress after trauma. *Br J Clin Psychol* 1996; **35**: 517–30
104. Joseph S, Dalgleish T, Williams R, Yule W, Thrasher S, Hodgkinson P. Attitudes towards emotional expression and post-traumatic stress in survivors of the Herald of Free Enterprise disaster. *Br J Clin Psychol* 1997: **36**: 133–8
105. Leventhal H, Meyer D, Nerenz D. The common sense representation of illness danger. In Rachman (ed) *Contributions to Medical Psychology*, vol II. Oxford: Pergamon, 1980
106. Leventhal H, Nerenz DR, Steele DJ. Illness representations and coping with health threats. In Baum A, Taylor S, Singer J (eds) *Handbook of Psychology and Health, vol IV, Social Psychological Aspects of Health*. Hillsdale, NJ: Erlbaum, 1984
107. Eysenck MW, Keane MJ. *Cognitive Psychology*. Hillsdale, NJ: Erlbaum, 1990
108. Diabetes Control and Complications Trial Research Group. The effect of intensive treatment on the development and progression of long-term complications in insulin-dependent diabetes mellitus. *N Engl J Med* 1993; **329**: 977–86
109. Bradley C. Contributions of psychology to diabetes management. *Br J Clin Psychol* 1994; **33**: 11–21
110. Bandura A. Self efficacy: toward a unifying theory of behavioural change. *Psychol Rev* 1977; **84**: 191–215

111. Beck AT, Rush AJ, Shaw BF, Emergy G. *Cognitive Therapy of Depression*. New York: Guilford, 1979
112. Padesky CA, Greenberger D. *Clinicians' Guide to Mind over Mood*. New York: Guilford, 1995
113. Schafer LL, Glasgow RE, McCaul KD. Increasing the adherence of diabetic adolescents. *J Behav Med* 1982; **5**: 352–62
114. Lowe K, Lutzher J. Increasing compliance to a medical regime with a juvenile diabetic. *Behav Ther* 1979; **10**: 57–64
115. Yue DK, Dunn SM, Fowler PM. The compliance of diabetic patients: relationship between subjective assessment by physicians and objective measurement of patient performance. *Diabet Res* 1984; **1**: 39–43
116. Marlott GA, Gordon JR. *Relapse Prevention: Maintenance Strategies in the Treatment of Addictive Behaviours*. New York: Guilford, 1985
117. Schachter S. Recidivism and self-cure of smoking and obesity. *Am Psychol* 1982; **37**: 436–44
118. Pill R, Stott NCH, Rollnick SR, Rees, M. A randomized controlled trial of an intervention designed to improve the care given in general practice to type II diabetic patients: patient outcomes and professional ability to change behaviour. *Family Pract* 1998; **15**(3): 229–35
119. Wanigaratue S, Wallace W, Pullin J. *Relapse Prevention for Addictive Behaviours*. Oxford: Blackwell Scientific, 1990

6

Medical Office-based Interventions

RUSSELL E. GLASGOW and ELIZABETH G. EAKIN
AMC Cancer Research Center, Denver, CO, USA

THEORETICAL BACKGROUND

When one thinks of the role of psychology in diabetes or other types of health care, the image that comes to mind is that of a patient discussing emotional difficulties with a therapist or counsellor in a mental health setting. This stereotype, based on a referral system for behavioural health care, was generally accurate for many years. Today, however, the face of psychology and behavioural science in diabetes is changing, spurred on by both the development of brief behavioural interventions and the information technology revolution[1–3].

Both the range of issues addressed by psychology and the modalities of intervention have expanded significantly. Psychologists and other health professionals are increasingly involved in diabetes care. In some instances, they are part of multidisciplinary teams providing direct patient care in medical offices. In other cases, they supervise practice innovations, design computer-assisted intervention programmes or instruct other health professionals in behaviour change principles and strategies.

There is an important need for psychologists to be more involved in the diabetes care that takes place in medical offices, for three primary reasons. First, many patients will not or cannot avail themselves of psychological

Psychology in Diabetes Care. Edited by Frank J. Snoek and T. Chas Skinner.

assistance offered via the traditional referral system. Patients frequently have many barriers to following through on referrals, including cost, lack of familiarity with behavioural science, convenience and time commitment required, and anticipated stigma associated with 'seeing a shrink'. Second, the quality of care provided for diabetes patients in most medical settings is substantially suboptimal[4–6]. Almost all population-based studies of the level of recommended 'best practices' received by patients have revealed much lower than desired rates of clinical services and screening measures[4,5]. The rates of preventive services, and especially lifestyle change interventions, are even lower[5,6]. Third, patient-centred, motivational interviewing, and patient activation/empowerment approaches have consistently been found to produce beneficial effects, yet such strategies are seldom employed in either primary care or specialty endocrinological settings. Thus, there is a compelling need and great opportunity for the application of behavioural science in medical office settings.

From a conceptual and social-environmental influence perspective[7,8] the medical office setting occupies a strategic position in the 'pyramid of social-environmental influences' on patient self-management and decision-making processes (see Figure 6.1). As can be seen in Figure 6.1, health care system encounters fall midway between the more proximal influences, such as personal actions and family and friends, on the one hand, and more distal factors, such as community and media/policy influences, on the other. Because of this position and the enormous credibility accorded to physicians and other health care professions in our society, interventions in medical settings have great potential also to leverage the other levels of social-environmental factors.

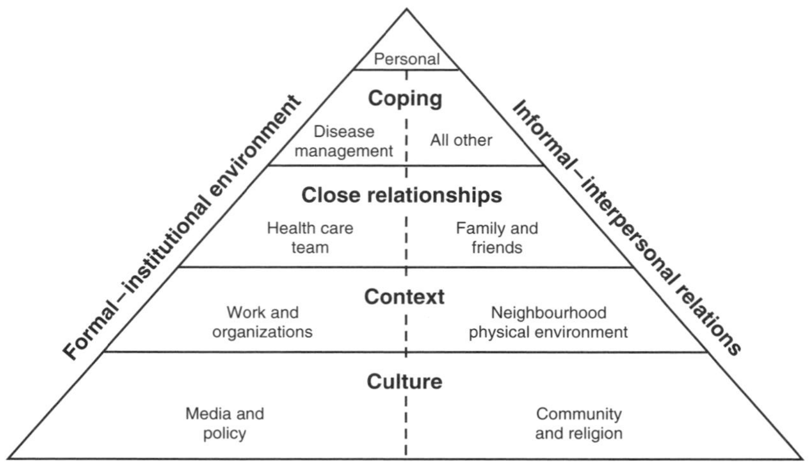

Figure 6.1. Pyramid of psychosocial factors

The medical office setting also has much to recommend it, due to the frequent contact most diabetes patients have with their health care providers. On average, patients with diabetes see their doctor for several visits per year. This repeated, ongoing contact provides a potent context within which to work with patients to collaboratively set goals, develop strategies, collect information, provide feedback, and modify goals or set new ones[1,9,10]. Another important asset from a public health perspective is the availability of medical records, and the increasing prevalence of diabetes registries, which permit population-based disease management activities[11].

To take advantage of these opportunities, however, psychologists will have to change how they do business[1]. In particular, they will need to adapt their assessment and intervention strategies to be compatible with, and to fit into, medical settings. In addition, they need to understand the world views and training of physicians (as well as nurses, dieticians and other health care professionals) and how these frequently differ from those to which psychologists have been acculturated in their own training and practice.

CLINICAL AND LOGISTICAL RATIONALE FOR OFFICE-BASED INTERVENTION

As noted above, the majority of patients with diabetes do not attend psychosocial disease management programmes, neither do most attend traditional diabetes education programmes[12]. Thus, we must look for other avenues via which to deliver behavioural interventions. The physician office visit is one such avenue, as most patients with diabetes (with access to health care) make frequent, often quarterly, visits to a health care provider. Even in the context of a brief office visit, the physician has a key role in helping the patient to manage his/her diabetes better[13–15]. The physician is seen as the expert. Anderson and Funnell[14] describe the office visit as a 'teachable moment', a time when patients are very motivated to listen to and act on the advice of the physician (and other health care team members). This is especially true if the visit represents something novel for the patient; for example, if the patient is newly diagnosed, beginning to experience chronic complications, started on insulin, or is referred to an endocrinologist for expert consultation. Thus, the physician office visit provides an opportunity to reach the majority of patients with diabetes and to do so with a highly credible source of information. This said, it is also the case that providers are often overwhelmed by multiple demands and time pressures, and are reticent to add yet another protocol into the busy office setting. In addition, studies of physician barriers to delivering behavioural interventions indicate that many physicians feel ill-equipped to counsel patients regarding behaviour change[2,16]. Commonly reported physician barriers include lack of training in behavioural counselling, lack of time, lack of reimbursement for such counselling, and doubts as to the efficacy of such interventions.

Tremendous opportunities for behavioural science contributions exist, given the complexity of the biopsychosocial issues in diabetes, the frequency of contact with diabetes patients, and the relatively low level of adherence to recommended guidelines[17–20] by both patients and providers[5,21]. To impact diabetes management, behavioural and psychological assessments, interventions and models should be practical and efficient, be readily understood by non-psychologists, and address issues that diabetes patients and providers (rather than psychologists) perceive as important[22,23]. Behavioural assessments and interventions must also be brief and integrated into the regular clinic flow. The use of interactive computer-based health care technology, which collects and immediately scores key behavioural assessment information and delivers, in full or in part, behavioural interventions, addresses this issue. Other ways to achieve this goal involve transferring management responsibilities to non-physician (and likely non-mental health professional) members of the health care team, such as nurses, dieticians or diabetes educators. Specific suggestions for incorporating brief, behavioural assessments and interventions into primary care settings are discussed later in this chapter.

RESEARCH FINDINGS FROM OFFICE-BASED INTERVENTIONS

There are at least four types of psychosocial research directly related to medical office practices, as well as a much broader array of psychosocial assessment and treatment activities, such as referral to lifestyle behaviour change or mental health services, reviewed elsewhere. These four types of research are: (a) data collection in the medical office setting that is used for designing later behavioural interventions; (b) psychosocial interventions conducted during the course of regular office visits; (c) training interventions to change the behaviour of physicians, nurses or other health professionals; and (d) systems interventions to alter the health care setting. A brief summary of key illustrative research is provided for each of these topics.

We also describe briefly relevant medical office applications conducted with other chronic illnesses to illustrate opportunities in cases where similar research in diabetes has not yet been conducted. First, however, we need to introduce the framework that we will use to evaluate the extant literature. Termed the RE-AIM model, this framework focuses attention on important applicability issues and a real world, effectiveness perspective[24,25] compatible with the realities of medical office treatment of diabetes at the beginning of the 21st century. There are five component dimensions to the RE-AIM model, which combine to determine the overall public health impact of an intervention: (a) Reach, or the percentage and representativeness of patients who are willing to participate in a given procedure; (b) Efficacy, or the impact of an intervention on important outcomes, including behavioural, biological, quality of life, and economic outcomes. There are also three less often studied, but equally important outcomes, which concern impact at the level of a medical office or health care system. These 'AIM' dimensions are: (c) Adoption, or the percentage and representativeness of settings that are willing to adopt or try an office innovation; (d) Implementation, or how consistently an intervention or procedure is delivered as intended; and (e) Maintenance, or the extent to which a programme or policy becomes institutionalized or part of the routine practice of medical settings. These five factors interact to determine the overall 'population-based' or public health impact of a programme as illustrated in Table 6.1.

An example may help to illustrate how the RE-AIM evaluation framework can lead to surprising conclusions about the wisest use of scarce health care resources. The basic assumption is that an intervention's impact is an interaction—represented as a multiplicative relationship in Table 6.1. Therefore, an intervention which is highly efficacious—say 0.7 (see Table 6.1)—such as intensive insulin management, but has very limited reach or appeal (0.1) may prove to have little overall impact ($0.7 \times 0.1 = 0.07$) and less population-wide benefit than a more modest intervention that has less efficacy (0.3) but higher reach (0.5) ($0.3 \times 0.5 = 0.15$).

This way of thinking about the population-based or public health impact of programmes is new for many psychologists, as well as physicians and other health care professionals. With the increasing emphasis on cost containment and accountability, evaluation criteria like those in the RE-AIM model become paramount. Most of our professional training has upheld the traditional double-blind randomized clinical trial as the 'gold standard' method for evaluating interventions. While such trials have certainly advanced our knowledge, they often oversimplify clinical realities and emphasize internal validity (efficacy)[24] at *the expense of* external validity. We need much more research conducted on representative patient samples in representative clinical settings, conducted under 'real-world' conditions, to help guide important policy and resource allocation decisions.

DIABETES-SPECIFIC OFFICE-BASED INTERVENTIONS

There have been relatively few studies of psychological or other behavioural science programmes that have been carried out in the medical office/care

Table 6.1. Component dimensions and related characteristics of the RE-AIM evaluation framework

Evaluation dimension	Units and level of measurement	Prevalence of research
% Reach (what proportion of the panel of patients will receive or be willing and able to participate in this intervention?)	Percentage and representativeness of members of a population that participate (0–1.0)	Modest
× % Efficacy (success rates if implemented as in guidelines: defined as positive outcomes minus negative outcomes)	Magnitude or percentage of improvement on outcome(s) of interest (0–1.0)	Substantial
× % Adoption (how many settings, practices and plans will adopt this intervention?)	Percentage and representativeness of organizations or settings that try an intervention (0–1.0)	Minimal
× % Implementation (to what extent is the intervention implemented as intended in the real world?)	Consistency and quality of intervention delivery under real world conditions (0–1.0)	Moderate
× % Maintenance (extent to which a programme is sustained over time)	Extent to which individuals or implementation agents continue to deliver a programme over time (0–1.0)	Little
= Public health impact (population-based effect)	End result of interaction of factors above (0–1.0)	None to our knowledge

setting. More often, behavioural, lifestyle and mental health counselling has been conducted on a referral basis. Table 6.2 and this section summarize the few reports of behaviour change intervention initiated or delivered in the office setting solely with diabetes patients, and uses the RE-AIM model to evaluate results.

One of the earlier psychological intervention studies to take place during regular office visits was conducted by Barbara Anderson *et al.*[26] with type 1 adolescents and their family members. Adolescents randomized to the intervention attended five group visits with peers, once every 3–4 months, conducted as part of their usual medical visits, while their parents participated in concurrent group sessions with other parents. Content of the

Table 6.2. Summary of diabetes medical office research literature by RE-AIM issues

RE-AIM dimension	Conclusions re: state of science	Amount of research	Example of diabetes references	Other chronic illness examples
Reach	Fairly broad—better than traditional education or referral	Moderate	Glasgow *et al.*[12]	Eakin *et al.*[84]
Efficacy	Variable—Moderate; better for personalized treatment	Good	Glasgow *et al.*[31] McNabb[86] Greenfield *et al.*[29]	Green *et al.*[85] Strecher[87] Brug[88] Lorig[48]
Adoption	Unknown	Little/None	None found	Goodman and Steckler[89]
Implementation	Unknown	Little	Litzelman *et al.*[35]	
Maintenance	Poor—especially unless follow-up support provided	Moderate at individual level; little at clinic level	Weinberger *et al.*[36]	Wasson *et al.*[38]

meetings focused on problem-solving and using blood glucose self-monitoring (BGSM) data for self-regulation. After 18 months, participants in the intervention condition showed significantly greater reductions in HbA_{1C} (adjusted differences of about 1%) then those in usual care, and more intervention than usual care adolescents (60% vs. 33%) reported using BGSM information when they exercised. More research is needed on similar approaches to aiding adolescents, as well as on group approaches to clinic visits for adults, which have been used with success in other areas[27,28].

An example of research using a patient-activation paradigm was reported by Greenfield *et al*[29]. In this randomized trial, a research assistant met with patients for 20 minutes just prior to two regular quarterly office visits to review their medical records, discuss medical decisions and self-management issues likely to arise during that visit, and rehearse negotiation and information-seeking skills. At 12 week follow-up, this patient activation intervention produced significant improvements in both glucose control (adjusted differences of approximately 2% HbA_{1C}), days lost from work and quality of life relative to controls. Patients in the experimental condition were also significantly more active during their visit with their physician, asked more questions, and elicited more information from their doctor.

A more recent high-tech approach to patient-centred self-management by our research group[30,31] focused on enhancing dietary self-management. This study began by contacting all adult diabetes patients who had an upcoming visit with one of two internists. Sixty-one per cent of eligible patients agreed to participate in the study and, importantly, there were no differences between participants and non-participants on demographic or medical characteristics collected[12]. The intervention package involved a sequence of: a 15-minute touchscreen computer assessment which helped patients identify dietary goals and barriers to accomplishing this goal; immediate scoring and printing of two tailored feedback/goal print-outs summarizing the information—one for the patient and one for the physician; a 20-second motivational message from the physician emphasizing the importance of the goal the patient had selected; a 15–20 minute meeting with a health educator to review the patient's goal and collaboratively develop barriers-based intervention strategies; and finally, two brief follow-up telephone calls from the health educator to check on progress. This sequence was repeated at a regular 3-month follow-up visit. Compared to a stringent, randomized control condition that received the same touchscreen computer assessment (but no tailored feedback) and physician encouragement, the intervention produced significantly greater improvements on a variety of dietary behaviour measures, as well as serum cholesterol levels. More importantly, these results were maintained at essentially the same level (e.g. adjusted difference of 16 mg/dl in serum cholesterol) at a 12-month follow-up, and the intervention was found to be cost-effective: an average, annual incremental cost over usual care of $115–139 per patient and $8.40 per unit reduction in serum cholesterol level.

We are currently replicating and expanding this intervention to assess its effectiveness across a wider range of primary care offices, health educators and patients. We are also investigating the cost-effectiveness of the telephone follow-up calls and of a brief intervention component to engage patients in more community support and self-management resource activities.

Bob Anderson and colleagues[32] have reported on the results of a training programme for diabetes educators to help them learn patient empowerment strategies for working with their patients. They evaluated a 3-day skills-based workshop (these authors have subsequently also developed shorter training programmes), which included following a simulated diabetes care regimen prior to the workshop training, demonstrations and practice in empowerment counselling skills, and finally a videotape review of counselling sessions. Following training, participants in the workshop showed significant improvement from baseline in counselling skills (on both videotape simulations and audio recordings of actual counselling sessions), and in their attitudes toward supporting patient autonomy on the Diabetes Attitudes Scale[32]. An interesting outcome of the study was that several of the educators who participated in the programme have, in turn, presented counselling skills in-service programmes to colleagues. The empowerment approach has been demonstrated to produce better patient outcomes than usual care in a randomized trial[33]. More research on the empowerment model and related approaches, such as motivational interviewing[34], are needed, especially studies that evaluate the adoption (who participates in such training), implementation and maintenance of counselling skills.

Litzelman et al.[35] have provided a good example of a very low-cost, office-based systems intervention which focused on enhancing foot care practices by both patients and providers. Their patient intervention involved nurse-clinician meetings with 1–4 patients to cover foot care education, individualized behavioural contracts, telephone follow-ups at 2 weeks, and mailed postcard reminders at 1 and 3 months. The office systems intervention consisted of colourful patient folders with foot decals to identify intervention patients, prompts to ask patients to remove their footware, and a guidelines-based flowsheet for physicians. One year after initiating the intervention, Litzelman *et al.*[35] found that this intervention package produced significant reductions in foot lesions (odds ratio = 0.4), increases in appropriate foot self-care behaviours, and increases in office foot examinations (68% vs. 28%), compared to randomized controls. The helpfulness of follow-up support was demonstrated by Weinburger *et al.*[36] who found that brief telephone calls conducted by nurses led to reductions in glycosylated haemoglobin (GHb). In a randomized study with older type 2 VA patients, they found that calls conducted once a month, on average, significantly decreased GHb levels (adjusted difference of 0.6%) relative to usual care. These results are consistent with studies demonstrating the efficacy and cost-effectiveness of telephone calls for enhancing maintenance and even serving as alternatives to office visits for non-diabetes health-related issues[37,38].

Finally, the Diabetes Control and Complications Trial (DCCT)[39] provides an interesting example of the power of systematically reorganizing office practices and patient self-management support activities. Although often interpreted solely as a demonstration of the efficacy of intensive insulin management, the DCCT obtained its incredibly good adherence and low attrition rates by providing an impressive array of ongoing patient support activities[1,40]. The DCCT is also interesting because it is probably the best example of a well-conducted and extremely influential efficacy trial in diabetes. It unquestionably produced impressive clinical outcomes. However, review of the controversies and differences of opinion regarding the applicability of DCCT-like procedures[41,42] illustrate the difficulties of making practice guideline and resource allocation decisions based solely on efficacy trials. From the RE-AIM perspective, the DCCT maximized Efficacy results, but would receive very low scores on Reach (percentage and representativeness of patients participating) and Adoption (conducted predominantly in unrepresentative, specialized tertiary care centres and with very high levels of clinical expertise and resources). More effectiveness trials conducted in primary care settings using population-based approaches are needed[9,25].

EXAMPLES FROM OTHER AREAS

Although the evidence from medical office-based intervention with diabetes patients is promising, it is still preliminary. Therefore, it is useful to consider interventions that have been successful in utilizing or supplementing the medical office encounter to enhance patient outcomes in other chronic illnesses. Below, we review several such examples that we think are transferable to diabetes.

The work of the Stanford Cardiac Rehabilitation Programme[43] with patients who have suffered a recent heart attack serves as a model of how integrated, home-based self-management support can be provided. Their programme is based on the social-cognitive theory[44] components of individualized goal setting, feedback and follow-up support integrated with medical care and coordinated by a nurse case manager.

This study evaluated computer-assisted goal setting, self-management planning, and follow-up telephone calls conceptually similar to the programme employed in diabetes by Glasgow *et al.*[31,45] This multiple risk factor programme was found to be significantly better in facilitating smoking cessation (70% vs. 53%, $p = 0.03$), physical fitness increases (9.3 vs. 8.4 metabolic equivalents, $p = 0.001$) and lipid reduction (LDL cholesterol, 107 vs. 132 mg/dl, $p = 0.001$) compared to a usual care condition in a randomized trial with 585 recent heart disease patients.

An innovative approach to redesigning the medical office visit has been employed with older chronic illness patients by Beck *et al.*[28] in the Denver Kaiser Permanente system. Rather than seeing patients in the usual 10–15 minute individual session, primary care is provided via monthly 90 minute group visits. These sessions, run by the physician and nurse coordinator, incorporate vital sign assessments, medication checks and other elements of care into the group session, which also permits discussion of various self-management topics of interest to the group, and much opportunity for peer support. Beck *et al.*[28] evaluated this approach relative to traditional physician–patient dyadic care in a 1 year randomized trial with 321 seniors having chronic illnesses. They found that the group visit participants had fewer emergency room visits, visits to subspecialists and repeat hospitalizations. Both patients and physicians reported greater satisfaction with the group visits, which cost an overall average of $15 per month less per member.

Approaches to extending the self-management support provided in the office have been developed by Lorig *et al.*[46] and Leveille *et al.*[47] Lorig *et al.*[46] have developed a peer-led arthritis, self-management programme and found it to be superior to usual care in a series of randomized trials. Recently, they have reported 4 year follow-up results indicating lasting reductions in pain, physician visits and cost relative to comparison conditions, and adapted their programme, which emphasizes self-efficacy enhancement[44], for diabetes patients and for patients having a variety of chronic illnesses, with similar impressive results on health care utilization[48].

Leveille *et al.*[47] demonstrated the value of community support to complement primary care in a randomized trial of 201 chronically ill, frail adults age 70 and older. Their disability prevention, disease self-management intervention, conducted in a senior centre in collaboration with primary care providers, produced less decline in function on standardized instruments and fewer disability days than controls. In addition, the intervention condition participants became more physically active, significantly reduced their psychoactive medication use, and had fewer inpatient hospital days.

Finally, two recent studies using computer technology to supplement usual care provide examples of cost-effective strategies for providing tailored goal setting, skills training and support. Skinner *et al.*[49] had primary care patients complete telephone interviews. Female patients aged 40–65 who had visited their primary care provider within the past 2 years were randomized to receive a tailored health communication based on their mammography history, beliefs, risk status and perceived barriers, or to a standardized letter encouraging mammography. This brief, single contact intervention improved mammography rates among women who were due for screening compared to standardized letters (44% vs. 31%, overall) and significant interaction effects revealed that the intervention appeared especially effective with African–American women and with lower-income women[49]. A similar approach to enhancing adherence to diabetes care guidelines might readily be applied.

In a recent article, Gustafson *et al.*[50] presented the first randomized outcome evaluation of an Internet health information/support system for patients. Their CHESS (Comprehensive Health Enhancement Support System) interactive computer support system, which has also been applied with breast cancer, heart disease and problem-drinking patients, was evaluated for its ability to provide support for HIV-positive patients. Half of the 204 patients had computers linked to the CHESS system placed in their homes for 3 or 6 months; controls received no intervention beyond usual care. The CHESS system was used daily, and produced significant improvements in several quality-of-life dimensions and fewer and shorter hospitalizations than were seen in control patients.

The above interventions have been validated in large-scale randomized studies with patient populations traditionally considered to be challenging (heart disease, older adults with multiple illnesses, arthritis, HIV/AIDS patients). Common elements across these diverse interventions seem to be a patient-centred approach that individualizes self-management and goal setting, provides strategies and models for coping with barriers and, importantly, some form of follow-up support that either changes or supplements that available through usual primary care. In our opinion, these

Collaborative
goal setting
Patient,
health care team,
health care system
Follow-up
support
ID barriers
Personalized
problem-solving

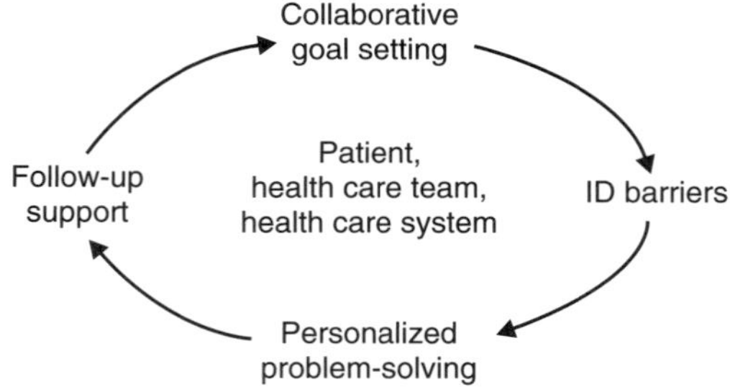

Figure 6.2. Cycle of self-management

strategies are the key components of 'the cycle of self-management' (see Figure 6.2), and should also be successful, with appropriate adaptation, in diabetes.

TARGET GROUPS FOR INCLUSION/EXCLUSION

From the existing literature, it is not possible to draw firm conclusions about subgroups for whom office-based interventions are most effective. Clearly, more research is needed, both on patient characteristics and also, equally importantly, on characteristics of the patient's social and physical environment[1,51,52] and of the office setting and medical staff characteristics associated with success.

Our clinical impressions are that there are probably some subsets of patients who have very complex or challenging issues to address that require more intensive intervention than is usually possible in the typical office visit. Such groups would include newly diagnosed patients, those with major psychological disorders such as clinical depression, and those being started on intensive insulin management regimens. Referral to appropriate specialists or more intensive programmes is warranted in such cases.

It is encouraging that the studies conducted to date have generally found office-based behavioural strategies to be equally effective across gender, age, education and medical/diabetes history and severity levels. To our knowledge, only the Anderson *et al.*[26] study has been conducted with adolescents and family members in the office setting. More research on this approach, and on group visit formats[28] for delivering primary care, is recommended (as contrasted with separate referrals to outside diabetes education groups, which are not well attended and have numerous barriers to participation).

In general, it appears that office-based behavioural assessment and counselling strategies can be effective for the vast majority of diabetes patients. Office-based psychosocial interventions can be used as the first stage in a stepped care programme[53] and have few, if any, contraindications.

ASSESSMENT AND CLINIC FLOW

As discussed below and depicted in Figure 6.3, there are many factors that influence diabetes self-management and its outcomes. The left side of Figure 6.3 illustrates the multiple levels of factors that influence diabetes self-management. The centre of the figure contains the various components of diabetes self-management. These component tasks are listed separately to illustrate that there is usually little relationship between the extent to which a patient follows one aspect of the regimen and his/her level of self-care in other areas. Finally, the right-hand side of the figure depicts the consequences of self-management, including physiological, quality-of-life and health care utilization outcomes. It is important to stress that self-care and diabetes control are not the same; self-management is one of the multiple determinants of health outcomes (along with genetics, regimen and medication prescriptions, stress, co-morbidities, disease severity and other variables)[54–56] The point is that one cannot judge a patient's level of self-management from his/her HbA_{1c} level. Poor metabolic control indicates that something is wrong, but it does not give specific information about what is wrong[13]. A second important point is that good diabetes outcomes and adjustment involve more than just low HbA_{1c} levels: variables such as the patients cardiovascular risk factors (smoking status, blood pressure, lipids), mental health status, and social, physical and role functioning (i.e. health-related quality of life) are equally or more important outcomes[57–61].

PATIENT FACTORS

The most important factors in developing self-management goals are the patient's perspective on the diabetes regimen and what changes she/he considers reasonable and realistic. Two important beliefs are that patients: (a) consider their diabetes to be serious; and (b) believe that what they do makes a difference[62–64]. Patients who do not hold these beliefs will likely not be motivated to engage in diabetes self-management behaviours. Such patients may need additional personalized feedback on the specific implications of diabetes for their health, as well as education on the potential benefits of specific self-management behaviours. The books *The Human Side of Diabetes* by Michael Raymond[15] and *Psyching Out Diabetes* by Rubin *et al.*[65] are useful resources for both patients and practitioners in illustrating how common experiences in living with diabetes can either promote or interfere with

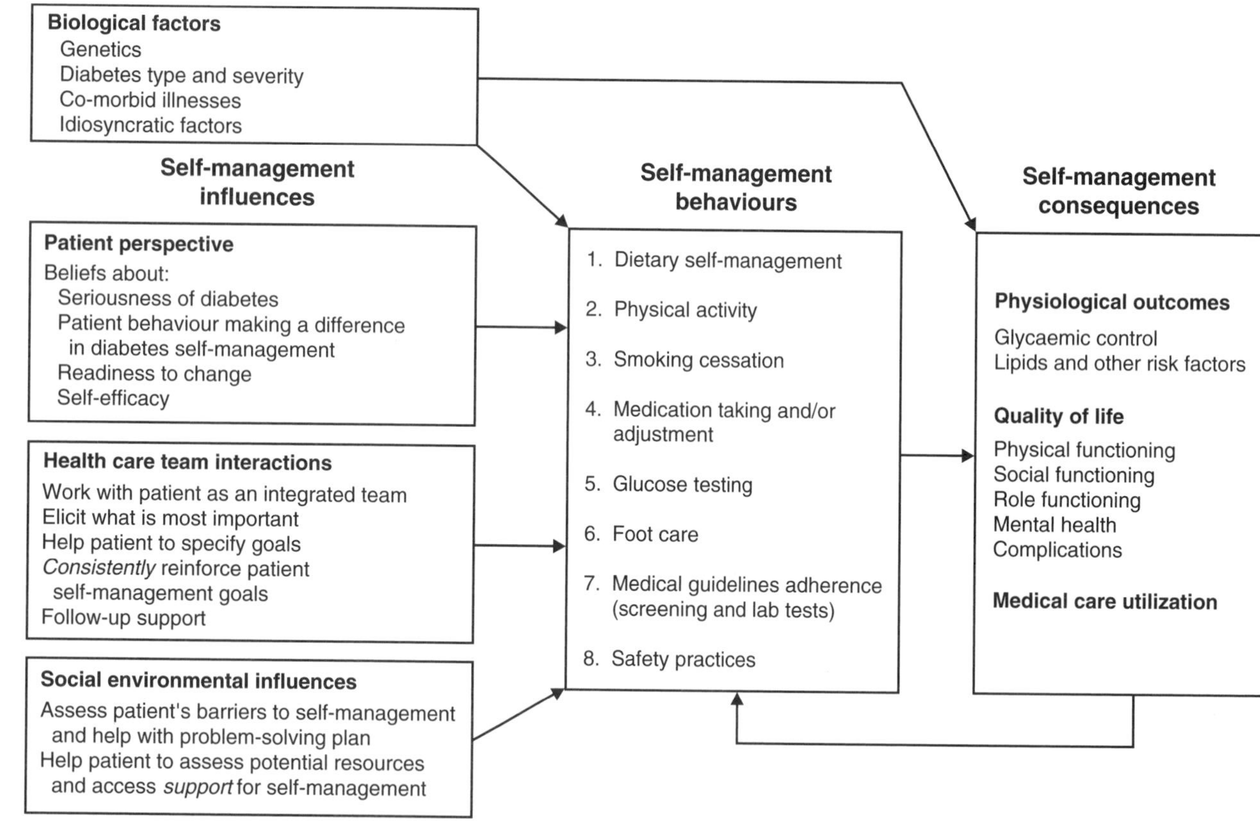

Figure 6.3. Multiple influences on diabetes self-management

establishment of such beliefs. In particular, it is important to see if a patient considers lifestyle aspects of diabetes management (e.g. diet and exercise) as important as medical aspects (e.g. medication taking and glucose testing). If they do not, they will be unlikely to follow-through with the challenges of lifestyle modification. Other important and related cognitive factors are a patient's readiness to adopt different self-management guidelines[66] and his/her self-efficacy or confidence that he/she can achieve specific goals.

HEALTH CARE TEAM ISSUES

The core issue here is consistency and reinforcement of patient goals across different health care team members. Rather than having the physician emphasize medication, the nurse stress glucose testing, and the nutritionist recommend major dietary changes, all team members need to reinforce a common self-management behaviour for that visit. The Litzelman *et al.*[35] study previously discussed provides a good example of how to coordinate preventive foot care activities, including brief education while patients are waiting to see the physician, having the nurse ask the patient to remove his/her shoes and socks before the physician arrives, followed by a physician foot examination and reinforcement of the patient education message about foot care. The patient needs to leave a given visit with a clear idea (and if possible a written 'goal' or 'contract sheet') of the key goal(s) for the next visit, and an understanding of why the goal is important to the management of his/her diabetes (see example, Figure 6.4). When patients are given assignments, it is particularly important, at the next visit or contact, to review and comment on any records that the patient has kept. The 1994 issue of *Diabetes Spectrum*, edited by Anderson and Jenkins,[67] on educational innovations provides discussion of other issues in system-wide interventions, as does the special supplement to *Diabetes Care* edited by Mazze and Etzwiler[68] and the conceptual article by Jenkins[57].

THE SOCIAL ENVIRONMENT

It is important to assess and incorporate both the patients' anticipated barriers to self-management and their available resources, at the level of (a) family and friends and (b) broader community influences, including work and neighbourhood factors (see Table 6.1)[69]. This can be accomplished by asking the patient what he/she thinks might interfere with the identified self-management goal(s) for the next visit (e.g. 'Ms Smith, what things do you think might make it difficult for you to follow the eating plan we discussed today?'). The clinician can then help the patient develop possible solutions, focusing on the use of available family, friend or community resources. Most

Overcoming barriers to healthy eating

For: **Test sample** Date: **12/12/99**

Personalized dietary goal for next few months:

To: **Substitute low-fat foods for high-fat foods**
(for example, use non-fat mayonnaise instead of regular mayonnaise)

Specific plans for accomplishing this goal:

1. ______________________________
2. ______________________________
3. ______________________________

Type of situation that is most challenging:
Moods and feelings that lead to eating

Specific situations:

I feel down or blue
I am bored or restless and feel like snacking

Other situations which make it difficult for you to follow your diet:

I have difficulty finding low-fat food items where I shop
I have junk food around the house

How you can prepare for problem situations

1. ______________________________
2. ______________________________
3. ______________________________

Figure 6.4. Overcoming barriers to healthy eating

communities have available a series of free or low-cost support or reinforcement activities (e.g. ADA meetings, hospital or HMO lectures or education programmes, newsletters) that can extend the motivation patients receive during office visits. Anderson and Funnell[14] have provided a useful discussion and examples of community support options to reinforce physician messages about diabetes management, and Anderson *et al.*[70] have described a series of publicly available, camera-ready, two-page, single-issue newsletters that can be sent to patients to reinforce a selected goal.

Self-management activities do not occur in a vacuum, but rather in a social context. If maintenance of self-management is to be expected, follow-up support must be arranged in the form of family and community social support, and follow-up contacts with members of the health care team[38]. The flow chart (Figure 6.5) and text below address how these suggestions might work into the flow of a busy practice.

PRIOR TO THE VISIT

Materials or reminders mailed to the patient prior to the visit can help focus attention on the importance of patient behaviour. One such example is a reminder to the patient to bring to an upcoming visit information which was supposed to be monitored between visits (e.g. blood glucose, food intake, or exercise logs) and to have him/her update his/her status on ADA recommended guidelines[71] or other 'best practices'.

THE WAITING ROOM

The focus on self-management can begin while the patient is in the waiting room. The patient's attention can be drawn to the importance of self-care activities by having various pamphlets, posters and notices placed in the waiting room. These might include notices from the hospital or clinic regarding diabetes education or information classes, support groups, as well as pamphlets on diet, exercise or smoking cessation.

While the patient is waiting, he/she could complete a brief form assessing the current level of diabetes self-management activities. An example of such a form is in Figure 6.6. This assessment could be easily conducted using a computer set up in a corner of the waiting room. The assessment information could also be incorporated into an interactive health technology intervention. Information from the self-management form is then used during the remainder of the visit, as described below.

THE EXAMINATION ROOM AND VITAL SIGNS

When the nurse or other office staff member takes the patient to the examination room and assesses vital signs (which should include smoking

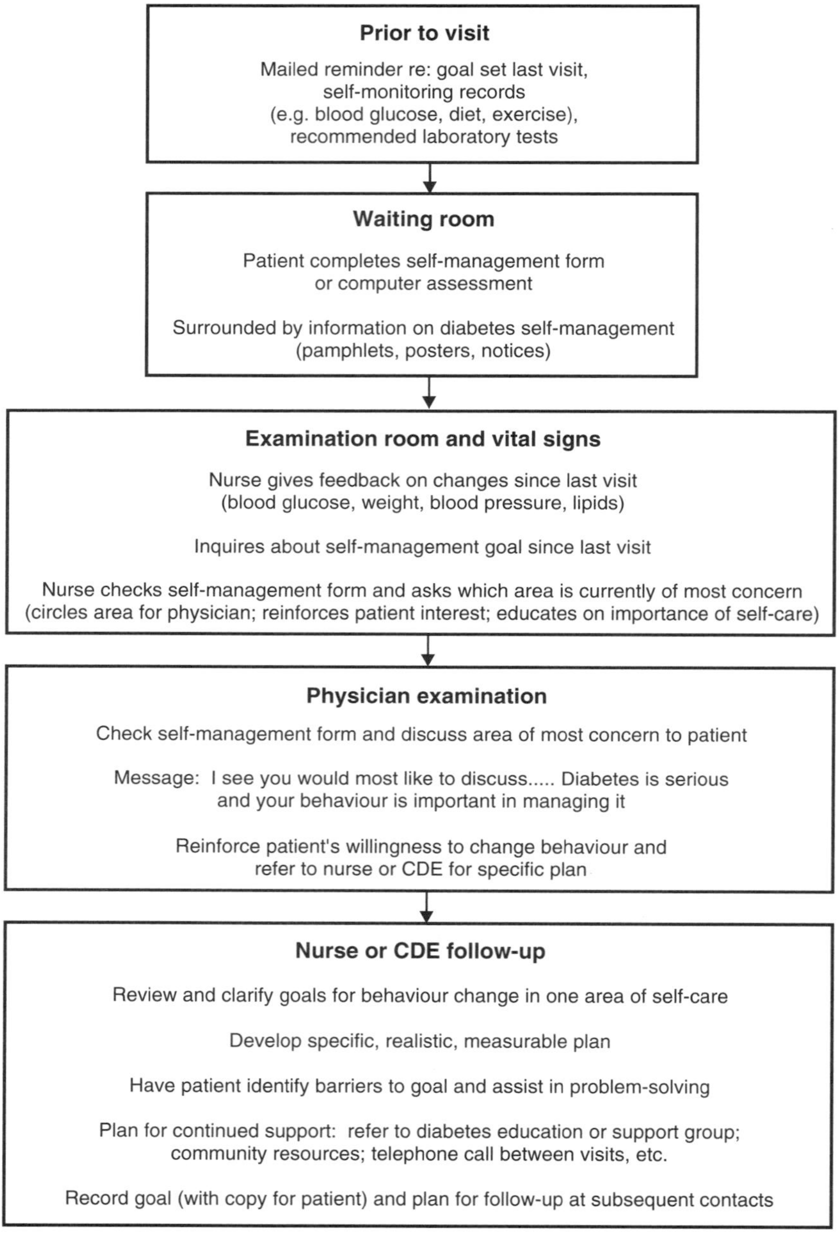

Prior to visit

Mailed reminder re: goal set last visit,
self-monitoring records
(e.g. blood glucose, diet, exercise),
recommended laboratory tests

↓

Waiting room

Patient completes self-management form
or computer assessment

Surrounded by information on diabetes self-management
(pamphlets, posters, notices)

↓

Examination room and vital signs

Nurse gives feedback on changes since last visit
(blood glucose, weight, blood pressure, lipids)

Inquires about self-management goal since last visit

Nurse checks self-management form and asks which area is currently of most concern
(circles area for physician; reinforces patient interest; educates on importance of self-care)

↓

Physician examination

Check self-management form and discuss area of most concern to patient

Message: I see you would most like to discuss..... Diabetes is serious
and your behaviour is important in managing it

Reinforce patient's willingness to change behaviour and
refer to nurse or CDE for specific plan

↓

Nurse or CDE follow-up

Review and clarify goals for behaviour change in one area of self-care

Develop specific, realistic, measurable plan

Have patient identify barriers to goal and assist in problem-solving

Plan for continued support: refer to diabetes education or support group;
community resources; telephone call between visits, etc.

Record goal (with copy for patient) and plan for follow-up at subsequent contacts

Figure 6.5. Flow of brief office-based diabetes self-management intervention

status)[72,73], this provides an opportunity to give the patient feedback on key issues, such as weight gain or loss and changes in blood glucose, cholesterol or blood pressure since the last visit. The nurse can also briefly check the self-management form and any other monitoring records for completeness and ask the patient which self-care area he/she would most like to focus on during this visit (circling the area for the physician and reinforcing the

1. Which of the following has your health care team (doctor, nurse, dietician, or diabetes educator) advised you to do? Please check all that apply:
   __a. Follow a low-fat eating plan.
   __b. Reduce the number of calories you eat.
   __c. Eat 5 or more servings per day of fruits and vegetables.
   __d. Eat very few sweets.
   __e. Other (specify): ______________________________
   __f. I have not been given any advice about my diet.

2. How often did you follow your recommended eating plan since your last visit?
   ___ Always ___Usually ___Sometimes___Rarely ___Never

3. Which of the following has your health care team (doctor, nurse, dietician, or diabetes educator) advised you to do? Please check all that apply:
   __a. Do low to moderate level activity (such as walking) on a daily basis.
   __b. Exercise continuously for at least 20 minutes at least 3 times a week.
   __c. Fit physical activity into your daily routine (take stairs instead of elevators, park a block away and walk, etc.).
   __d. Other (specify): ______________________________
   __e. I have not been given advice about physical activity.

4. How often did you follow your exercise plan recommendations since your last visit?
   ___ Always ___Usually ___Sometimes___Rarely ___Never

5. Which of the following has your health care team (doctor, nurse, dietician, or diabetes educator) advised you to do? Please check all that apply:
   __a. Test your blood glucose (sugar) using a drop of blood from your finger.
   __b. Test your blood glucose using a machine to read the results.
   __c. Test your urine for sugar.
   __d. Other (specify): ______________________________
   __e. I have not been given advice about testing my blood glucose.

6. How often are you supposed to test your blood glucose level?
   __ times per day or __ times per week

7. How often did you follow your blood glucose testing recommendations since your last visit?
   ___ Always ___Usually ___Sometimes___Rarely ___Never

Figure 6.6. Diabetes self-management and patient involvement assessment form. © 1995, Oregon Research Institute and Group Health Cooperative.

8. Which of the following medications for your diabetes has your doctor prescribed? Please check all that apply:
   __a. An insulin shot 1 or 2 times a day.
   __b. An insulin shot 3 or more times a day.
   __c. Diabetes pills (sulfa drugs) to control your blood glucose level.
   __d. Glucophage (Metformin tablets)
   __e. Other (specify): ____________________
   __f. I have not been prescribed medication for my diabetes.

9. How often did you take your diabetes medication as prescribed since your last visit?
   ___ Always ___Usually ___Sometimes ___Rarely ___Never

10. Which of the following has your health care team (doctor, nurse, dietician, or diabetes educator) advised you to do? Please check all that apply:
   __a. Check your feet daily for sores, cuts, calluses, infection, etc.
   __b. Check inside your shoes daily for loose objects or rough edges.
   __c. Not to go barefoot either inside or outdoors.
   __d. Wash your feet daily, remembering to dry between your toes.
   __e. Other (specify): ____________________
   __f. I have not been given advice about foot care.

11. How often did you follow your foot care recommendations since your last visit?
   ___ Always ___Usually ___Sometimes ___Rarely ___Never

12. Have you smoked, even a puff, during the past 7 days?
   ___Yes ___No (skip to Question #15)

13. Has anyone from your health care team advised you to stop smoking?
   ___Yes ___No

14. Are you seriously considering stopping smoking in the near future?
   ___Yes ___No

15. Has your health care team instructed you what to do if your blood glucose is too low or too high?
   ___Yes ___No

16. How confident are you that you know what to do if your blood glucose is too low?
   Not confident Confident
   1 2 3 4 5 6 7

17. How confident are you that you know what to do if your blood glucose is too high?
   Not confident Confident
   1 2 3 4 5 6 7

(NOTE: We recommend assessment of barriers to achieving goals in the area(s) in which patients are having difficulty)

Figure 6.6. *(continued)*

patient for willingness to work on diabetes self-care, or educating the patient about the importance of self-care if he/she is not initially interested). This is also an excellent opportunity to flag often neglected issues, such as depression, stress, smoking or foot care, for both patients and physicians.

PHYSICIAN EXAMINATION

The physician should begin by asking the patient what he/she would most like to discuss at that visit[14,30]. The two most important messages from the physician have to do with the seriousness of diabetes and the importance of patient behaviour in managing the disease. Following-up on the self-management form, the physician should address the area of greatest concern to the patient. This is an opportunity to both reinforce the patient's intention to make behaviour changes and educate the patient on the importance of diabetes self-care (e.g. 'Mrs. Gonzales, I'm glad to see that you'd like to focus on your diet. Following a low saturated fat diet will help you to manage your diabetes better and will also reduce your risk of heart disease'). The physician can then let the patient know that the nurse, nutritionist or diabetes educator will meet with him/her briefly after the examination to help them develop a specific plan for addressing changes in the self-care area.

NURSE OR DIABETES EDUCATOR FOLLOW-UP

Following the examination, the nurse, nutritionist, or diabetes educator meets briefly with the patient to review and clarify specific goals for behaviour change and develop problem-solving strategies. It is critical—and often inadequately implemented—to consider the patient's perspective and readiness to change during this process. Anderson and colleagues have written extensively on patient empowerment and patient-centred approaches to enhancing diabetes self-management[14,32]. Patients will be unlikely to make behaviour changes if: (a) they are not motivated to do so; (b) they do not understand the importance of the recommended behaviour in managing their diabetes; or (c) they do not have the necessary skills to carry out the behaviour. Optimally, the goal(s) should be generated by the patient and then worked into a specific behavioural plan in collaboration with the nurse or educator. Using principles of behaviour change, this means that the goal(s) should be specific, manageable and measurable, that the patient should understand the importance of the behaviour in managing diabetes, and that he/she should be educated in the skills necessary to perform the behaviour[74–79].

Once a plan for a specific behaviour change is agreed upon, the next step is to ask the patient to identify the things that are most likely to interfere with following the plan. Help the patient to come up with at least two practical solutions to these barriers. One of the most common barriers to self-care, even for the most motivated patients, is returning to a home, work, and neighbourhood environment that does not support the self-management goal (there are brief questionnaires that can be used to structure this discussion)[80,81]. A number of studies have evaluated patients' 'barriers' to self-management[80,82]. Rather than labelling the patient as 'non-compliant', an attempt should be made to understand the factors that interfere with the identified goal. Commonly reported barriers include lack of family support, stress, being busy, being away from home, lack of insurance reimbursement (e.g. for glucose testing strips), and lack of convenient, safe, low-cost places to exercise. Glasgow *et al.*[82] and Glasgow[81] have reported that most patients experience the highest frequency of barriers to dietary and exercise adherence and the fewest to medication taking, and that patients' self-reported barriers to adherence are prospectively predictive of their level of diabetes self-care. These findings suggest that helping patients to identify barriers to self-management and develop strategies to overcome these barriers should increase the success of their diabetes self-management activities.

Finally, it is also important to assist the patient in accessing support for his/her new behaviour. This might entail referral to diabetes education classes or a support group, related reading materials, and often a follow-up telephone call to check on progress between visits. Finally, the self-management goal and plan for achieving it should be recorded (Figure 6.4), with a copy given to the patient and another placed in the chart so that it can be followed-up during the next visit.

LINKS TO MEDICAL MANAGEMENT

One of the key advantages to office-based psychosocial interventions is that the potential exists for coordination with, and integration into, regular clinical practice. Behavioural and psychological issues can be treated by health care staff and seen by patients as a regular part of patient care. This is in contrast to the situation that currently exists in most settings, in which a 'psychological or diabetes education/self-management' referral is seen as stigmatizing, separate from usual patient care, and something that is often poorly connected with the medical management of diabetes.

Still, just because an intervention is conducted in the office setting is no guarantee that it will be integrated with, or consistent with, other aspects of a patient's care. It is essential that all health care team members be aware of what other team members are working on with a patient, that they reinforce each other's efforts, and that they do not overwhelm the patient with too many goals and priorities at once. Such coordination and mutual support is much more likely to happen if it is programmed into the office practice and prompted by the use of patient goal setting and strategy forms (see Figure 6.4) rather than left to chance.

As reviewed above, there are different models for determining which staff member implements the behavioural strategies, and advantages and limitations to each. In terms of consistent and quality implementation, it makes most sense to have behavioural interventions delivered either by behavioural specialists experienced in diabetes and working in health care settings, by diabetes educators trained in behavioural intervention, or by user-friendly, highly interactive multi-media computer-based applications. The present-day reality, however, is that few offices, and especially few primary care settings responsible for treating the patients most in need, will have the resources to adopt such strategies.

It is also clear that one does not need to be a highly trained psychologist to deliver most of the behavioural intervention strategies that have been reviewed above. The few studies that have evaluated counsellor characteristics have not found one type of health professional to be more effective than others at producing behaviour change. This of course assumes that staff members are well trained and receive adequate supervision and feedback. From a social influence perspective, it makes most sense to have a physician deliver the intervention. In practice, this is seldom possible due to the extreme time limitations and lack of training of physicians in behavioural intervention[83]. The doctor is probably best utilized as a motivator, who can briefly emphasize the importance of behavioural goals and of working with the interventionist. The most generalizable model, especially in managed care settings, is probably to have some form of automated assessment, followed by a motivational message from the physician, and then intervention and follow-up conducted by a nurse or case manager.

The greatest opportunity for linking to medical management and improving overall quality of diabetes care lies in the area of tracking guidelines for preventive care, such as those developed by the American Diabetes Association and various other organizations, for all patients in an office practice. This assumes an accurate diabetes registry and a list of guidelines or best practices that includes behavioural, psychosocial and patient-focused issues[6] in addition to medical and laboratory screening activities. The second most important issue, and one that has impressive empirical support, is to conduct brief follow-up contacts with patients, as discussed above.

UNANSWERED QUESTIONS, NEW DIRECTIONS

Good progress has been made in medical office-based psychosocial interventions during the few years that this has been an area of investigation, but much more remains to be done. As summarized in Table 6.1, studies are particularly needed of the extent and characteristics of practices that adopt, implement and maintain such interventions. This conclusion is not unique to medical office-based interventions, but also applies to much of health psychology[25]. As research shifts to a broader focus that includes not only individual and intrapersonal determinants of health and behaviour, but also broader social-environmental determinants, setting and organization factors become an important area of investigation.

As this field of inquiry advances, the issues studied will shift from basic questions, such as 'Does this type of intervention work?', to more sophisticated questions, such as 'which types of intervention are most effective, for what purpose (e.g. increasing participation; producing immediate behaviour change; enhancing maintenance), with which type of patient, in which type of setting and when implemented by which type of interventionist?' Given the inherent advantages of consistent delivery, freeing staff time for other duties, automated and immediate scoring and feedback, and the high degree of individualization possible, we are likely to see much more application of interactive computer-based applications in medical settings. It is hoped that these applications will be evidence-based, and that they will be developed with a focus on the RE-AIM dimensions discussed above.

The final and most important challenge for the future remains optimal ways in which to integrate psychosocial assessments and interventions into regular medical office-based diabetes care, and to do so in a way that enhances quality of care and patient-centred outcomes.

REFERENCES

1. Glasgow RE, Fisher E, Anderson BJ *et al.* Behavioral science in diabetes: contributions and opportunities. *Diabet Care* 1999; **22**: 832–43
2. Glasgow RE, McKay HG, Boles SM *et al.* Interactive technology, behavioral science, and health care: progress, pitfalls, and promise. *J Fam Pract* 1999; **48**(6): 464–70
3. Street RL Jr, Gold WR, Mannning TE. *Health Promotion and Interactive Technology: Theoretical Applications and Future Directions*. London: Erlbaum, 1997
4. Harris MI. Medical care for patients with diabetes: epidemiologic aspects. *Ann Intern Med* 1996; **124**: 117–22
5. Marrero DG. Current effectiveness of diabetes health care in the U.S. *Diabet Rev* 1994; **2**: 292–309
6. Glasgow RE, Boles SM, Calder D *et al.* Diabetes care practices in primary care: results from two samples and three performance measure sets. *Diabet Educ* 1999; **25**
7. Glasgow RE. A practical model of diabetes management and education. *Diabet Care* 1995; **18**: 117–26
8. Winett RA, King AC, Altman DG. *Health Psychology and Public Health: an Integrative Approach*. New York: Pergamon, 1989
9. Glasgow RE, Wagner E, Kaplan RM *et al.* If diabetes is a public health problem, why not treat it as one? A population-based approach to chronic illness. *Ann Behav Med* 1999; **21**(2): 159–70

10. Funnell MM, Anderson RM. Patient education in the physician's office. *Pract Diabetol* 1993; 22–25
11. Wagner EH. Population-based management of diabetes care. *Patient Educ Counsel* 1995; **26**: 225–30
12. Glasgow RE, Eakin EG, Toobert DJ. How generalizable are the results of diabetes self-management research? The impact of participation and attrition. *Diabet Educ* 1996; **22**: 573–85
13. Johnson SB. Regimen adherence: roles and responsibilities of health care providers. *Diabet Spectrum* 1993; **6**: 204–5
14. Anderson RM, Funnell MM. The role of the physician in patient education. *Pract Diabetol* 1990; 10–12
15. Raymond M. *The Human Side of Diabetes: Beyond Doctors, Diets and Drugs.* Chicago: Noble, 1992
16. Orlandi MA. Promoting health and preventing disease in health care settings: an analysis of barriers. *Prevent Med* 1987; **16**: 119–30
17. Oregon Diabetes Project. *Measuring Quality of Care in Health Systems: Population-based Guidelines for Diabetes Mellitus.* Portland, OR: State of Oregon, 1997; 1–45
18. American Diabetes Association Task Force to Revise the National Standards. - National standards for diabetes self-management education programs. *Diabet Care* 1995; **18**: 141–43
19. American Diabetes Association. Standards of medical care for patients with diabetes mellitus. *Diabet Care* 1995; **18**: 8–15
20. American Diabetes Association. *Mission Statement*, Alexandria, VA: American Diabetes Association, 1995
21. Harris MI, Eastman RC, Siebert C. The DCCT and medical care for diabetes in the U.S. *Diabet Care* 1994; **17**: 761–64
22. Anderson BJ, Rubin RRE. *Practical Psychology for Diabetes Clinicians: How to Deal with the Key Behavioral Issues Faced by Patients and Health Care Teams.* Alexandria, VA: American Diabetes Association, 1996
23. McCulloch DK, Glasgow RE, Hampson SE *et al.* A systematic approach to diabetes management in the post-DCCT era. *Diabet Care* 1994; **17**: 765–69
24. Flay BR. Efficacy and effectiveness trials (and other phases of research) in the development of health promotion programs. *Prevent Med* 1986; **15**: 451–74
25. Glasgow RE, Vogt TM, Boles SM. Evaluating the public health impact of health promotion interventions: the RE-AIM framework. *Am J Public Health* 1999; **89**: 1322–7
26. Anderson BJ, Wolf FM, Burkhart MT *et al.* Effects of peer-group intervention on metabolic control of adolescents with IDDM: randomized outpatient study. *Diabet Care* 1989; **12**: 179–83
27. Wagner EH. Care of older people with chronic illness. In Calkins E, Boult C, Wanger EH, Pacala J (eds) *New Ways to Care for Older People.* New York: Springer, 1998
28. Beck A, Scott J, Williams P *et al.* A randomized trial of group outpatient visits for chonically ill older HMO members: the cooperative health care clinic. *J Am Gerontol Soc* 1997; **45**: 543–49
29. Greenfield S, Kaplan SH, Ware JE *et al.* Patients' participation in medical care: effects on blood sugar control and quality of life in diabetes. *J Gen Intern Med* 1988; **3**: 448–57
30. Glasgow RE, Toobert DJ, Hampson SE. Effects of a brief office-based intervention to facilitate diabetes dietary self-management. *Diabet Care* 1996; **19**: 835–42

31. Glasgow RE, La Chance P, Toobert DJ *et al.* Long-term effects and costs of brief behavioral dietary intervention for patients with diabetes delivered from the medical office. *Patient Educ Counsel* 1997; **32**: 175–84
32. Anderson RM, Funnell MM, Barr PA *et al.* Learning to empower patients: results of professional education program for diabetes educators. *Diabet Care* 1991; **14**: 584–90
33. Anderson RM, Funnell MM, Butler PM *et al.* Patient empowerment. Results of a randomized controlled trial. *Diabet Care* 1995; **18**: 943–49
34. Miller WR, Rollnick S. *Motivational Interviewing: Preparing People to Change Addictive Behavior.* New York: Guilford, 1991
35. Litzelman DK, Slemenda CW, Langefeld CD *et al.* Reduction of lower extremity clinical abnormalities in patients with non-insulin-dependent diabetes mellitus: a randomized, controlled trial. *Ann Intern Med* 1993; **119**: 36–41
36. Weinberger M, Kirkman MS, Samsa GP *et al.* A nurse-coordinated intervention for primary care patients with non-insulin-dependent mellitus: impact on glycemic control and health-related quality of life. *J Gen Intern Med* 1995; **10**: 59–66
37. Lichtenstein E, Glasgow RE, Lando HA *et al.* Telephone counseling for smoking cessation: rationales and review of evidence. *Health Educ Res* 1996; **11**: 243–57
38. Wasson J, Gaudette C, Whaley F *et al.* Telephone care as a substitute for routine clinic follow-up. *J Am Med Assoc* 1992; **267**: 1788–93
39. DCCT Research Group. The effect of intensive treatment of diabetes on the development and progression of long-term complications in insulin-dependent diabetes mellitus. *N Engl J Med* 1993; **329**: 977–86
40. Fisher EB Jr, Arfken CL, Heins JM *et al.* Acceptance of diabetes in adults. In Gochman DS (ed) *Handbook of Health Behavior Research, II: Provider Determinants.* New York: Plenum, 1997; 189–212
41. Eastman RC, Siebert CW, Harris M *et al.* Clinical review: implications of the diabetes control and complications trial. *J Clin Endocrinol Metab* 1993; **77**: 1105–7
42. Fisher EB Jr, Heins JM, Hiss RG *et al.* *Metabolic Control Matters: Nationwide Translation of the Diabetes Control and Complications Trial: Analysis and Recommendations*. National Institute of Diabetes, Digestive and Kidney Diseases (NIH Publication No. 94-3773). Bethesda, MD: National Institute of Diabetes and Digestive and Kidney Diseases, 1994
43. DeBusk RF, Miller NH, Superko HR. A case-management system for coronary risk factor modification after acute myocardial infarction. *Ann Intern Med* 1994; **120**: 721–9
44. Bandura A. *Self-efficacy: The Exercise of Control*. New York: W.H. Freeman, 1997
45. Glasgow RE, Toobert DJ, Hampson SE *et al.* A brief office-based intervention to facilitate diabetes self-management. *Health Educ Res Theory Pract* 1995; **10**: 467–78
46. Lorig KR, Mazonson PD, Holman HR. Evidence suggesting that health education for self-management in patients with chronic arthritis has sustained health benefits while reducing health care costs. *Arthritis Rheum* 1993; **36**: 439–46
47. Leveille SG, Wagner EH, Davis C *et al.* Preventing disability and managing chronic illness in frail older adults: a randomized trial of a community-based partnership with primary care. *J Am Gerontol Soc* 1998; **46**: 1–9
48. Lorig KR, Sobel DS, Stewart AL *et al.* Evidence suggesting that a chronic disease self-management program can improve health status while reducing hospitalization. *Med Care* 1999; **37**: 5–14
49. Skinner CS, Strecher VJ, Hospers H. Physicians' recommendations for mammography: do tailored messages make a difference? *Am J Publ Health* 1994; **84**: 43–9

50. Gustafson DF, Hawkins R, Boberg E *et al.* Impact of a patient-centered, computer-based health information/support system. *Am J Prev Med* 1999; **16**: 1–8
51. Sallis JF, Owen N. Ecological models. In Glanz K, Lewis FM, Rimer BK (eds) *Health Behavior and Health Education: Theory, Research and Practice*. San Francisco, CA: Jossey-Bass, 1996; 403–24
52. Stokols D. Establishing and maintaining healthy environments: toward a social ecology of health promotion. *Am Psychol* 1992; **47**: 6–22
53. Abrams DB, Orleans CT, Niaura RS *et al.* Integrating individual and public health perspectives for treatment of tobacco dependence under managed health care: a combined stepped care and matching model. *Ann Intern Med* 1996; **18**: 290–304
54. Johnson SB. Compliance and control in insulin-dependent diabetes: does behavior really make a difference? In Krasnegor NA, Epstein L, Johnson SB, Yaffe SJ (eds) *Developmental Aspects of Health Compliance Behavior*. Hillsdale, NJ: Erlbaum, 1993; 275–97
55. Glasgow RE, McCaul KD, Schafer LC. Self-care behaviors and glycemic control in type I diabetes. *J Chron Dis* 1987; **40**: 399–412
56. Rost KM, Flavin KS, Schmidt LE *et al.* Self-care predictors of metabolic control in NIDDM patients. *Diabet Care* 1990; **13**: 1111–13
57. Jenkins CD. An integrated behavioral medicine approach to improving care of patients with diabetes mellitus. *Behav Med* 1995; **21**: 53–65
58. Kaplan RM. Behavior as the central outcome in health care. *Am Psychol* 1990; **45**: 1211–20
59. Glasgow RE, Osteen VL. Evaluating diabetes education: are we measuring the most important outcomes? *Diabet Care* 1992; **15**: 1423–32
60. Glasgow RE. Behavioral and psychosocial measures for diabetes care: what is important to assess? *Diabet Spectrum* 1997; **10**: 12–17
61. UK Prospective Diabetes Study Group. Intensive blood-glucose control with suphonylureas or insulin compared with conventional treatment and risk of complications in patients with type 2 diabetes (UKPDS 33). *Lancet* 1998; **352**: 837–53
62. Hampson SE, Glasgow R, Toobert DJ. Personal models of diabetes and their relations to self-care activities. *Health Psychol* 1990; **9**: 632–46
63. Hampson SE, Glasgow RE, Foster L. Personal models of diabetes among older adults: relation to self-management and other variables. *Diabetes Educ* 1995; **21**: 300–307
64. Glasgow RE, Ruggiero L, Eakin EG *et al.* Quality of life and associated characteristics in a large diverse sample of adults with diabetes. *Diabetes Care* 1997; **20**: 562–7
65. Rubin RR, Biermann J, Toohey B. *Psyching Out Diabetes: A Positive Approach to Your Negative Emotions*. Los Angeles: RGA, 1992
66. Ruggiero L, Glasgow RE, Dryfoos JM *et al.* Diabetes self-management: self-reported recommendations and patterns in a large population. *Diabet Care* 1997; **20**: 568–76
67. Anderson LA, Jenkins CM. Educational innovations in diabetes: where are we now? *Diabet Spectrum* 1994; **7**: 89–124
68. Mazze RS, Etzwiler DD, Strock E *et al.* Staged diabetes management. *Diabet Care* 1994; **17**: 56–66
69. Glasgow RE, Eakin EG. Issues in diabetes self-management. In Shumaker SA, Schron EB, Ockene JK, McBee WL (eds) *The Handbook of Health Behavior Change*. New York: Springer, 1998; 435–61

70. Anderson RM, Fitzgerald JT, Funnell MM *et al.* Evaluation of an activated patient diabetes education newsletter. *Diabet Educ* 1994; **20**: 29–34
71. Joyner L, McNeeley S, Kahn R. ADA's provider recognition program. *HMO Practice* 1997; **11**: 168–70
72. Fiore MC. The new vital sign. Assessing and documenting smoking status [commentary]. *J Am Med Assoc* 1991; **266**: 3183–4
73. Haire-Joshu D, Glasgow R, Tibbs TL. American Diabetes Association technical review on smoking and diabetes. *Diabet Care* 1998
74. Orleans CT, Glynn TJ, Manley MW *et al.* Minimal-contact quit smoking strategies for medical settings. In Orleans CT, Slade J (eds) *Nicotine Addiction: Principles and Management*. New York: Oxford University Press, 1993; 181–220
75. Karoly P. Self-management in health-care and illness prevention. In Snyder CR, Forsyth DR (eds) *Handbook of Social and Clinical Psychology*. New York: Pergamon, 1991
76. Karoly P. Goal systems: an organizing framework for clinical assessment and treatment planning. *Psychol Assessment* 1993; **5**: 273–90
77. Hampson SE, Glasgow RE, Zeiss AM. Coping with osteoarthritis by older adults. *Arthritis Care Res* 1996; **9**: 133–41
78. Bandura A. *Social Foundations of Thought and Action: A Social Cognitive Theory*. Englewood Cliffs, NJ: Prentice Hall, 1986
79. Nouwen A, Gingras J, Talbot F *et al.* The development of an empirical psychosocial taxonomy for patients with diabetes. *Health Psychol* 1997; **16**: 263–71
80. Irvine AA, Saunders JT, Blank MB *et al.* Validation of scale measuring environmental barriers to diabetes—regimen adherence. *Diabet Care* 1990; **13**: 705–11
81. Glasgow RE. Social-environmental factors in diabetes: Barriers to diabetes self-care. In Bradley C (ed) *Handbook of Psychology and Diabetes Research and Practice*. Chur, Switzerland: Harwood Academic, 1994; 335–49
82. Glasgow RE, McCaul KD, Schafer LC. Barriers to regimen adherence among persons with insulin-dependent diabetes. *J Behav Med* 1986; **9**: 65–77
83. Beaven DW, Scott RS. The organisation of diabetes care. In Alberti KGMM, Krall LP (eds) *The Diabetes Annual*, vol 2. New York: Elsevier, 1986; 39–48
84. Eakin EG, Gasgow RE, Whitlock EP, Smith P. Reaching those most in need: participation in a planned parenthood smoking cessation program. *Ann Behav Med* 1998; **20**(3): 216–20
85. Green LW, Richard L, Potvin L. Ecological foundations of health promotion. *Am J Health Promotion* 1996; **10**: 270–81
86. McNabb WL. Adherence in diabetes: can we define it and can we measure it? [commentary]. *Diabet Care*, 1997; **20**(2): 215–18
87. Strecher VJ, Kreuter M, Den Boer DJ, Kobrin S, Hospers HJ, Skinner CS. The effects of computer-tailored smoking cessation messages in family practice settings. *J Fam Pract* 1994; **39**: 262–8
88. Brug J, Glanz K, van Assema P, Kok G, van Breukelen GJ. The impact of computer-tailored feedback and iterative feedback on fat, fruit, and vegetable intake. *Health Educ Behav* 1998; **25**: 517–31
89. Goodman RM, Steckler A. A model for the institutionalization of health promotion programs. *Fam Commun Health* 1987; **11**: 63–78

7

Blood Glucose Awareness Training

LINDA GONDER-FREDERICK, DANIEL COX, WILLIAM CLARKE and DIANA JULIAN
University of Virginia Health Sciences Center, Charlottesville, VA, USA

INTRODUCTION AND THEORETICAL BACKGROUND

This chapter provides an overview of the conceptual development, empirical investigation, content and clinical application of Blood Glucose Awareness Training (BGAT), a psycho-educational intervention designed for patients with type 1 diabetes. The purpose of BGAT is to improve patients' ability to recognize, predict, avoid and respond to extreme fluctuations in blood glucose (BG) levels. Training focuses on learning how to use both internal 'cues' to BG (physical symptoms, mood changes, deterioration in mental function) and external cues (insulin action, food intake, physical activity) to improve glucose awareness. In its current form (BGAT-III), BGAT is an 8-week intervention which can be conducted on an individual basis or in group format with weekly sessions lasting from 1–2 hours. An eight-chapter manual serves as a guide for active self-learning and homework exercises. BGAT is both an empirically and theoretically-derived intervention. The current version is the product of over 18 years of research into the symptomatology, recognition, impact and treatment of hypo- and hyperglycaemia in type 1 diabetes. Each version of BGAT has been evaluated empirically and its efficacy has been demonstrated repeatedly by research conducted at divergent geographical locations with divergent patient populations. At present, BGAT is being used across the world and its manual has been translated into Japanese, German and Dutch. Because of the need to

Psychology in Diabetes Care. Edited by Frank J. Snoek and T. Chas Skinner.

incorporate new research findings relevant to our training goals, we do not view BGAT as a 'finished' product but rather as a constantly evolving intervention.

Theoretically, BGATs conception and development arose within the framework of psychological models of health-related behaviours, most importantly theories of self-regulation. Self-treatment of diabetes has been described as a process of behavioural self-regulation by several authors[1–4]. In this self-regulatory process, feedback about extreme BG fluctuations leads to behavioural attempts to normalize glycaemic status. In the absence of diabetes, a negative feedback control system maintains euglycaemia automatically by monitoring current circulating glucose levels and responding hormonally to normalize BG when it deviates from a normal range. Thus, when BG levels rise dramatically after the intake of a large meal, pancreatic insulin production and secretion also increase to promote glucose transport and metabolism. When BG levels are low due to lack of food intake or high utilization of metabolic fuel, glucagon secretion increases to stimulate glycogenolysis and gluconeogenesis. Since these endogenous hormonal reactions are inadequate or absent in type 1 diabetes, this normally automatic physiological regulatory system cannot regulate glycaemic status. Instead, patients with type 1 diabetes must behaviourally regulate glucose metabolism. This requires the patient to monitor BG levels, inject insulin into the body and adjust the timing and amount of food intake and physical activity to match BG and insulin levels. Because it is quite difficult to duplicate normal glucose metabolism with this behavioural regimen, patients with type 1 diabetes frequently experience hypo- and hyperglycaemia which, when detected, require additional behavioural adjustments to re-regulate BG.

In the self-regulatory model of diabetes management, appropriate behavioural responses to regulate BG levels depend on feedback concerning current BG levels. There are three primary types of feedback for the patient with type 1 diabetes: self-measurement of BG (SMBG), perception of physical symptoms indicating hypo- or hyperglycaemia, and feedback from others regarding symptoms they notice. In addition, patients obtain feedback by estimating the impact of their previous insulin, food and physical activity on current BG. The fundamental goal of BGAT is to improve patients' ability to utilize the information available to them as feedback about their BG levels which will, in turn, improve their ability to detect and predict extreme fluctuations in BG accurately. However, BGAT does not minimize the critical role of feedback from SMBG in diabetes management, but rather encourages frequent self-testing, not only at routine times to monitor fasting, preprandial, postprandial, or bedtime BG, but also as a tool to *verify* objectively patients' subjective impressions that BG is too low or high. But since patients can only use SMBG a limited number of times each day (8–10 times/day for the most motivated patients), they must rely on other types of feedback much of the time, primarily physical symptoms that signal hypo- or hyperglycaemia.

Psychological theories of health care and illness behaviour have long emphasized the critical role of symptom feedback in processes of physiological self-regulation and disease management[5–7]. At the most basic level, this process includes eating when the sensations of hunger occur, sleeping to alleviate exhaustion, and seeking medical help for illness or injury. However, even these basic self-regulatory behaviours are not always simple, as evidenced by the high rate of eating and sleep disorders. Self-regulation via perceived symptoms can become quite complex because there is not a one-to-one correspondence between physiological change and symptom perception. Symptom perception also requires the *interpretation* of physiological feedback which, in turn, involves a myriad of complex psychological phenomena, including attention mechanisms, information processing, affective responses and contingency factors. For this reason, symptom perception and interpretation does not always accurately parallel physiological reality. Whether accurate or not, people tend to trust their perceptions of physical symptoms. In their studies of hypertensive patients, Howard Leventhal and his colleagues elegantly demonstrated the primary role of symptoms in the 'commonsense models of illness' that guide health care beliefs and behaviours[8,9]. In these studies, even when told that changes in blood pressure were asymptomatic, patients continued to monitor and rely on symptoms for information about their hypertension. Patients with type 1 diabetes report that, when they 'feel' hypoglycaemic, their first response is to treat themselves before using SMBG to verify the low BG.[10] Symptoms have several attributes that make them compelling and convincing. The are readily available, immediate and experiential, and past experience has taught most people that symptoms can provide valuable and accurate information about physical status. The problems arise when symptoms are not easily recognized or are interpreted inaccurately.

From a clinical perspective, then, two critical questions determine the usefulness of physical symptoms as accurate feedback and guides to self-regulatory behaviour. First, does the physiological parameter being regulated produce detectible symptoms that reliably co-vary with deviations from normal function? And if so, are patients able to perceive and accurately recognize these symptoms as cues that they need to regulate their health status behaviourally? The fact that BG fluctuations in type 1 diabetes can be quite symptomatic is well-documented, and patients are taught to monitor themselves for certain symptoms as signs of hypo- or hyperglycaemia. This education is based, of course, on the assumption that patients detect and recognize these symptoms accurately, an assumption long-held by most diabetes researchers and practitioners. However, prior to 1980, there was virtually no systematic research into the nature of glycaemic symptomatology and the ability of type 1 patients to discriminate BG levels accurately. Since then, a plethora of studies have been conducted, demonstrating that BG symptomatology and detection are far more complex than originally believed.

BG SYMPTOMATOLOGY—EMPIRICAL FINDINGS

Several characteristics of BG symptoms contribute to their complexity. One of these is the lack of specificity of many of the symptoms caused by glycaemic changes[7]. In other words, while both hypo- and hyperglycaemia can cause numerous physical symptoms, many of these are not exclusively related to glycaemic changes and, in fact, co-occur with a number of other physiological states (e.g. hunger, fatigue, weakness, trembling, dry mouth). The list of potential symptoms that can be caused by hypo- and hyperglycaemia is quite long, because extremes in BG levels can have an impact on nearly every organ system, including a dramatic impact on the central nervous system. Table 7.1 lists the symptoms most commonly associated with hypo- and hyperglycaemia.* It is important to emphasize, however, that a given individual patient will not experience all of these symptoms. This is because BG symptomatology is highly *idiosyncratic*. Early studies found that no one symptom was associated with hypo- and hyperglycaemia for all patients[11]. Instead, the symptoms that most reliably co-vary with BG can differ greatly from patient to patient. This symptom idiosyncracy has been repeatedly demonstrated across all age groups—in children and adolescents, as well as adults with type 1 diabetes[12–17]. As Table 7.1 indicates, some symptoms can also occur with both hypo- and hyperglycaemia which means that, for one patient, a symptom such as fatigue may signal low BG while, for another patient, fatigue is a sign that glucose levels are high. Several factors appear to contribute to the idiosyncracy of BG symptomatology, including individual differences in physiological responses to glucose changes (e.g. hormonal reactions), as well as psychological differences in symptom perception (e.g. attentional biases).

In addition to those sensations typically viewed as physical symptoms (e.g. pounding heart, dry mouth), Table 7.1 shows that both hypo- and hyperglycaemia can cause changes in mood, mental/motor function, and behaviour. These sequelae are also idiosyncratic in nature. For example,

*The symptoms listed in Table 7.1 represent those which have been demonstrated empirically to relate to BG levels. Empirically-related symptoms are identified using a repeated-measures procedure in which patients rate the extent to which they are experiencing symptoms on a checklist, then measure their BG and record this value. Symptom ratings and BG values can be recorded on paper checklists or entered into handheld computers. This procedure is repeated several times each day over a several-week period.

Table 7.1. Blood glucose symptoms in type 1 diabetes

Hypoglycaemia	Hyperglycaemia
Trembling	Dry mouth, throat
Sweating	Thirst
Pounding heart	Need to urinate
Fast pulse	Stomach pain
Changes in body temperature	Nausea
Heavy breathing	Vomiting
Slowed thinking	Weakness
Difficulty concentrating	Blurred vision
Mental confusion	Headache
Slurred speech	Tingling/pain in extremities
Blurred vision	Fatigue
Incoordination	Lethargy
Fatigue/sleepiness	Mental confusion
Dizziness	Alertness
Weakness	Energetic
Hunger	Sadness
Headache	
Nausea	
Anxious	
Irritability	
Sadness	
Crying	
Pessimistic thinking	
Arguing	
Euphoria	
Giddiness	

hypoglycaemia is associated with negative changes in mood (e.g. anxiety, irritability), thinking (e.g. pessimistically orientated), and behaviour (e.g. arguing) in the majority of patients[18,19]. However, some patients experience positive changes (e.g. giddiness, euphoria, friendly behaviour). Patients also vary greatly in the degree to which they become symptomatic in response to glycaemic extremes. Individual differences have been found in the number of different symptoms experienced, the intensity of symptoms, and the glycaemic threshold at which physiological responses and subsequent symptoms occur. Thus, some patients become quite symptomatic with relatively mild hypoglycaemia or hyperglycaemia, while others notice nothing until their BG is extremely low or high. Idiosyncratic symptom clusters are stable over relatively short periods of time, such as 3–6 months[12], but may also change dramatically over time. In fact, symptoms may vary across different episodes of hypo- and hyperglycaemia for an individual patient.

In general, hypoglycaemia is more symptomatic than hyperglycaemia, which tends to be associated with symptoms which are less intense perceptually and slower in onset. The aetiology for many hyperglycaemic symptoms is unclear. Some are caused by osmotic diuresis as the kidneys attempt to excrete excess glucose and ketones, including thirst, dry mouth and frequent urination. Gastro-intestinal symptoms, such as nausea and abdominal pain, are probably caused by ketosis and/or acidosis. The effects of hyperglycaemia on cognitive and motor functioning has not been studied extensively, and research has yielded conflicting results, with some finding deterioration in performance and others showing no effect on the CNS with moderately high BG[20,21]. However, severe and prolonged hyperglycaemia certainly causes changes in mentation, including disorientation and eventual coma. Mood changes occur with moderate hyperglycaemia, but these appear to be more subtle than those associated with hypoglycaemia and tend to be positively valenced, such as feeling alert, energetic or cheerful[19].

In contrast, hypoglycaemic symptoms often onset suddenly and can be quite aversive. Hypoglycaemia causes two major physiological reactions that underlie most symptoms—*hormonal counter-regulation* and *neuroglycopenia*. In both non-diabetic and diabetic glucose regulation, abnormally low BG levels trigger the release of hormones, including glucagon and epinephrine, which increase glycogenolysis and inhibit insulin action, causing BG to stop falling and begin to rise. In type 1 diabetes, glucagon secretion and action grows progressively less effective, so epinephrine becomes the primary mechanism of hormonal counter-regulation. Counter-regulatory symptoms (also referred to as autonomic, adrenergic and neurogenic symptoms) include trembling, pounding heart, sweating and feeling 'jittery' or tense. Neuroglycopenic symptoms are caused by insufficient glucose available for brain metabolism and function. Early signs include difficulty concentrating, thinking clearly and performing fine motor tasks, as well as a general slowing of problem solving and reaction time. If BG continues to fall to moderate or severe hypoglycaemia, symptoms can progress to disorientation, mental stupor, unconsciousness, seizure and, in extreme cases, even death. One recent study found that 10% of deaths in patients with type 1 diabetes under the age of 40 appeared to be caused by nocturnal hypoglycaemia[22].

There is some controversy concerning the glycaemic threshold for counter-regulatory vs. neuroglycopenic symptoms. Traditionally, counter-regulatory symptoms were believed to occur first, providing the best early warning signs of mild hypoglycaemia. Neuroglycopenic symptoms, in contrast, were believed to onset only after BG fell quite low and to be of little use as early warning cues. However, several studies[16,23–25] have shown that counter-regulatory and neuroglycopenic symptoms occur at similar thresholds, and that neuroglycopenic symptoms occur as frequently with hypoglycaemia as hormonal symptoms. In addition, significant deterioration in task performance, including driving, can occur at relatively mild (3.0–3.9 mM) hypoglycaemic levels[26–28]. The degree of impairment associated with hypoglycaemia varies across patients but appears to be somewhat reliable across time[28,29].

While some patients become obviously impaired with relatively moderate drops in BG, others show only minor deficits with extreme hypoglycaemia. Subjective awareness of these early signs of impairment also differs greatly across individual patients. Some do not recognize these symptoms until they are severely impaired and others never recognize them. The progressive impairment in mental function caused by neuroglycopenia can severely interfere with patients' ability to recognize low BG symptoms and self-treat appropriately. For this reason, patients sometimes exhibit resistant behaviour toward others, denying that their BG is low and refusing carbohydrate treatment. Inability to recognize neuroglycopenia and self-treat appropriately can also lead to accidents and injury.

A significant number of type 1 patients are classified as 'hypoglycaemic unaware', a condition in which the hormonal counter-regulatory response and symptoms are dampened or delayed[30–32]. Until relatively recently, decreased ability to counter-regulate and hypoglycaemic unawareness were believed to be secondary to the development of autonomic neuropathy, a common long-term complication of type 1 diabetes. However, studies of patients suffering from hypoglycaemic unawareness found that many did not show evidence of autonomic neuropathy or diabetes of long duration[23,30,32]. More recent research has focused on the impact of recurrent hypoglycaemia on hormonal response. There is now strong evidence that even a relatively mild hypoglycaemic episode can decrease the glycaemic threshold for hormonal counter-regulation in response to episodes occurring in the next few days[31,33]. Thus, BG levels fall lower before counter-regulation and symptoms occur, increasing the probability of significant neuroglycopenia, inability to recognize that BG is low and self-treat, and an episode of severe hypoglycaemia.* It is important to emphasize, however, that even though patients classified as hypoglycaemic unaware have reduced hormonal symptoms, they are not completely asymptomatic[30]. Hypoglycaemic symptomatology is best described as a continuum on which some patients show *reduced* hypoglycaemic awareness.

The above findings have several implications for the clinical use of symptoms in regulating type 1 diabetes. First, because many symptoms are subtle and non-specific to glycaemic changes, it may not always be easy for patients to discriminate those symptoms that are indicative of BG level from those related to other changes in physiological state. This problem is exacerbated by the number of different symptoms that can correlate with BG. These findings suggest that patients may not always accurately recognize glucose symptoms and, consequently, may make errors in BG detection

---

*Severe hypoglycaemia, as defined by the Diabetes Control and Complications Trial, occurs when a patient is unable to self-treat due to neuroglycopenia, leading to progressive cognitive deterioration, unconsciousness and possible seizure.

which could, in turn, lead to errors in self-treatment In addition, the idiosyncratic nature of BG symptoms has implications for diabetes education. Patients need to be taught about the idiosyncracy of BG symptoms and helped to identify those that are personally most reliable. In clinical settings, assessment of symptoms typically involves asking patients to describe which symptoms they experience with BG extremes. This method of symptom assessment is based on the notion that patients' *beliefs* about their symptoms are accurate. An early study[15] tested this assumption by asking patients to rate the extent to which potential symptoms co-occurred with their hypo- and hyperglycaemic episodes, then empirically testing the relationship.

While symptom beliefs were generally accurate, there were also large individual differences in accuracy and a significant number of patients held erroneous symptom beliefs. The most common type was false-positive beliefs (i.e. false alarm symptoms), but patients also made false-negative errors (i.e. missed symptoms). Both types of errors have potential clinical implications. For example, the patient who erroneously believes that hunger is a reliable sign of hypoglycaemia (false alarm) may often treat him/herself for low BG unnecessarily, leading to hyperglycaemia. In contrast, the patient who is unaware that unusual fatigue is a sign of low BG (missed symptom) may fail to self-treat when needed, causing glucose to fall more precipitiously and increasing the risk of severe hypoglycaemia. A more recent study tested patients' symptom beliefs in a laboratory study during which BG levels were manipulated via insulin and glucose infusion[25] and found a similar pattern of errors. Fewer than half of the patients who reported sweating as a reliable sign of hypoglycaemia actually experienced this symptom during hospital testing (false alarm symptom), and half of the patients who did not report sweating as a reliable symptom experienced it.

ACCURACY OF BG DETECTION

The above studies suggest that BG symptoms are not always recognized accurately. Thus, the next question of critical clinical importance is: how well can patients with type 1 diabetes detect hypo- and hyperglycaemia? Even though patients do not always recognize symptoms, ability to estimate BG could conceivably be accurate if patients are adept at using external cues, including information about time of day, timing and amount of recent insulin, food and physical activity. To address this question empirically, the issue of measurement of accuracy needs to be considered. The use of traditional measures of accuracy, such as correlations and deviation scores, is problematic for several reasons[34–36]. For example, the correlation between subjective BG estimates and objective measures can be quite high, and the

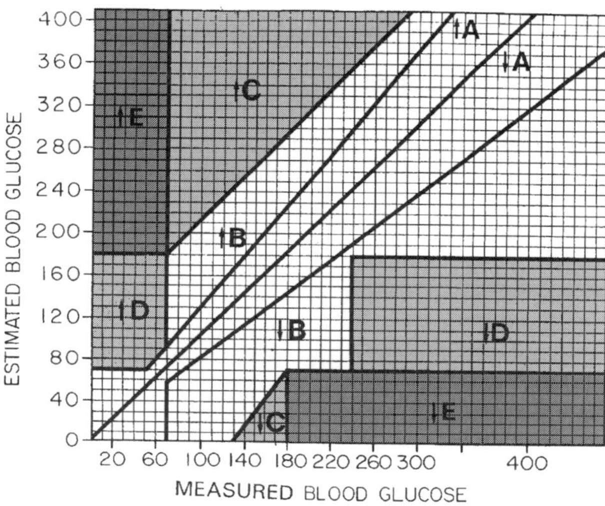

Figure 7.1. Error Grid analysis (EGA). Blood glucose measured in mg/dl

average deviation between the two can be low, even when patients make errors with potentially serious clinical implications. To address the question of the impact of BG detection on diabetes regulation, we developed a classification procedure, the Error Grid Analysis[34], which quantifies the *clinical significance* of patient accuracy.* Figure 7.1 shows the Error Grid Analysis (EGA), which involves plotting patients' BG estimates (y axis) in comparison to measured BG (x axis), so that each estimate falls into one of 10 categories or zones. Each zone represents the potential clinical outcome of taking action to adjust BG based on the subjective estimate.

The Error Grid is divided by a regression line that represents perfect agreement between estimated and actual BG. Data points falling above and below this line represent overestimates and underestimates of actual BG, respectively. The upper and lower A zones include estimates considered to be clinically acceptable; that is, the estimate is either within 20% of actual BG or both estimated and actual BG are below 3.9 mM (70 mg/dl). Estimates falling into the upper and lower B zones deviate more than 20% from actual BG, but are considered to be *benign* errors, since it is unlikely that patients would take action that was clinically dangerous based on these estimates, if action were taken, the clinical implications would be minimal. The C, D and E zones are considered to be clinically significant errors. C zone errors represent potential unnecessary *corrections* of BG because it estimated to be

*Information concerning the purchase of computer software for Error Grid Analysis is available from the author.

too high (upper C zone) or too low (lower C zone) when actual glucose is in an acceptable range. Taking action to treat BG based on these estimates could result in hypo- or hyperglycaemia. D zone errors occur when estimated BG is in an acceptable range but actual BG is too low (upper D zone) or high (lower D zone). These failures to *detect* hypo- or hyperglycaemia can lead to a failure to provide needed self-treatment. Finally, E zone estimates can lead to *erroneous* self-treatment, such as taking action to lower BG when hypoglycaemic (upper E zone) or to raise BG when hyperglycaemic (lower E zone).

Our first study of BG detection assessed patient accuracy under two conditions*, during hospital testing (while BG levels were manipulated via insulin and glucose infusion) and at home (while following normal daily routines)[34]. During hospital testing and BG manipulation, external cues such as time of day were irrelevant, forcing patients to rely on symptom feedback to estimate BG. In contrast, during home testing patients had access to external cues. As Figure 7.2 shows, patients made significantly more accurate estimates during home testing (A zones = 61%) as compared to hospital testing (A zones = 46%). Although the majority of estimates were clinically acceptable or benign errors, patients also made a substantial number of clinically significant errors. A total of 19% and 13% of estimates fell in the C, D and E zones in the hospital and home conditions, respectively. By far the most common error was failure to detect extreme BG levels (D zones), with C and E zone errors being rare. Unawareness of hypoglycaemia occurred more frequently than unawareness of hyperglycaemia, with patients detecting BGs < 3.9 mM only about 50% of the time. However, in a more recent laboratory study[25], BG levels were raised to a more extreme hyperglycaemic range (21.1 mM). These researchers found more errors in detecting high BG as compared to low BG. While only 17% of patients made clinically significant errors in detecting hypoglycaemia, 66% made these errors in their detection of hyperglycaemia—errors that included unawareness that BG levels were high (lower D zone) and believing BG was hypoglycaemic when it was quite high (lower E zone).

Other studies, by our research group and others, have used the EGA to assess BG detection, often employing a summary measure of the EGA called the *accuracy index* (AI). The AI is computed by subtracting the percentage of clinically significant errors (C, D and E zones) from the percentage of A zone estimates. In studies of adults with type 1 diabetes and a history of using SMBG, AI scores have ranged from 35% to 60%[37–39]. Accuracy appears to be

*The basic method for assessing accuracy of detection involves asking the patient, who is blind to actual glucose level, to estimate current BG on the basis of available cues, followed by an objective measure of glucose. BG estimates and measures can be recorded on paper forms or entered directly into computers. In the hospital assessment, BG estimates and measures were obtained every 10 minutes over a period of several hours and entered into a hand-held computer. In the home assessment, patients recorded their estimates on paper forms before SMBG several times each day over a period of 1–2 weeks.

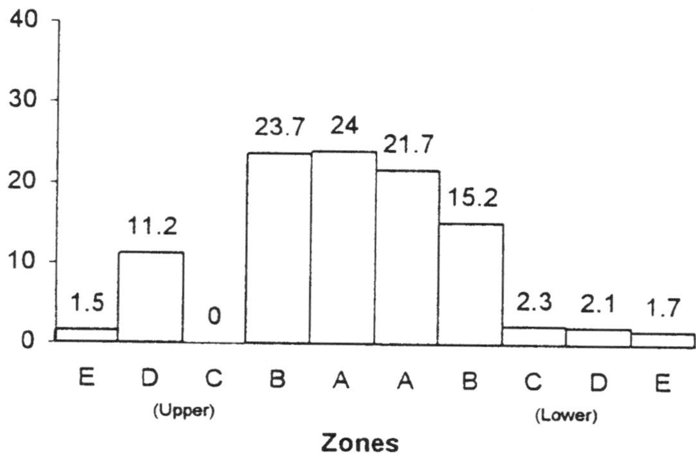

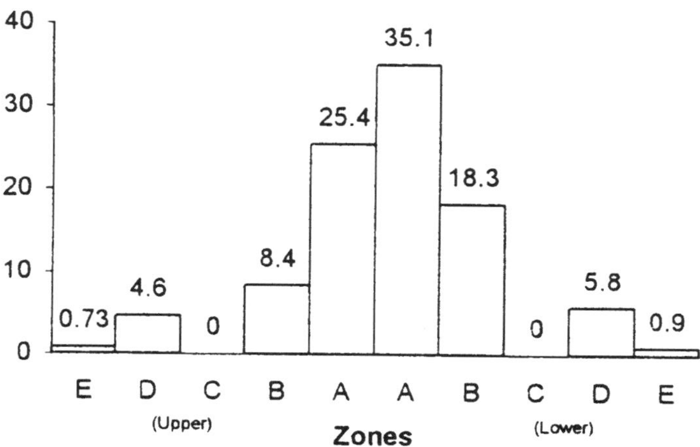

FIgure 7.2. Percentage of patient blood glucose (BG) estimates falling into each EGA zone

significantly poorer in younger age groups. For example, the first study of adolescents[14] found that 55% of BG estimates were clinically accurate; however, since that study did not compute clinically significant errors, AI scores could not be computed. A subsequent study[40] found poorer accuracy in both young adults (AI = 32%) and adolescents (AI = 7%). Children with type 1 diabetes and their parents exhibit even poorer accuracy, with average AI scores of − 1.05% and 5.0%, respectively[41]. This means that children and parents make clinically serious errors almost as often as clinically accurate estimates. Children also differed from adult patients in the types of errors they made. As Figure 7.3 shows, children made a much higher rate of lower E zone errors than adult patients. Thus, children often believed they were hypoglycaemic when in fact their BG was high, which could lead them to take action to raise BG when it is already too high. Several factors likely contribute to children's poor ability to detect BG extremes and the tendency to make more lower E zone errors; for example, developmental differences in the cognitive skills involved in discriminating physical symptoms. In addition, parental concern about and focus on immediate treatment may increase the salience of hypoglycaemia, and there are important reinforcement contingencies, since children typically are given some sort of sweet food or drink to treat low BG.

Patients who report reduced hypoglycaemic awareness also show poorer accuracy[30]. They detect only about 33% of BG readings below 3.9 mM, compared to adults without reduced awareness who detect, on average, 50% of their low BGs. Overall accuracy (AI) is also significantly lower (15%), closer to that seen in younger patient groups.

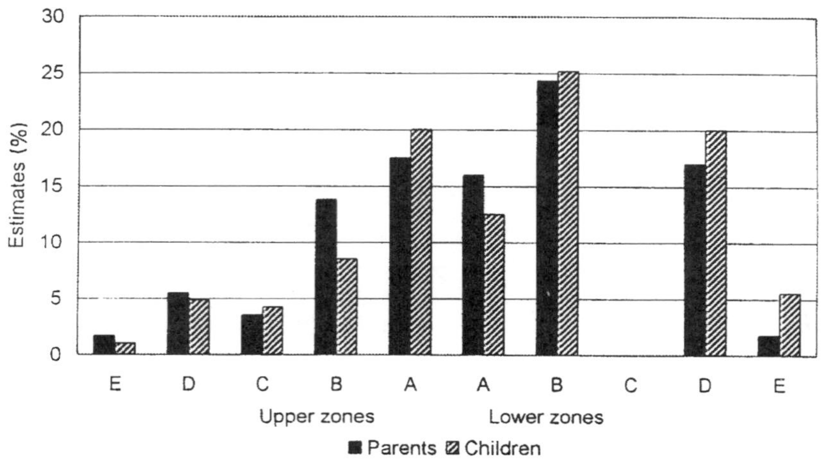

Figure 7.3. Frequency (total %) of estimates falling into each Error Grid zone for parents and children

Regardless of demographic and other differences in patient population, several findings have consistently emerged from studies of BG detection. First, ability to detect both hypo- and hyperglycaemia varies greatly across individual patients[14,25,35,41,43]. However, few patients demonstrate clinically acceptable accuracy at every BG range. Weinger *et al.*[25], for example, found that only one of 31 patients tested could accurately discriminate low, normal and high BG levels 100% of the time during hospital manipulations of glucose. Unfortunately, studies have repeatedly found that patients' *confidence* in their ability to detect BG fluctuations does *not* predict objectively-measured accuracy, meaning that clinicians cannot take self-reports of accuracy at face value[25,34,41,43]. Across studies, patients also show a consistent pattern in the types of errors made, the most common being failure to detect extreme low and high BG levels. Patients show a strong tendency to 'normalize' glucose fluctuations; that is, to overestimate the value of low BGs and to underestimate high BGs[25,34,41,43,44]. Normalization in BG estimates appears to be, in part, due to a tendency for patients to be 'overly optimistic' about their glucose control, as well as to a tendency to believe that, in the absence of symptoms, BG is likely to be euglycaemic.

The above research clearly demonstrates that the assumption that patients can 'tell' when their BG levels are too low or too high, based on symptoms and other cues, is problematic. Rather, studies repeatedly show that patients often make potentially serious errors in symptom perception and subjective BG estimations. Based on these findings, it might seem that clinicians should discourage patients from monitoring themselves for symptoms of extreme BG and basing treatment decisions on subjective estimations of glucose level. Instead, perhaps patients should be encouraged to use SMBG as often as possible and to rely solely on this objective feedback as a guide to self-regulation. However appealing, this is not a practical solution for several reasons. First, there is much evidence from previous symptom research[7–10] demonstrating the tenacity of patients' tendency to rely on subjective symptoms and illness beliefs. In short, even if patients are told that they cannot monitor symptoms and other cues for accurate information about their BG, they are likely to continue believing they can and doing so. Another reason is that only the minority of patients are willing to test their BG more than four times each day and even the most motivated test no more than eight to ten times daily. Thus, SMBG feedback is not obtained frequently enough to guide all self-treatment decisions. There are occasions when patients *must* rely on symptom feedback and subjective BG estimations to make treatment decisions; for example when hypoglycaemic symptoms onset suddenly, immediate treatment is needed and a meter is not available for SMBG.

An alternative solution, and the one represented by BGAT, is to develop interventions to train patients in skills that enhance glucose awareness and improve the ability to use symptoms and other subjective cues as accurate

Table 7.2. Goals of an effective intervention to improve BG awareness

Intervention goals
Test symptom beliefs
Correct erroneous symptom beliefs
Identify predictive/misleading symptoms
Identify diabetes management behaviours that lead to BG extremes
Objectively assess individual ability to estimate BG
Identify types of detection errors made
Objectively assess personal BG profiles
Outcome goals ↓
Increase frequency of clinically accurate estimates of current/future BG
Decrease frequency of clinically significant errors in estimating current/future BG
Outcome goals ↓
Increase frequency of appropriate self-treatment decisions and behaviours
Decrease frequency of extreme BG fluctuation

feedback about glycaemic changes. The results of research into BG symptoms and detection has obvious implications for the development of such a training programme. For example, because of errors in symptom perception and beliefs, patients need to identify objectively those symptoms and other cues that are most *sensitive* and *specific* in relationship to their BG changes. Because patients tend to normalize estimated BG, representing errors in beliefs about the range of daily glucose fluctuations, they need to assess objectively the frequency and extent of their own hypo- and hyperglycaemia. Table 7.2 summarizes the major goals of BGAT, each of which is derived empirically. We quantify success in achieving these goals by measuring the accuracy of BG detection as the outcome variable; specifically, increasing the rate of clinically accurate estimates and decreasing the rate of clinically significant errors. Of course, the ultimate desired outcome, which is more difficult to operationalize, is to improve ability to make wise self-treatment decisions and take appropriate behavioural actions. In the next section, the general content and format of BGAT in its current form is described, as well as some of the specific interventions developed to achieve these goals.

BGAT—A DESCRIPTION OF THE INTERVENTION

BGAT is structured into eight weekly classes* which follow an eight-chapter manual. Each chapter and class focuses on a different type of *internal*

*Although we use the term 'classes' to describe the eight weekly meetings, this is somewhat misleading since BGAT is not designed to be implemented in a lecture format. Rather, weekly meetings involve group discussions about the personal implications of the material and exercises, and how to apply newly-learned information to improve accuracy of BG detection and diabetes management.

Table 7.3. BGAT-III Table of Contents

Table of Contents

(physical symptoms, mental–motor function and moods) or *external* (insulin, food and physical activity) cue that can provide information about current or future BG fluctuations. Table 7.3 shows the table of contents from the current BGAT manual (BGAT-III). While a different topic and different material is presented each week, certain learning tools are incorporated throughout the entire intervention. BGAT is based on the teaching methods of active learning and self-experimentation. Therefore, each chapter of the manual contains exercises which require patients to stop reading and actively apply the information they have just learned. There are several different types of exercises, but most require patients to reflect on the personal implications of the material or to test their understanding of the information just read. Each chapter also contains 'key concepts' which summarize critical facts and ideas, as well as case studies (taken from actual patient experiences) describing the relevance of the information to daily self-management of diabetes. At the end of each chapter, there is a quiz to assess mastery of the material covered, and 'homework' assignments designed to provide opportunities to practise new skills, learn more about personal BG cues and fluctuations, and monitor progress.

The cornerstone of BGAT homework is the weekly BG Awareness Diary, which patients keep throughout the entire 8 weeks of training. This diary provides patients with a way to use daily SMBG readings to obtain systematic feedback about their most reliable symptoms, symptom beliefs, ability to use external cues, and the impact of different self-management behaviours on BG. Some form of the BG Awareness Diary has been included in every version of BGAT, including the original version. Figure 7.4 shows the current version of the Diary form, which is presented in Chapter 1 of the BGAT manual. Patients make Diary entries at least four times each day—before their routine SMBG and whenever they believe, because of internal or external cues, that their BG may be too high or too low. After recording the date and time of the entry, patients 'scan' themselves for internal cues. They are asked to record any internal cue they perceive, regardless of whether or not they believe it is related to BG. Patients then consider their recent insulin,

BG Diary Sheet
Introduction
Chapter 1

Name: ______________________

Cues: Scan your body for changes in your:
Head, Thinking, Vision, Dryness in mouth and nose,
Taste, Balance, Sweating, Breathing, Heart rate,
Coordination, Urination, Hunger, Energy, Tension,
Tolerance, Insulin, Food, Activity, Others: ______________________

Date	Time	BG cues, Internal and External	Est	Actual	Zone	High & Low BG Causes

Figure 7.4. Blood glucose (BG) awareness diary (BGAT)

food, and physical activity, as well as any other external cues they think might be having an impact on their BG (e.g. illness, medication, psychological stress), and record these. Based on the cues recorded, patients estimate their current glucose level, then measure actual BG. Patients evaluate the accuracy of their estimate by plotting it on the EGA, which is printed on the back of each Diary form, and recording the zone into which the estimate falls (i.e. upper or lower zone A, B, C, D, or E). Finally, if actual BG is lower than 3.9 mM or higher than 10 mM, patients consider possible causes for their hypo- or hyperglycaemia, and record these.

During the first week of BGAT, patients are taught how to use the Diary and EGA and why homework completion, including frequent Diary entries, is critical to success. They also list those symptoms they believe are reliable signals of hypo- and hyperglycaemia for ongoing evaluation of symptom beliefs. Beginning the second week, patients review and summarize the information contained in their Diary forms by following structured exercises to evaluate their use of cues and accuracy. Figure 7.5 shows a sample of the Summary Sheet used for this purpose. Briefly, patients identify the symptoms and other cues that were recorded when clinically accurate estimates of hypo- and hyperglycaemia were made (A zones), as well as those cues that were present but disregarded when they failed to detect BG extremes (D

Summary Sheet – Front

Name: ______________________

Date start: ______________ Date end: ______________

	# 1 Best hypo cues As < 70 ↑ Ds	BG	# 2 Misleading low BG cues ↓ Cs ↓Es	# 3 Causes (low BG)	# 4 Best hyper cues As > 180 ↓ Ds	BG	# 5 Misleading high BG cues ↑ Cs ↑Es	# 6 Causes (high BG)
Week 1								
Week 2								
Week 3								
Week 4								

Figure 7.5. BGAT-II summary sheet

zones). They then identify those cues which misled them to think their BG was too low or high when it was actually in an acceptable range (C zones) or to think their BG was too low when it was actually too high, and vice versa (E zones). The Summary sheet is completed at the end of each week throughout the remainder of BGAT and can be done either individually before the weekly meeting or at the beginning of a group meeting.

The next three weeks of BGAT focus on internal cues—physical symptoms, neuroglycopenic symptoms and mood changes. Chapter 2 describes the physiological mechanisms underlying counter-regulatory symptoms and hyperglycaemic symptoms (e.g. fluid loss, build-up of ketones). Factors that can interfere with symptom occurrence and perception are also reviewed, including behavioural (alcohol or caffeine consumption), physiological (inadequate counter-regulation due to frequent low BG) and psychological (inattentiveness, denial) factors. Patients learn about the idiosyncracy of BG symptoms and the importance of identifying personally reliable ones. Homework includes listening to a 'symptom awareness' audiotape each day, which includes exercises to promote sensitivity to internal cues.

Week 3 is devoted to neuroglycopenic symptoms, called 'Performance Cues' in BGAT. The primary goal is to increase patient sensitivity to the often-ignored, subtle and early signs of deterioration in mental and motor function due to mild hypoglycaemia. Patients learn to use *self-tests* to assess their own ability to function. These include 'Formal self-tests' (e.g. mental arithmetic, coin flipping) derived from tests which have been shown to deteriorate empirically with mild hypoglycaemia[28]. Patients also learn to use 'informal tests' that involve monitoring their ability to perform routine daily tasks (e.g. following conversations, reading, counting money, typing, remembering phone numbers), as compared to their usual skill level. Since there are individual differences in which routine tasks are relevant, patients compile a list of informal self-tests they believe will be personally useful and assess these during the next week. For example, a restaurant server might find it useful to monitor his/her ability to keep track of several different food orders, while a carpenter might monitor coordination when using certain tools. Research has shown that mild hypoglycaemia tends to cause a slowing down of cognitive–motor performance, but not necessarily more errors in performance[20,28,45]. For this reason, patients are taught to monitor how long it takes to perform tasks, as well as the degree of effort they have to expend to complete the task compared to their usual speed and difficulty in performing it. The effects of neuroglycopenia on driving ability are also described in Chapter 3, emphasizing that even mild hypoglycaemia may cause deficits in driving ability and the importance of avoiding driving when BG is low[26,46].

In Class 4, patients learn about the impact of extreme BG fluctuations on emotions and moods, and how to use these as internal cues. Mood changes are often more difficult to recognize as signs of BG extremes, primarily because moods tend to be attributed to socio-environmental factors, including the actions of other people, rather than physiological status. Thus, patients are taught to monitor themselves for emotional over-reactions or times when their affective response seems to be 'over-amplified' compared to their typical response to a similar situation. Since mood state appears to change in a negative direction for most people, the impact these reactions can have on relationships and interpersonal interaction is also reviewed, with special emphasis on emotional reactions to others during hypoglycaemic episodes (e.g. refusing help with treatment from others). Exercises to identify personal problems with BG-related mood changes and to work on improving communication with others about this issue are included in this chapter, and patients are encouraged to have their loved ones who participate in their diabetes care read this chapter of the manual. In response to patient requests, this chapter also includes a section on the effects of psychological stress on BG in type 1 diabetes.

Internal cue training during the first 3 weeks of BGAT provides patients with skills and practice to recognize hypo- and hyperglycaemic symptoms and episodes when they occur. During the next 3 weeks, patients work on building skills at using external cues—insulin, time of day, food, and physical activity—to anticipate extreme BG fluctuations. External cues are unique in that they can help patients to predict the likelihood of *future* hypo- and hyperglycaemia, as well as to estimate current BG more accurately. A major goal of external cue training is to teach patients to recognize 'mismatches' in the action of their insulin, food and physical activity on BG levels, which are the cause of most episodes of hypo- and hyperglycaemia. To do this, patients first have to understand the impact of their personal diabetes regimen and routine self-care behaviours on daily BG fluctuations. In the insulin chapter, patients begin by learning about the kinetics (duration and intensity of action) of the different types of insulin they take. They then complete exercises with step-by-step guidelines for computing the start time, peak time, peak intensity of action, and end time for each of their daily insulin doses. Using this information, patients plot their own 'insulin curves' which graphically depict the action of their insulin throughout the day.

Figure 7.6 shows a sample insulin curve from Chapter 5 of BGAT. The dotted lines represent rapid- or short-acting insulin and the dashed lines represent long- or intermediate-acting insulin. The time course of an insulin's action is represented by placing an 'I' at the time of injection (or basal rate change, or bolus for insulin pump users), a 'S' at the time the insulin starts working, a 'P' at the beginning and end of the insulin's peak action period, and a 'D' at the end of the insulin's duration of action. Curves are plotted in a downward direction toward peak intensity of action to reflect visually the BG-lowering effects of insulin throughout the day. One major goal of Class 5

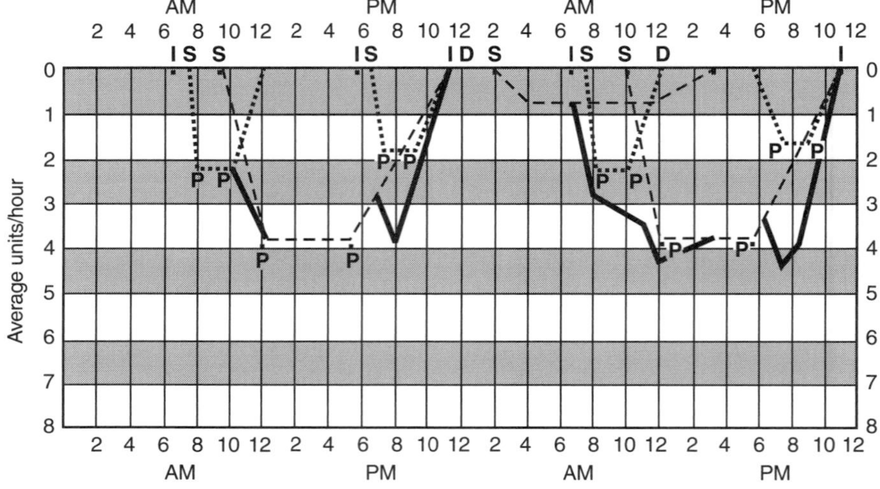

Figure 7.6. Insulin curve

is to help patients identify those times of the day or night when their BG is most likely to be too low or too high due to changes in the availability and intensity of insulin's action. Patients also plot curves to determine the effects on daily BG fluctuations when they change the timing and/or amount of their insulin dose. Patients often find the insulin chapter to be the most challenging, because it requires mathematical computations and the plotting of insulin curves can seem complex initially. However, after BGAT, many patients rate this material as one of the most valuable components of training.

In Chapter 6, patients learn about the impact of food on their BG and use carbohydrate counting to estimate the extent to which meals and snacks will increase glucose levels. Patients learn to monitor the fat content of their food, since high-fat foods can cause a significant increase in digestion time, which can dampen and/or delay BG increase. The implications of this for use of high-fat foods to treat hypoglycaemic episodes are emphasized; specifically, the danger of BG not increasing quickly enough. Patients plot the time course of their foods' effects on BG levels using 'food curves' such as the example one shown in Figure 7.7. They also keep a carbohydrate diary for several days to assess the extent to which the carbohydrate content of their meals and snacks varies from day to day, then plot these changes on food curves to determine the expected impact on BG. After plotting food curves for several days, patients compare these to their insulin curves to identify mismatches in the timing or intensity of food and insulin action; for example, a difference in the time of peak action for insulin and food. This type of mismatch is

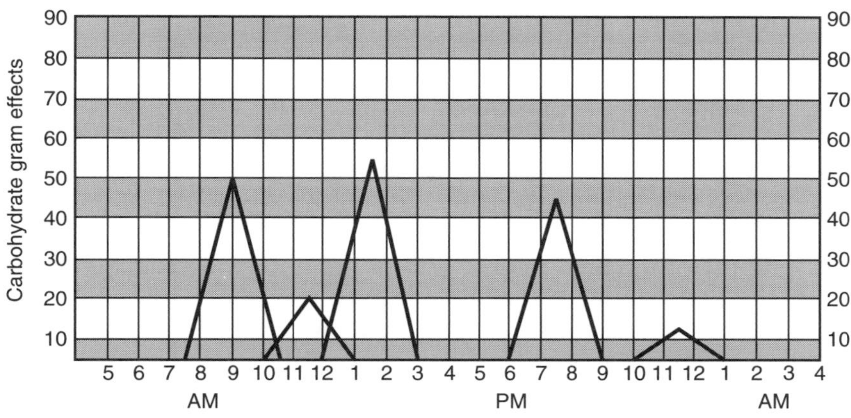

Figure 7.7. Food curve

common, such as when pre-breakfast short-acting insulin peaks mid-morning after the BG-raising effects of breakfast have ended, and no snack has been eaten.

The last external cue chapter focuses on physical activity. The term 'physical activity' is used instead of 'exercise' to emphasize the fact that *any significant change* in metabolic demand can alter BG. This includes unanticipated increases in activity during routine tasks (e.g. housework, gardening, child care, running errands, shovelling snow), as well as scheduled physical exercise. These unanticipated, and often unnoticed, increases in routine activity are a common cause of hypoglycaemic episodes. Unnoticed decreases in activity can also be problematic, leading to hyperglycaemia if food intake remains the same. To increase awareness of physical activity, patients monitor the *intensity* of their daily activity levels, categorizing them as low, moderate or high in intensity. Patients learn to plot physical activity curves that graphically summarize changes in intensity throughout the day (see Figure 7.8). Curves are plotted for several days during the week to

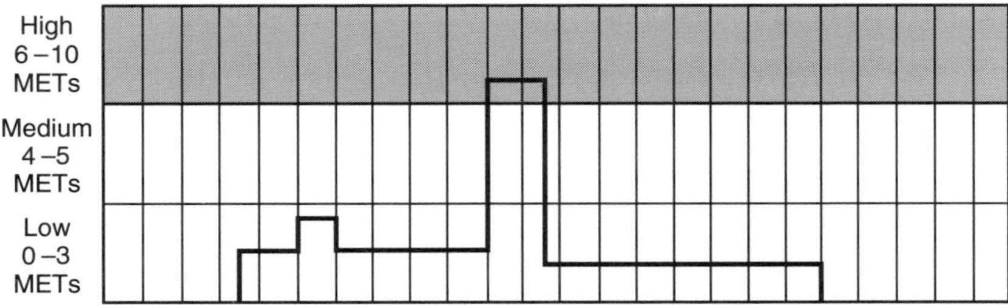

Figure 7.8. Physical activity curve

determine the extent to which activity varies from day to day, and for weekdays and weekends when schedules and activity levels often change. To complete external cue training, patients compare their insulin, food and physical activity curves to identify mismatches in these three basic aspects of diabetes management. Throughout external cue training, patients engage in an ongoing evaluation of how self-care behaviours contribute to mismatches in insulin, food and activity, and how they can change their behaviour to produce better matches and thereby avoid predictable BG extremes.

The purpose of the final chapter of BGAT is to provide patients with an opportunity to review what they have learned over the past weeks, receive positive reinforcement for completing training, and prepare to continue improving BG awareness on their own without the structure and support of the manual and weekly meetings. The chapter summarizes the most important didactic material from each chapter, and includes exercises requiring patients to reflect on what they have learned about themselves. Patients also review their Summary Sheet information from the past 7 weeks and evaluate their own symptoms, beliefs, accuracy and behavioural changes.

BGAT—EARLY STUDIES

While some aspects of BGAT have remained consistent over consecutive revisions (e.g. Awareness Diaries, weekly meetings), the intervention in its current form bears little resemblance to early versions. In the original version[37] (Study I) there was no structured manual or BG Awareness Diary. Patients recorded their symptoms, BG estimates, and actual BG measurements on paper, then reviewed and discussed these diaries in meetings held for 10 consecutive weeks. The goals for these meetings included identifying reliable and misleading symptom cues, as well as systematic biases in BG estimation (e.g. underestimating hyperglycaemia). A control group met for 10 weekly classes in stress management training. Pre-treatment and post-treatment accuracy of BG estimation was assessed in both an inpatient setting, where glucose levels were manipulated[34], and at home. After BGAT, both hospital and home estimates showed a significant improvement, with an increase in A zone estimates and a decrease in D zone errors. However, home estimates were more accurate than hospital estimates, providing further evidence that external cues play an important role in BG awareness. The control group showed no change in A zone estimates from pre- to post-treatment, and an increase in clinically serious errors.

The next BGAT study (Study II)[37] included only a treatment group and tested a revised version of BGAT which included a structured, six-chapter,

57-page manual and reduced the number of weekly meetings from 10 to six. The manual focused primarily on internal cues, with four chapters devoted to physical symptoms, mood changes, neuroglycopenic symptoms and perceptual changes, but one chapter was devoted exclusively to external cues. In addition, a structured Diary form was used to encourage more frequent and detailed entries. Again, pre- to post-treatment results showed an increase in clinically accurate estimates and a decrease in D zone errors. More patients showed improvements in accuracy (87%) in Study II as compared to Study I (70%), suggesting that the more structured training and increased emphasis on external cues enhanced BGAT's efficacy. In both studies, there was no association between improvement in accuracy and demographic/clinical variables, such as age, gender, age of onset or duration of diabetes. The only variable that predicted improvement was pre-treatment accuracy, with those patients who showed poorer accuracy before training improving more.

For the next two studies, BGAT was again revised by expanding the manual to seven chapters and 105 pages (BGAT-I) and increasing the number of weekly meetings to seven. BGAT-I also incorporated the EGA into training, allowing patients to evaluate their accuracy and errors in BG estimation on an ongoing basis. These studies utilized more sophisticated data procurement methods for pre- and post-treatment assessment in the home environment. Memory meters were used to determine SMBG frequency and patients carried pagers which 'beeped' on a random schedule four times/day for 10 days to prompt them to record estimated and actual BG level. The first study[38] tested whether BGAT-I improved metabolic control and whether frequency/duration of SMBG predicted improvement in accuracy of glucose detection. A control group met for seven weekly sessions to discuss topics relevant to diabetes that did not overlap with BGAT- I material. As in earlier studies, BGAT increased clinically accurate estimates and reduced clinically significant errors, while the control group showed no improvements. AI scores were higher (mean = 60%) after BGAT-I compared to the previous version (mean = 53%), indicating that the revised intervention was more effective. In addition, glycosylated haemoglobin improved in the BGAT group, decreasing from 12.2% at recruitment to 10.8% after training. SMBG history (frequency or duration) did not predict improvement but, as in the previous study, pre-treatment accuracy of BG estimation did, providing further evidence that BGAT is most beneficial for those patients who need it the most, i.e. those patients who were most inaccurate at baseline. Post-training accuracy and glycosylated haemoglobin measures were unrelated, indicating that improvement in BG detection does not necessarily lead to better metabolic control.

The next study of BGAT-I used similar methods to assess the impact of a more intensive intervention, which included *in vivo* symptom discrimination training prior to BGAT[39]. Half of the BGAT patients underwent an inpatient training procedure, during which their BG was lowered (mean nadir = 2.7 mM), then raised (mean apex = 13.3 mM). Throughout this procedure, patients were asked to rate their symptoms, then estimate their current BG level, every 10 minutes. They were then given their actual BG measurement and asked to pay attention to any symptoms or other internal cues present. After this training procedure, these patients underwent BGAT-I. The remaining BGAT patients did not receive this intensive training procedure before the intervention. Both the intensive and standard training groups showed improvements in accuracy after BGAT-I (mean AI scores = 67% and 56%, respectively), while the control group (who met for seven weekly diabetes discussions) showed no improvement (mean AI = 36%). Both BGAT-I groups showed a decrease in undetected hyperglycaemia, and there was a trend toward a reduction in undetected hypoglycaemia. Table 7.4 summarizes the improvements in accuracy found in both studies of BGAT-I[38,39].

However, in the second study of BGAT-I[39], only the intensive training group showed an improvement in glycosylated haemoglobin with a decrease of 2.5%. Neither SMBG frequency or diabetes knowledge related to improvement in accuracy, but poorer baseline accuracy was again predictive of more improvement. Memory meter data demonstrated that frequency of SMBG did not decrease after BGAT, suggesting that patients did not become overconfident in their ability to recognize glucose extremes.

Table 7.4. BGAT-I studies: summary of results

Study	AI scores (%)	Undetected hyperglycaemia (%)	Undetected hypoglycaemia (%)
Cox *et al.*, 1989			
BGAT	41 pre	18 pre	48 pre
	60 post	6 post	25 post
Control	51 pre	8 pre	50 pre
	43 post	13 post	67 post
Cox *et al.*, 1991			
Standard BGAT	41 pre	19 pre	46 pre
	56 post	8 post	36 post
Intensive BGAT	45 pre	13 pre	51 pre
	67 post	3 post	24 post
Control	42 pre	12 pre	62 pre
	36 post	16 post	61 post

BGAT—RECENT STUDIES

The above studies demonstrate clearly the efficacy of BGAT and also suggest that certain patients may be especially likely to benefit from the intervention, i.e. those patients who have more difficulty recognizing BG symptoms and other cues. To further enhance the efficacy of BGAT for this patient population, the next version (BGAT-II) made two significant changes: (a) the addition of three chapters devoted exclusively to external cues (insulin, food and physical activity) and (b) more structured training in the use of neuroglycopenic symptoms, including the use of self-tests to assess mental and motor function. The decision to increase the emphasis on external cues was based on our growing appreciation of their critical role in BG awareness, especially their potential value in helping patients to predict glucose extremes which should, in turn, lead to improved ability to avoid these. In addition, research from Spain[44] had suggested that external cue training alone could improve ability to estimate BG. There were several reasons for deciding to expand training on neuroglycopenic cues to detect hypoglycaemia, not the least of which were patients' self-reports that they use this type of feedback frequently; for example, noticing incoordination when items were dropped, inability to remember familiar phone numbers, and difficulty reading the newspaper. Patients who have lost the ability to counter-regulate effectively are often still able to recognize hypoglycaemia during hospital testing, suggesting the use of neuroglycopenic cues[23,24]. Our research had also shown that performance of routine tasks can be disrupted by mild hypoglycaemia[26,28]. Subsequent research has shown that perception of personal impairments in task performance make a major contribution to the recognition of hypoglycaemia[47].

BGAT-II included a 132-page, seven-chapter manual that followed the format shown in Table 7.3 with the exception of no summary chapter. This revision introduced the use of graphic plots of insulin, food and physical activity curves to: (a) understand the impact of these factors on daily BG fluctuations; (b) identify times of day when risk for hypo- or hyperglycaemia is high; and (c) evaluate how well these aspects of diabetes management are matched throughout the day. The method for weekly review of BG Awareness Diaries was revised, providing a structured form and exercises to summarize information about cues and accuracy. BGAT-II also increased the amount of active interaction with manual material by incorporating more exercises, self-tests and case reports, as well as more structured homework assignments to facilitate practice and skill acquisition.

To test BGAT-II[42], patients with reduced hypoglycaemic awareness (RHA) were compared to patients who were hypoglycaemic-aware (HA) in a repeated baseline design. This allowed us to assess whether BGAT would benefit a patient population (RHA) who have significant deficits in ability to recognize hypoglycaemia. Patients were also tested at three different geographical sites (University of Virginia, Vanderbilt University and Joslin Diabetes Institute, Boston) by four separate trainers to assess the generalizability of the intervention. Figure 7.9 shows the repeated baseline design of the study. Patients underwent assessment at study entry, after a 6-month baseline and just before entering BGAT, 1 month after BGAT, 6 months later, and 1 year post-treatment. At each assessment, patients used a handheld computer (Psion P-250) containing a programme which required them to enter symptom ratings, perform cognitive-motor tasks, rate their task impairment, record recent insulin, food and physical activity, estimate BG level, indicate whether they would drive or raise/lower their BG based on this estimate, then measure actual BG and enter that value. Four to six entries were made each day over a 3–4 week period for a total of 70 trials. Patients also completed a battery of psychosocial questionnaires (e.g. Diabetes Quality of Life, Fear of Hypoglycaemia, Beck Depression Inventory, and Dyadic Adjustment Scale) at assessments, and had blood drawn for glycosylated haemoglobin analysis. During the 6-month baseline period, patients recorded episodes of severe hypoglycaemia, as well as any automobile accidents or traffic violations, on a diary which was mailed in on a monthly basis. Patients again completed these monthly diaries after BGAT until 1 year follow-up.

During the 6 month baseline period, there were no changes in estimation accuracy, BG profiles, metabolic control or psychosocial status. One month after BGAT-II, both HA and RHA patients showed significant improvements in accuracy, although the RHA group, who were significantly less accurate at baseline, showed the most improvement. While both groups reduced the number of undetected hyperglycaemic episodes, only RHA patients reduced the number of undetected hypoglycaemic episodes. Changes in BG profiles were assessed by computing the 'Low BG Index' and 'High BG Index', measures that reflect the frequency and severity of glucose fluctuations into

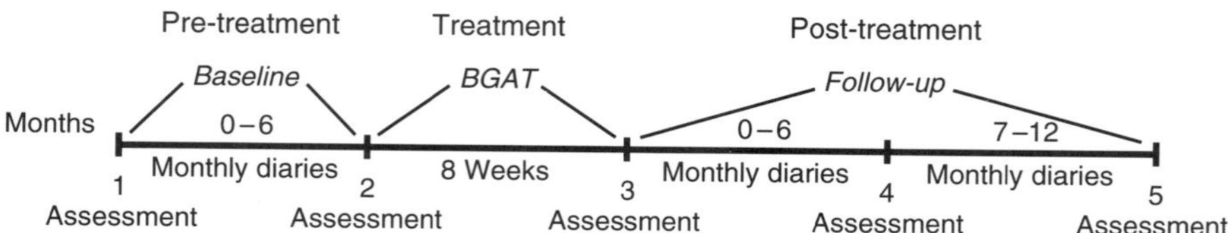

Assessments: Hand-held computer, HbA1, Psychosocial Questionnaire

Monthly Diaries: Severe hypoglycaemia, motor vehicle violations, missed work days

Figure 7.9. Repeated baseline design for study of BGAT-II

extreme levels[48], from the handheld computer data. A reduction in Low BG Index indicates that hypoglycaemic episodes have decreased in frequency and/or severity. After BGAT-II, the HA group showed a reduction in the Low BG Index, while the RHA group showed a reduction in the High BG Index. Thus, even though BGAT-II improved detection of hypoglycaemia, it did not appear to reduce the frequency and severity of low BG fluctuations in patients with RHA. The number of symptoms related to hypo- and hyperglycaemia did not increase after training, suggesting that patients were not identifying new symptoms but rather using pre-existing symptoms and external cues more effectively. Glycosylated haemoglobin did not change in either group. Importantly, there were no differences between the three different training sites, indicating that BGAT can be effectively generalized to other patient populations, geographic regions and trainers.

Even though BGAT-II improved detection of hypoglycaemia in RHA patients, its failure to decrease the frequency and severity of low BG excursions was somewhat disappointing. To address this problem, BGAT-II was revised to include training specifically targeted toward reducing the frequency of hypoglycaemia. This revision (BGAT-III) incorporated more information on the impact of frequent hypoglycaemia on counter-regulation and hormonal symptoms. Research was included that showed that avoidance of hypoglycaemia, even for only a few days to a week, can improve counter-regulation and strengthen symptoms[49,50], and patients were given explicit instructions to try to reduce the frequency of SMBG readings < 3.9 mM. BGAT-III is currently being used by hundreds of patients in several different countries. However, only one controlled study testing its efficacy has been published[51]. Researchers at the Joslin Diabetes Center at Harvard University assessed BGAT in patients undergoing intensive insulin therapy to improve diabetes control which, as shown by the DCCT and subsequent studies, greatly increases the risk for severe hypoglycaemia[52,53], presumably because the increase in frequency of low BG impairs counter-regulation. These researchers tested whether BGAT would reduce this risk. After intensive therapy training, half of the patients were assigned to BGAT-III and the other half were assigned to a control group who attended a class on cholesterol awareness. Before intensive therapy training and after BGAT, patients underwent a hypoglycaemic clamp study to assess symptoms, counter-regulation and ability to detect extreme BGs, then used the handheld computer for 70 home trials to assess symptoms, accuracy and glucose profiles.

The results of this study are exciting, albeit somewhat mixed. As expected, intensive insulin therapy improved metabolic control in both the BGAT and control groups. However, the frequency of low BG readings also increased equally in both groups, indicating that BGAT-III did not reduce this risk factor for severe hypoglycaemia. In terms of ability to recognize hypoglycaemia, BGAT patients did not show an improvement in accuracy compared to the control group during inpatient testing. However, when hand-held computer data were analysed, BGAT patients showed the expected improvements in detection of low glucose levels and had fewer undetected low BG readings than control patients. Perhaps most importantly, this study yielded the first evidence that BGAT can have an impact on physiologic response. Even though intensive insulin therapy improved metabolic control and increased frequency of low BG, BGAT patients did *not* show the expected reduction in epinephrine response to hypoglycaemia. In contrast, control patients showed the well-documented decrease and delay in counter-regulation. Because BGAT did not improve ability to reduce the frequency of low BG readings, the mechanism by which counter-regulatory integrity was preserved is unclear. Nonetheless, this study provides intriguing preliminary evidence that BGAT, through some indirect mechanism, can maintain the efficiency of hormonal counter-regulation during intensive therapy.

Another question of recent interest is the long-term effects of BGAT. In other words, do the benefits of BG persist over time? To test this question[54], we recruited 28 BGAT patients and 12 control group patients from the first study[37] an average of 4.9 years after their original participation. Half of the BGAT group received 'booster training', which involved keeping BG Awareness Diaries for 2 weeks prior to assessment of accuracy. The remaining BGAT patients, as well as the control group, received no booster training before accuracy assessment. Patients also had blood drawn for glycosylated haemoglobin measurement, and filled out a questionnaire asking them how many days of work they had missed due to hypoglycaemia or DKA, as well as how many automobile accidents they had had since their participation in the original study. BGAT + booster patients demonstrated significantly more accuracy in BG detection than either the BGAT + no booster or control patients, and BGAT + no booster showed a trend toward better accuracy than control patients. There were no group differences in lost work days, but BGAT patients reported significantly fewer automobile accidents than control patients. Only 15% of BGAT patients reported accidents, while 42% of control patients reported one or more. There were no differences in metabolic control.

More recently, we have analysed follow-up data from the multi-center study of BGAT-II reported previously[42] (see Figure 7.9)*, which offers the most comprehensive evaluation of long-term effects to date, with hand-held computer assessments, prospective monthly diaries, and psychosocial measures 1 month, 6 months, and 1 year following training. Table 7.5 summarizes these results, which we find quite encouraging. Improvements in ability to estimate BG were maintained across the year for both HA and

---

*Manuscript in preparation.

Table 7.5. BGAT II: 1-year follow-up results

	Improvements maintained	Improvements *not* maintained	No improvement
Accuracy	AI score Increased A zone estimates Decreased D zone estimates Low BG detection	High BG detection	
Decision making	To treat when actual BG <70 Not to drive when actual BG is <70 Not to drive when estimated BG <70		To treat when estimated BG is <70
Risk factors	High BG risk index Number of severe hypoglycaemia episodes Number of nocturnal hypoglycaemia episodes Number of automobile violations		Low BG risk index Daytime severe hypoglycaemia
Psychosocial	Diabetes quality of life Diabetes knowledge		Dyadic adjustment scale Beck Depression Inventory
Metabolic			Glycosylated haemoglobin

RHA patients on nearly every measurement of accuracy—AI scores, A zone estimates, D zone estimates, and percentage low BG episodes detected. Improvements in detection of high BG, however, were not maintained. BGAT did not reduce the Low BG Index; however, there were significant decreases in severe hypoglycaemia, nocturnal hypoglycaemia, and traffic violations after intervention. One perplexing finding, for which we have no explanation, was a decrease in the number of symptoms related to hypoglycaemia over time.

This study also provides the first evidence that BGAT has beneficial effects on decision-making and judgement. Hand-held computer data showed that decisions to self-treat actual BG levels <3.9 mM increased in frequency, as did decisions *not* to drive when BG was low. RHA and HA patients differed, however, in changes in decision-making when BG was believed to be low (estimated BG <3.9 mM). Decisions to self-treat when BG was estimated to be low increased in RHA patients but decreased in HA patients. This may reflect increased awareness in RHA patients that, whenever they feel symptoms, they are likely to be quite hypoglycaemic and in need of immediate treatment. In contrast, HA patients may learn that they cannot always trust subjective estimations of BG and, consequently, that they need to verify these with SMBG before taking action. The frequency of decisions *not* to drive when BG was believed to be low increased in HA patients but, unfortunately, did not change in RHA patients.

Taken together, these studies provide encouraging evidence that BGAT has benefits beyond simply improving BG detection, such as improvements in decision-making and reduced risk for severe hypoglycaemia and motor vehicle violations, and that many of these benefits are maintained over time, although some sort of booster training may be needed to preserve them over several years. Furthermore, these studies provide preliminary evidence that BGAT may improve counter-regulation and reduce the risk of severe hypoglycaemia *without* jeopardizing metabolic control. However, there remains 'room for improvement' to optimize the effects of this intervention. As yet, we have not been able to reduce the frequency of low BG excursions, a major risk factor for future severe hypoglycaemia, or the frequency of daytime episodes of severe hypoglycaemia. The frequency of low BG and severe hypoglycaemia depends, in large part, on the decisions patients make and the actions they take to manage their diabetes. For example, deciding to delay a meal can precipitate low BG, while deciding to delay treatment of low BG can lead to severe hypoglycaemia. Even though BGAT reduced risky decisions about treatment and driving when patients *knew* they were hypoglycaemic, RHA patients did not become less willing to drive when they *believed* their BG might be low. Unfortunately, the handheld computer program used in these studies did not assess whether or not patients planned to *measure* their BG to verify their subjectively perceived hypoglycaemia. This methodological limitation, which has been corrected in our current research, restricted our ability to make definitive conclusions about self-treatment decisions when BG is believed to be low. Nonetheless, these findings provide empirical evidence that decision-making and behavioural response play an important role in reducing the risk of hypoglycaemia and its negative consequences, and that these areas may be important targets for future intervention.

IMPLICATIONS AND FUTURE DIRECTIONS

Given the solid body of empirical evidence that BGAT is effective, the next important question from a clinical perspective is: what types of patients should be considered for this intervention? The specific effects demonstrated in studies of BGAT suggest that several patient groups are most likely to benefit, which are shown in Table 7.6. For example, BGAT improves detection of low BG, reduces the frequency of severe hypoglycaemia, and may preserve the integrity of hormonal counter-regulation after the implementation of intensive insulin therapy. Therefore, it should be considered for patients who have reduced hypoglycaemic awareness, are using intensive insulin therapy, and have a history of recurrent severe hypoglycaemia. Since

Table 7.6. Patient groups likely to benefit from BGAT

Poor ability to recognize/predict BG extremes
Using intensive insulin therapy
Reduced hypoglycaemic awareness
History of recurrent severe hypoglycaemia
High fear of hypoglycaemia
Recurrent DKA
Poor metabolic control

there is some evidence that BGAT can reduce emotional fear of hypoglycaemia, patients with a history of traumatic experiences related to low BG or high levels of anxiety about their ability to cope with hypoglycaemia may benefit. BGATs potential effects on hyperglycaemia detection, frequency and severity of high BG excursions and metabolic control also suggest that it may be useful for patients with poor diabetes control. Finally, BGAT studies have repeatedly shown that those patients who are very poor at estimating glucose levels can benefit greatly. Therefore, it should be useful for patients who are frequently 'surprised' to find out that their BG is far too low or high, or who are unaware of the extreme range of their glucose fluctuations.

There are also patient groups who are not likely to be good candidates. BGAT requires a large investment of time and effort (e.g. daily Diary entries, homework exercises) and patients who are not highly and intrinsically motivated will have difficulty completing the intervention. Patients who are unwilling to self-test their BG several times daily are also likely to be unsuccessful, since this is necessary to obtain the systematic feedback from diary entries which are integral to training. Even though BGAT can teach patients a great deal about diabetes and improves knowledge, it should not be considered as a form of or replacement for general diabetes education. In fact, only patients who already have a good foundation of knowledge about their illness and its treatment should be considered. For this reason, we do not recommend it be used with newly-diagnosed patients who are struggling to assimilate all the information they need to manage diabetes on a daily basis. Finally, even though BGAT contains elements of cognitive-behavioural therapy, it should not be considered a substitute for psychological intervention for patients who are having significant difficulty with emotional and/or behavioural adjustment to diabetes.

The research suggests that BGAT would be beneficial for other patient groups but, unfortunately, the intervention has not yet been modified for appropriate use with these. For example, children with type 1 diabetes and their parents show very poor BG detection and a tendency to make a high rate of errors, with potentially dangerous clinical implications, such as mistaking hyperglycaemic symptoms for hypoglycaemia[41]. Our hope is to adapt and test BGAT for children and their parents in the near future. The current version of BGAT also needs to be revised and tested with adolescent populations. One previous study[40] tested an intervention similar to BGAT with adolescents in an inpatient setting using three sessions for training. Accuracy of BG detection improved significantly, with AI scores increasing from 7% before training to 30% afterwards, but we would expect to see more improvement with the more intensive intervention provided by BGAT. A related, ongoing effort is to simplify BGAT; for example, by lowering the required reading level and reducing patient effort. However, the impact of such alterations on training benefits must also be assessed carefully. Finally, although BGAT has been translated into several other languages and is being employed in studies around the world, we do not yet have data to demonstrate that it is effective in other cultures.

Another important future direction is to improve BGAT's ability to reduce the risk of severe hypoglycaemia in patient groups who are vulnerable to this dangerous condition. Severe hypoglycaemia appears to a recurrent problem for a highly specific group, with the majority of episodes occurring in a small percentage of patients. While there are no studies to document it, we would expect that this subset of patients are also those at highest risk for accident, injury and even death due to hypoglycaemia. To increase BGATs effectiveness for this population, we have recently developed a new intervention, Hypoglycaemia Anticipation, Awareness and Treatment Training (HAATT), specifically designed to reduce risk factors for severe hypoglycaemia. The content and goals of HAATT are derived both from BGAT and a biopsychobehavioural model of the occurrence of severe hypoglycaemia[55].

Figure 7.10 presents a simplified version of the biopsychobehavioural model*, showing that it extends beyond self-regulation via symptom awareness and BG detection to incorporate processes of decision making and self-treatment behaviour. At every step of the model, the risk that severe hypoglycaemia will occur can increase or decrease. For example, precursor self-care behaviours (Step 1) either increase or decrease the probability that insulin levels will be too high relative to recent food intake and physical activity. Thus, precursors determine the likelihood of low BG, a necessary prerequisite to severe hypoglycaemia (Step 2). If low BG occurs, the person may or may not react physiologically with hormonal counter-regulation and neuroglycopenia (Step 3). Even if counter-regulation and/or neuroglycopenia occur, the person may or may not be aware of the symptoms caused by

---

*In reality, this is a non-linear model of transitional probabilities, with numerous possible pathways and outcomes that lead to the avoidance or occurrence of severe hypoglycaemia. However, for the purposes of understanding its relevance to the structure and content of HAATT, a simplified linear version is presented here.

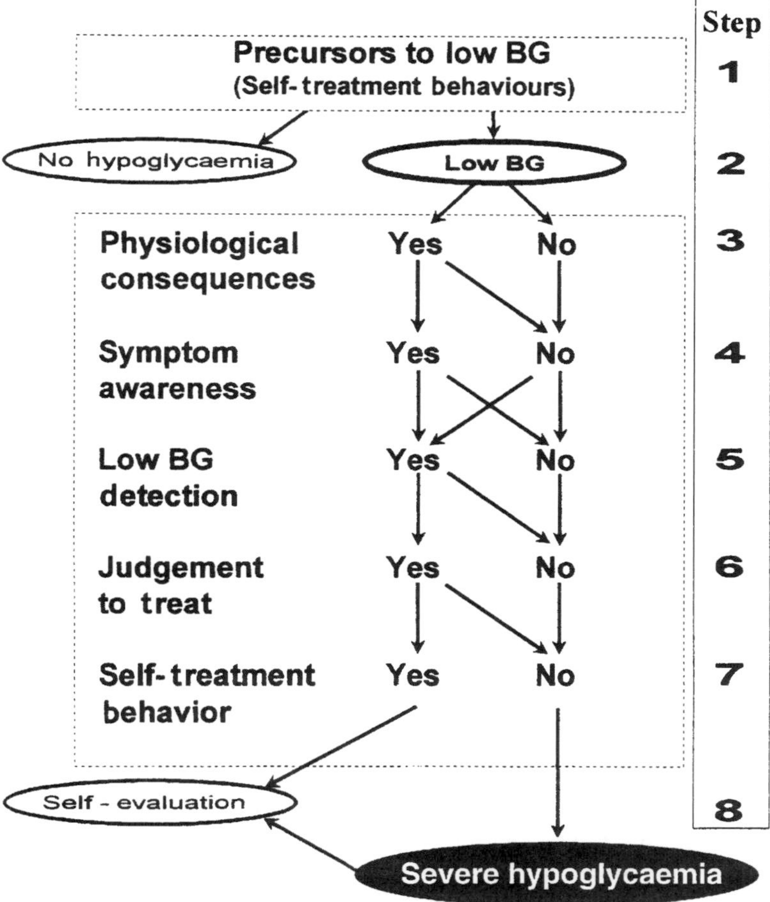

Figure 7.10. Biopsychobehavioural model of severe hypoglycaemia

these physiological changes (Step 4). If symptoms are perceived, they may or may not be attributed to low BG, leading to accurate detection (Step 5). Also, even if low BG is detected, the person may or may not make appropriate decisions (Step 6); for example, he/she may decide that treatment is not needed or can be delayed. Finally, even if a decision to treat is made, the person may or may not follow through behaviourally (Step 7); for example, an appropriate food or drink to raise BG may not be immediately available.

The structure and content of HAATTs seven-chapter training manual follows this model. Three chapters are devoted to precursor self-care behaviours (insulin, food, physical activity) that lead to hypoglycaemia. In addition to identifying personal self-care behaviours that increase the risk of low BG, patients learn to use these components of diabetes management as external cues to current glucose levels as in BGAT. The next chapter is devoted to symptoms caused by counter-regulation and neuroglycopenia, as well as changes in mood related to low BG. Unlike BGAT, HAATT reviews the impact of these mood changes on behaviour and interpersonal relationships in detail, provides self-assessments for determining whether this is a personal problem area, and encourages patients to have their loved ones read this chapter to improve communication. Like BGAT, HAATT includes self-tests for impairment in mental/motor function and encourages increased attention to neuroglycopenic symptoms.

The next chapter is devoted to improving decision making and treatment of hypoglycaemia when it cannot be avoided. Self-assessments to identify personally risky attitudes and behaviours are included, with exercises to help alter these risk factors. Self-inquiries are provided to address the fears, beliefs and other feelings underlying these risky attitudes and behaviours. This chapter emphasizes the negative impact of neuroglycopenia on judgement and behaviour, including the effects of mental confusion on ability to recognize hypoglycaemia and willingness to accept assistance with treatment. Overall, the format of the manual and basic learning tools of HAATT are very similar to BGAT, with the use of diaries, interactive exercises, graphic plots of insulin, food and physical activity, and homework assignments. There is much more emphasis, however, on understanding and identifying personal risk factors, as well as training in problem-solving and coping skills to reduce these risks. Currently, we are testing the efficacy of HAATT in patients who have a history of recurrent severe hypoglycaemia in a controlled, multi-site study to determine whether or not it decreases the frequency of future episodes and related risk factors.

Clearly, BGAT has many implications for future directions in clinical application and research in patients with diabetes. As stated in the introduction, we do not consider BGAT to be a finished product. In fact, it requires almost constant revision to incorporate new research findings and training methods that are relevant to BGATs goals. More research is needed to understand the mechanisms of BGATs efficacy, its differential benefits across patient groups, and the exciting possibility that it may preserve the integrity of counter-regulatory hormonal response and symptoms without jeopardizing tight metabolic control. Just as importantly, BGAT needs to be adapted for younger type 1 populations and their care givers. Although research shows that BGAT can provide a wide range of benefits across many patient groups, one of its most important positive features may be the ability to evolve and accommodate discrete patient populations and problems in diabetes management. For this reason, BGAT may best be viewed as a 'parent' intervention, with well-documented efficacy and general clinical utility, but also the capacity to generate 'offspring' interventions designed specifically to target particular patients groups and outcome goals. BGAT stands as an example of both the effort required to develop and evaluate effective psycho-educational interventions for diabetes and the enormous benefits that can be reaped from such an effort. On a broader level, this body of research serves as an example of the concrete relevance and application of psychological theories and methods to the treatment of chronic illnesses.

REFERENCES

1. Cox D, Gonder-Frederick L. Major developments in behavioral diabetes research. *J Consult Clin Psychol* 1992; **60**(4): 628–38
2. Gonder-Frederick L, Cox D. Symptom perception, symptom beliefs, and blood glucose discrimination in the self-treatment of insulin-dependent diabetes. In Skelton JA, Croyle RT (eds) *Mental Representations in Health and Illness*. New York: Springer-Verlag, 1991; 221–46
3. Gonder-Frederick L, Cox D. Symptom perception and blood glucose feedback in the self-treatment of IDDM. In Holmes C (ed) *Neuropsychological and Behavioral Aspects of Diabetes*. New York: Springer-Verlag, 1990; 155–74
4. Wing R, Epstein L, Nowalk M, Lamparski D. Behavioral self-regulation in the treatment of patients with diabetes mellitus. *Psychol Bull* 1986; **99**(1): 78–89
5. Leventhal H, Meyer D, Nerenz D. The common sense representation of illness danger. In Rachman S (ed) *Medical Psychology*, vol 2. New York: Pergamon, 1980
6. Leventhal H, Zimmerman R, Gutmann M. Compliance: a self-regulation perspective. In Gentry D (ed) *Handbook Behav Med*. New York: Guilford Press, 1980; 369–436
7. Pennebaker J. *The Psychology of Physical Symptoms*. New York: Springer-Verlag, 1982
8. Baumann L, Leventhal H. 'I can tell when my blood pressure is up, can't I?' *Health Psychol* 1985; **4**: 203–18
9. Meyer D, Leventhal H, Gutmann M. Common-sense models of illness: the example of hypertension. *Health Psychol* 1985; **4**: 115–35
10. Gonder-Frederick L, Cox D. Behavioral responses to perceived hypoglycemic symptoms. *Diabet Educ* 1986; **12**: 105–7
11. Pennebaker J, Cox D, Gonder-Frederick L, Wunsch M, Evans W, Pohl S. Physical symptoms related to blood glucose in insulin-dependent diabetics. *Psychosom Med* 1981; **43**(6): 489–500
12. Cox D, Gonder-Frederick L, Pohl S, Pennebaker J. Reliability of symptom–blood glucose relationships among insulin-dependent adult diabetes. *Psychosom Med* 1983; **45**: 357–60
13. Cox D, Gonder-Frederick L, Pohl S, Carter W, Clarke W, Bennett-Johnson S, Rosebloom A, Bradley C, Moses J. Symptoms and blood glucose levels in diabetics. *J Am Med Assoc* 1985; **253**(11): 1558
14. Freund A, Bennett-Johnson S, Rosenbloom A, Alexander B, Hansen C. Subjective symptoms, blood glucose estimation, and blood glucose concentrations in adolescents with diabetes. *Diabet Care* 1986; **9**(3): 236–43
15. Gonder-Frederick L, Cox D, Bobbitt S, Pennebaker J. Blood glucose symptom

beliefs in type 1 diabetic adults: accuracy and implications. *Health Psychol* 1986; **3**: 327–41

16. Hepburn D, Deary E, Frier B, Patrick A, Quinn J, Fisher B. Symptoms of acute insulin-induced hypoglycemia in humans with and without IDDM. *Diabet Care* 1991; **14**(11): 949–57
17. McCrimmon R, Gold A, Deary I, Kelnar C, Frier B. Symptoms of hypoglycemia in children with IDDM. *Diabet Care* 1995; **18**: 858–61.
18. Deary I, Frier B, Gold A, Macleod K. Changes in mood during acute hypoglycemia in healthy participants. *J Personality Soc Psychol* 1995; **68**: 498–504
19. Gonder-Frederick L, Cox D, Bobbitt S, Pennebaker J. Changes in mood state associated with blood glucose fluctuations in insulin-dependent diabetes mellitus. *Health Psychol* 1989; **8**: 45–59
20. Holmes C, Hayford J, Gonzalez J, Weydert J. A survey of cognitive functioning at different glucose levels in diabetics. *Diabet Care* 1983; **6**: 180–83
21. Holmes C, Hayford J, Gonzalez J, Weydert J. A survey of cognitive functioning at different glucose levels in diabetic persons. *Diabet Care* 1983; **6** 180–85
22. Bloomgarden Z. International Diabetes Federation Meeting, 1997, and Metropolitan Diabetes Society of New York Meeting, November 1997—approaches to treatment and other topics in type 1 diabetes: genetic heterogeneity of diabetes. *Diabet Care* 1998; **21**(4): 658–65
23. Clarke W, Gonder-Frederick L, Richards F, Cryer P. Multifactorial origin of hypoglycemic symptom unawareness of IDDM association with defective glucose counter-regulation and better glycemic control. *Diabetes* 1991; **40**: 680–85
24. Cox D, Gonder-Frederick L, Antoun B, Cryer P, Clarke W. Perceived symptoms in the recognition of hypoglycemia. *Diabet Care* 1993; **16**: 519–27
25. Weinger K, Jacobson A, Draelos M, Finkelstein D, Simonson D. Blood glucose estimation and symptoms during hyperglycemia and hypoglycemia in patients with insulin-dependent diabetes mellitus. *Am J Med* 1995; **98**: 22–31
26. Cox D, Gonder-Frederick L, Clarke W. Driving decrements in type 1 diabetes during moderate hypoglycemia. *Diabetes* 1993; **42**: 239–43
27. Driesen N, Cox D, Gonder-Frederick L, Clarke W. Reaction time impairment in insulin-dependent diabetes: task complexity, blood glucose levels, and individual differences. *Neuropsychol* 1995; **9**(2): 246–54
28. Gonder-Frederick L, Cox D, Driesen N, Ryan C, Clarke W. Individual differences in neurobehavioral disruption during mild and moderate hypoglycemia in adults with IDDM. *Diabetes* 1994; **43**: 1407–12
29. Quillian W, Cox D, Gonder-Frederick L, Driesen N, Clarke W. Reliability of driving performance during moderate hypoglycemia in adults with IDDM. *Diabet Care* 1994 **17**(11): 1367–8
30. Clarke W, Cox D, Gonder-Frederick L, Julian D, Schlundt D, Polonsky W. Reduced awareness of hypoglycemia in IDDM adults: a prospective study of hypoglycemia frequency and associated symptoms. *Diabet Care* 1995; **18**: 517–22
31. Cryer P. Iatrogenic hypoglycemia as a cause of hypoglycemia-associated autonomic failure in IDDM: a vicious cycle. *Diabetes* 1991; **41**: 255–60
32. Hepburn D, Patrick A, Eadington D, Ewing D, Frier B. Unawareness of hypoglycaemia in insulin-treated diabetic patients: prevalence and relationship to autonomic neuropathy. *Diabet Med* 1990; **7**: 711–17
33. Ovalle F, Fanelli C, Paramore D, Hershey T, Craft S, Cryer P. Brief twice-weekly episodes of hypoglycemia reduce detection of clinical hypoglycemia in type 1 diabetes mellitus. *Diabetes* 1998; **47**: 1472–9

34. Cox D, Clarke W, Gonder-Frederick L, Pohl S, Hoover C, Snyder A, Zimbleman L, Carter W, Bobbitt S, Pennebaker J. Accuracy of perceiving blood glucose in IDDM. *Diabet Care* 1985; **8**: 529–36
35. Cox D, Gonder-Frederick L, Kovatchev B, Julian D, Clarke W. Understanding error grid analysis. *Diabet Care* 1997; **20**(6): 911–12
36. Dedrick R, Davis W. What do statistics really tell us about the quality of the data from self-monitoring of blood glucose? *Diabet Med* **6**: 267–73
37. Cox D, Carter W, Gonder-Frederick L, Clarke W, Pohl S. Blood glucose awareness training in IDDM patients. *Biofeed Self-Reg* 1988; **13**: 201–17
38. Cox D, Gonder-Frederick L, Lee J, Julian D, Carter W, Clarke W. Blood glucose awareness training among patients with IDDM: effects and correlates. *Diabet Care* 1989; **12**: 313–18
39. Cox D, Gonder-Frederick L, Julian D, Cryer P, Lee J, Richards F, Clarke W. Intensive versus standard blood glucose awareness training (BGAT) with insulin-dependent diabetes: mechanisms and ancillary effects. *Psychosom Med* 1991; **53**: 453–562
40. Nurick M, Bennett-Johnson S. Enhancing blood glucose awareness in adolescents and young adults with IDDM. *Diabet Care* 1991; **14**(1): 1–7
41. Gonder-Frederick L, Snyder A, Clarke W. Accuracy of blood glucose estimation by children with IDDM and their parents. *Diabet Care* 1991; **14**(7): 565–70
42. Cox D, Gonder-Frederick L, Polonsky W, Schlundt D, Julian D, Clarke W. A multicenter evaluation of blood glucose awareness training—II. *Diabet Care* 1995; **18**(4): 523–8
43. Moses J, Bradley C. Accuracy of subjective blood glucose estimation by patients with insulin-dependent diabetes. *Biofeed Self-Reg* 1985; **10**(4): 301–14
44. Roales-Nieto J. Blood glucose discrimination in insulin-dependent diabetics: training in feedback and external cues. *Behav Modification* 1988; **12**(1): 116–32
45. Cox D, Gonder-Frederick L, Schroeder D, Cryer P, Clarke W. Disruptive effects of acute hypoglycemia on speed of cognitive and motor performance. *Diabet Care* **16**: 1391–3
46. Cox D, Gonder-Frederick L, Kovatchev B, Julian D, Clarke W. Driving impairment during progressive hypoglycemia: occurrence, awareness and correction. *Diabet Care* (in press)
47. Kovatchev B, Cox D, Gonder-Frederick L, Schlundt D, Clarke W. Stochastic model of self-regulation decision making exemplified by decisions concerning hypoglycemia. *Health Psychol* 1998; **17**(3): 277–84
48. Kovatchev B, Cox D, Gonder-Frederick L, Young-Hyman D, Schlundt D, Clarke W. Assessment of risk for severe hypoglycemia among adults with IDDM. *Diabet Care* 1998; **21**(11): 1870–75
49. Cranston I, Lomas J, Maran A, Macdonald I, Amiel S. Restoration of hypoglycemia unawareness in patients with long duration insulin dependent diabetes mellitus. *Lancet* 1994; **344**: 283–7
50. Fanelli C, Epifano L, Rambotti A, Pampanelli S, Di Vincenzo A, Modarelli F, Lepore M, Annibale B, Ciofetta M, Bottini P, Porcellati F, Santeusanio F, Brunetti P, Bolli G. Meticulous prevention of hypoglycemia normalizes the glycemic thresholds and magnitude of most neuroendocrine responses to, symptoms of, and cognitive function during hypoglycemia in intensively treated patients with short-term IDDM. *Diabetes* 1993; **42**: 1683–9
51. Kinsley B, Weinger K, Bajaj M, Levy C, Quigley M, Simonson D, Cox D, Jacobson A. A blood glucose awareness and intensive diabetes treatment. *Diabet Care* 1999 (in press)

52. The Diabetes Control and Complications Trial Research Group. Hypoglycemia in the diabetes control and complications trial. *Diabetes* 1997; **46**: 271–86
53. Reichard P, Phil M. Mortality and treatment side-effects during long-term intensified conventional insulin treatment in the Stockholm Diabetes Intervention Study. *Diabetes* 1994; **43**: 313–17
54. Cox D, Gonder-Frederick L, Julian D, Clarke W. Long-term follow-up evaluation of blood glucose awareness training. *Diabet Care* 1994; **17**(1): 1–5
55. Gonder-Frederick L, Cox D, Kovatchev B, Schlundt D, Clarke W. A biopsychobehavioral model of risk of severe hypoglycemia. *Diabet Care* 1997; **20**: 661–9

8

Cognitive-Behavioural Group Training

NICOLE CW VAN DER VEN[a], MARLÈNE CHATROU[b] and FRANK J SNOEK[a]

[a]Vrije Universiteit Hospital, Amsterdam, The Netherlands; [b]Ignatius Ziekenhuis, Breda, The Netherlands

INTRODUCTION

While the benefits of intensive therapy and the importance of self-management in the treatment of diabetes are well established, it is clear that adhering to every aspect of the treatment regimen is hard for most, if not all, patients[1,2].

In the past decades, there has been a growing interest in the role of cognitive and motivational factors as determinants of self-management behaviour. Several social-cognitive models have been developed, of which the stress-coping model by Lazarus and Folkman[3] is a widespread example, that describes the way people cope with stressors in general. In this model, behavioural and emotional coping with a stressor (e.g. the demands of a chronic disease) are largely determined by evaluations of the personal meaning of these demands (e.g. how much of a threat is this to other important lifegoals) and an appraisal of one's own capacities to meet these demands (coping capacities). Other models are specifically developed to explain health-related behaviour, of which the Health Belief Model (HBM)[4,5] is the best known. The HBM is explained in more detail by Doherty and colleagues (this volume). Such models take into account beliefs patients hold about themselves, about the disease and about the treatment regimen. These beliefs include, for example: 'self-efficacy'[6], the belief that one is capable of

Psychology in Diabetes Care. Edited by Frank J. Snoek and T. Chas Skinner.

successfully performing the required behaviour, and 'locus of control'[7,8] or 'perceived control'[9,10], the degree to which people believe their lives are under their own control; beliefs about the disease and its treatment, including beliefs about benefits of and barriers to treatment, vulnerability to and severity of complications derived from the HBM; 'personal models' of diabetes[11,12], including beliefs about cause, symptoms, course and consequences of the disease; and beliefs about the effectiveness of treatment.

It is assumed that people are most likely to follow self-care recommendations when they believe: (a) that they are vulnerable and susceptible to chronic or acute complications; (b) that these complications will have a serious negative impact on their lives; (c) that following recommendations will be beneficial in reducing the threat or severity of diabetes and its complications; (d) that psychological costs or barriers associated with the treatment are outweighed by its benefits; (e) that they are capable of performing the required behaviour[13]; and that their own behaviour is responsible for their health, instead of others' behaviour (e.g. the doctor's) or luck or fate[8].

Studies into the relationship between health beliefs, on the one hand, and adherence to self-care recommendations in people with diabetes, on the other, have yielded varied results. In a number of studies, beliefs related to disease and treatment have been found to be associated with adherence[13–25], glycaemic control[26,27] or both[28–30]. Believing that one is capable of performing the behaviours required by the regimen, and that these behaviours are responsible for health-outcomes, are also positively associated with adherence to treatment recommendations[31–35] and glycaemic control[36–40]. Other studies however, have found no association between health beliefs and treatment outcome, or have found associations that appear counterintuitive. Brownlee-Duffeck and associates[29] found, for example, that greater perceived susceptibility was positively related to poorer control.

The varying results and sometimes unexpected directions of associations between health beliefs and behaviour are partly due to methodological inconsistencies. Samples are often small and non-random, most studies are retrospective in nature, and concepts have been operationalized and applied differently across studies. Furthermore, the psychometric properties of the questionnaires used are not always well-established, and generic as well as diabetes-specific instruments are applied. As McNabb[41] and others have demonstrated, adherence is a complex construct and difficult to assess. A specific problem when measuring patients' beliefs stems from the dynamic inter-relationships between beliefs and outcomes, with beliefs influencing outcomes and vice versa. Feelings of vulnerability, for example, may give rise to improvement of glycaemic control, which might in turn result in reduced feelings of vulnerability[42].

What becomes clear, however, is that thoughts people hold about their disease, their expectancies of the treatment regimen and self-efficacy strongly influence their intention to engage in self-management activities. A major difference with psychological trait variables, such as intelligence and personality, is that these beliefs are not static and universal but rather dynamic and susceptible to change[43]. This implies that self-management, and ultimately glycaemic control, could be enhanced by altering dysfunctional beliefs. This is in line with Lazarus[44], one of the founders of the stress-coping model, who states that cognitive evaluations and appraisals especially are important starting points in altering coping behaviour.

COGNITIVE-BEHAVIOURAL THERAPY

A clinical model that is used in psychotherapy to modify cognitions (the way a person interprets events), was developed by A.T. Beck, the founder of cognitive-behavioural therapy. This model can be helpful in understanding and modifying the beliefs of people with diabetes.

Cognitive therapy, originally developed to treat depression[45] and anxiety[46], has been successfully applied to a wide array of psychological problems, ranging from personality disorders to eating disorders and substance abuse[47]. Cognitive therapy is described as:

> ...an active, directive, time-limited, structured approach...based on an underlying theoretical rationale that an individual's affect and behaviour are largely determined by the way in which he structures the world. His cognitions (verbal or pictorial 'events' in his stream of consciousness) are based on attitudes or assumptions (schemas), developed from previous experiences.[45]

In other words, central to cognitive therapy is the assumption that behaviour and emotions are in constant interaction with cognitions. These cognitions or beliefs may be inaccurate, leading to excessive emotional reactions and a failure to cope effectively. The aim of cognitive therapy is to help patients identify their dysfunctional cognitions, test them against reality and alter them, thereby modifying emotional disturbances and improving coping behaviour.

The assignment of meanings, explanations and expectations to internal and external events is thought to be accounted for by 'cognitive schemata', also called 'core beliefs' or 'automatic thoughts'. Core beliefs are highly individual, are formed by past experiences, and are activated by particular events within or outside the person[48]. When underlying cognitive schemata are mainly negative in content, the processing of incoming information will be distorted, resulting in unpleasant, maladaptive feelings and behaviour. Depressed patients, for example, often show a characteristic cognitive pattern, consisting of a negative view of themselves, the future and the world surrounding them. This can result in feelings of inadequacy, worthlessness and blame directed at oneself, hopelessness and apathy with regard to the future and a world that is unjust and excessively demanding.

Cognitive techniques used in CBT to help patients alter these negative automatic thoughts involve monitoring negative automatic thoughts and recognizing the interactions between cognition, affect and behaviour. The patient is invited to examine the evidence for his/her automatic thoughts and to substitute distorted cognitions with more realistic ones. In effect, patients learn to identify and alter the underlying beliefs which lead them to think in a distorted way[45].

A therapeutic approach that is closely related to the work of Beck and stems from the same period, is rational-emotive therapy (RET), developed by Albert Ellis. Identical to CBT, Ellis states that thinking, feeling and acting are in constant interaction. One of the statements most central to Ellis's work is the phrase by the ancient Greek, Epictetus[49]: 'People are disturbed not by things, but by the views they take of them'. Dysfunctional beliefs in RET are termed 'irrational beliefs' and can, according to Ellis, be classified in three main categories: (a) demandingness towards the self ('I must, under all circumstances, perform well and have the approval of others; if not, that is awful and makes me an incompetent and unworthy person!'); (b) demandingness towards others ('You must treat me nicely, otherwise it is terrible and you are bad, unworthy people!'); and (c) demandingness towards the world ('The conditions under which I live must at all times be easy and enjoyable; if not, I can't stand it and life isn't worth living!'). Obviously, these beliefs can result in a variety of negative emotional states, including anxiety, self-hatred, anger, depression and dysfunctional behaviours such as procrastination, withdrawal, phobias and addictions[50]. RET has been applied to a wide variety of emotional and behavioural problems, and although there are various theoretical and philosophical differences between the two approaches, RET and CBT are not that different in clinical practice. An element important to note is the 'ABC Model' that is used in RET to identify and challenge irrational beliefs. This model is further explained in the section on content of CBGT.

COGNITIVE-BEHAVIOURAL THERAPY IN DIABETES AND OTHER SOMATIC DISORDERS

As CBT and RET have become well-established in the treatment of psychological disorders, their application has widened to the treatment of patients with various medical conditions. Information on the effect of psychosocial interventions in diabetes is meager, and often lacks systematic, quantitative evaluation[51]. Interventions that are described in the literature can be categorized either as psychotherapy, support groups or coping-oriented groups. To our knowledge there are no reports on cognitive-behavioural group interventions that are studied in a controlled randomized design.

Studies on the use of cognitive techniques in individual psychotherapy in diabetes include a study in which the effects of individual cognitive analytic therapy (CAT) are compared to diabetes education[52]. Glycaemic control improved in both conditions, but improvements were maintained in the longer term in the CAT group only. In addition, patients receiving CAT experienced fewer interpersonal difficulties in the longer term. To date, the only experience with CBT directed specifically at adults with diabetes is a randomized, controlled trial on the efficacy of CBT for type 2 patients suffering from depression[53]. In this study, the effects of CBT were compared to the effects of no specific antidepressant treatment in patients receiving diabetes education. Ten individual sessions of CBT proved to be an effective treatment for depression (85% of the treated patients achieved remission, compared with 27.3% of the controls). There were no direct effects on glycaemic control, but improvements were seen in the CBT group at 6 month follow-up. The prognosis for recovery was worse when complications of diabetes were present and when compliance with blood glucose monitoring was poorer[54]. The majority of patients with diabetes, however, do not suffer from depression, although affective disorders appear to be more prevalent than in the general population[55].

Many patients do have difficulty coping with the diabetes regimen. Various group interventions have been described, aimed at helping patients to cope more effectively with their diabetes. These coping-oriented group interventions typically consist of problem-solving and/or social skills training. The short and structured nature of these interventions seems to have positive effects on attendance[56] and assertiveness[57]. Uncontrolled studies with adolescents found increases in assertiveness[58] and problem-focused coping[59]. In controlled studies, a trend was found towards reduced depression, increased self-esteem and a greater use of emotion-focused coping[60], improved glycaemic control[61], improved coping abilities[62], and a reduction of diabetes-specific distress[63]. In two recent studies, a coping skills training (CST)[64] and a behavioural programme to improve adherence and stress management[65] were compared to standard medical care. Both interventions had positive effects on emotional well-being, which were maintained at follow-up. In participants of CST, glycaemic control also improved.

Beneficial effects of coping-oriented group interventions were demonstrated in adults, including improvements in self-reported compliance and self-confidence[66]. The number of participants in this study was, however, very small and there was no formal evaluation. A behavioural group programme developed by Zettler and colleagues[67], teaching participants strategies to cope with complications, was aimed at reducing anxiety and avoidance behaviour, encouraging adherence, and preparing patients with type 1 diabetes for crises. Analysis of dysfunctional health beliefs was used as a cognitive strategy. The intervention resulted in a reduction of fear and an enhanced acceptance of the disease. Rubin and colleagues[68] added two sessions of diabetes-specific coping skills training, focusing on attitudes and beliefs underlying self-care, to an outpatient education programme. This training, containing cognitive-behavioural elements, resulted in an improvement of emotional well-being and HbA1c, an increase in SMBG, and a decrease of bingeing 6 months after the intervention. Positive effects on self-esteem, anxiety, diabetes knowledge and self-efficacy were maintained at 12 months follow-up[69]. In a study by Anderson *et al.*[70], the effects of a six-session patient empowerment programme were evaluated in a randomized, waiting list-controlled trial. The aim of the programme was to improve goal setting, problem-solving skills, emotional coping, stress management, obtaining social support and motivation. The intervention resulted in improvements in self-efficacy in these domains and reduced HbA1c.

In a review of cognitive approaches in various somatic disorders, Emmelkamp and Van Oppen[71] found that though the relative contribution of cognitive therapy varies, positive effects are well established. In controlled studies, positive effects were found for patients with chronic pain, which were maintained at follow-up. Cognitive-based interventions also proved effective in the treatment of tension headaches. Reduction of emotional distress following cognitive programmes has been reported in HIV-seropositive men and patients with various forms of cancer. Applied to self-management training in patients with asthma, cognitive therapy resulted in improved coping behaviour, increased compliance to medication and less preoccupation with the disease in daily life. Patients with irritable bowel syndrome experienced a reduction of symptoms. The evidence for effects on risk factors for cardiovascular disorders (e.g. hypertension, components of type A behaviour, smoking) and on weight loss in obese patients remains inconclusive. In the treatment of bulimia, however, substantial changes in bingeing and vomiting and improvements in psychosocial problems are reported.

More recent randomized controlled trials of cognitive-behavioural-based group interventions continue to show encouraging results that vary for different somatic conditions and different groups of patients. For patients with chronic pain, beneficial effects are found[72,73]. Positive effects of a behavioural programme were magnified by adding a cognitive component[74]. For patients with fibromyalgia, this was not the case[75], possibly due to poor compliance and difficulty of the programme[76]. In patients with cancer, a cognitive approach led to decreased pain[77], reduced distress and improved psychosocial functioning[78]. In HIV-seropositive patients, improved cognitive coping and social support seemed related to enhanced psychological well-being and quality of life[79]. Two studies show a reduction of symptoms in patients with irritable bowel syndrome, and a reduction of signs of depression[80,81]. In patients with rheumatoid arthritis, a decrease in pain, emotional distress and disease activity eventually resulted in a reduction of clinic visits and hospitalization. Only minor changes in coping behaviour were found, possibly due to the progressive status of the illness[82]. In several studies, beneficial effects were maintained at long-term follow-up[83–86].

We can conclude that the application of cognitive approaches in diabetes and other somatic disorders show promising results. Additional advantages of CBGT-based programmes are that these interventions can be delivered by professionals with varying backgrounds (including psychologists, diabetes educators/nurse specialists, doctors and social workers), are relatively short and can be transferred to other centres. In the next section, the content and effects will be discussed of a group intervention based on cognitive-behavioural therapy that was developed and evaluated at our centre.

COGNITIVE-BEHAVIOURAL GROUP TRAINING (CBGT)

INTRODUCTION

Cognitive-Behavioural group training (CBGT) is a psycho-educational intervention developed by Snoek and colleagues[87] at the Vrije Universiteit Hospital, Amsterdam, in collaboration with Jacobson and associates at the Joslin Diabetes Center, Boston. CBGT was designed to be delivered in an outpatient setting, by a team of a diabetes nurse specialist and a psychologist. The overall goal of CBGT is to help patients to cope more effectively with their diabetes regimen, in order to improve glycaemic control, without compromising, and possibly enhancing, psychological well-being. CBGT is based on principles from cognitive-behavioural therapy (CBT) and rational emotive therapy (RET). Several cognitive and behavioural techniques (cognitive restructuring, stress-management, cueing) are used to help patients to diminish diabetes-related distress, to reduce perceived barriers to various aspects of self-management and to enhance coping skills. This should result in improved self-care behaviour and consequently in improved glycaemic control.

Rubin, Walen and Ellis[88] describe that in diabetes, apart from the regimen being demanding, unpleasant and having negative side-effects, a major reason for low adherence is the pessimistic belief that 'trying hard does not work'. Multiple failures to control the diabetes can give rise to feelings of frustration, hopelessness and anger. Feelings of guilt can develop from the patient's belief that he/she must have done *something* wrong. Such feelings of distress foster a negative attitude towards diabetes and self-care, encouraging people to 'let it all go' instead of keeping up the effort, thereby reinforcing the negative cycle of negative emotions leading to poor management and control, giving rise to even more negative feelings.

This view is in line with the cognitive model: past experiences with diabetes may give rise to cognitive distortions that colour present events. When these past experiences have been mainly negative, events in the present will easily trigger negative automatic thoughts that, in turn, result in unpleasant feelings towards diabetes and inadequate self-management. Examples of cognitive distortions that might occur in people with diabetes are: the belief that blood glucose levels depend on 'chance' and are beyond personal control; the belief that sticking to the treatment will have no positive effects on blood glucose levels or future complications; the conviction that one is not capable of meeting all the demands imposed by the regimen. Such beliefs can easily lead to unpleasant emotions and poor self-management.

CBGT is designed to deal with a broad range of problems, addressing various themes. To evaluate which patients benefit most, what problems are best resolved and what the effects of CBGT are in the longer term, this intervention was piloted in a 2-year study. In the following sections, formative and summative evaluations of four CBGT groups that took part in this study are described, preceded by an outline of the intervention[89].

FORMAT AND CONTENT OF THE TRAINING

CBGT comprises four consecutive weekly meetings of 2 hours, and is delivered in small groups of five to eight participants, by a psychologist and diabetes educator. During sessions, coffee, tea and snacks are available at no charge. A CBGT trainer's manual has been developed, and a set of brochures that are handed out the week prior to each class. Four themes are addressed in four sessions: (a) the way cognitions affect emotions and behaviour—developing a different view on diabetes and self-care; (b) stress and metabolic control—ways to cope with stressful situations; (c) diabetes, complications and the future—ways to cope with worries and insecurity; and (d) diabetes and social relationships—ways to obtain support from your environment. The content of the four sessions is summarized below.

Session 1: a cognitive-behavioural model of diabetes

At the beginning of the first session, it is emphasized that sticking to self-care recommendations all the time is difficult for most people. Following the *cognitive-behavioural model*, it is explained that when people do not succeed in maintaining normal glucose levels, this can give rise to negative thoughts (e.g. 'I will never get my diabetes under control'). Negative thoughts can result in negative feelings (e.g. frustration, hopelessness, disappointment), which can in turn be detrimental to (self-care) behaviour. This is illustrated by drawing upon the ABC method used in RET: the way Activating events (A) have emotional and behavioural Consequences (C), mediated by cognitive Beliefs (B). Then it is explained how rational (or 'helping') beliefs can be the underlying motive for good self-care, and irrational (or 'blocking') beliefs can make living with diabetes more difficult. To find out whether thoughts are irrational, four questions are considered—Is this belief true, is there proof for what I'm thinking? Does this belief help me to achieve my goals? Does it help me to avoid negative, unwanted feelings? Does it help me to avoid problems or conflicts with my social environment? Irrational beliefs are then challenged for Discussion (D) and replaced by more rational, helping beliefs, which lead to the Effect (E): the desired behaviour and adequate feelings in the activating situation. An example of a worksheet, filled out during CBGT, is given in Figure 8.1 (these worksheets are also used for homework assignments).

Participants practise in small subgroups with the RET principles by applying them to personal situations in which they were not satisfied with their behaviour or feelings towards their diabetes (e.g. a situation in which their self-care behaviour was not optimal or they felt anxious or depressed). Results are discussed in the larger group. At the end of the first session, homework assignments are given. Participants are asked to fill out ABC worksheets in the coming week regarding situations in which they are bothered by either their emotions or their behaviour towards diabetes. They are asked to write down as clearly as possible the Activating event, the unwanted Consequences, and the Beliefs that gave rise to this behaviour and feelings.

Session 2: Stress

Session two starts with discussing and 'harvesting' homework in pairs. Participants discuss their irrational beliefs and try to replace them by more rational, helping thoughts. This is followed by a plenary discussion with the aid of a flip-over board.

After a short break, the topic of '*stress and diabetes*' is introduced. The various ways in which stress can result in poor control (through physiological and behavioural pathways) are discussed, and how being in poor control can be a stressful experience in itself. Various sources of stress in daily life are discussed, and the effects on blood glucose levels that

Homework assignment session 1

We discussed thoughts that interfere with good control. To identify and change irrational or 'blocking'' thoughts, the ABC method is used.

This week, fill out three ABCs in situations in which you have difficulty getting your blood glucose in good control.

- In A: Give a short description of the activating event
- In C: write down the consequences: your feelings, and what you do/ don't do.
- Next, in **B**: write down your beliefs or thoughts in this situation. It might help to consider what you 'told yourself'.
- In **E**: write down how you would like to feel and what you would ideally do.
- In **D**: challenge the beliefs in B for discussion. Try to determine for each belief whether it is true, it helps you to reach your goal, it helps you to prevent unwanted feelings and if you can recognize any thinking-errors.

A. Activating event: 'I check my blood glucose and the reading is high '	
B. Beliefs: (what did you think/ tell yourself?) - 'I'll never be able to get it right'	**D. Discussion:**
C: Consequences: how did you feel? - nervous - tense - …………… **What did you do/didn't you do?**	**E. How would you like to feel?** **What would you ideally do?**

Figure 8.1. ABC worksheet for homework assignments during CBGT

participants have observed. After this, the role of irrational thoughts leading to stress is highlighted and stress-management techniques are reviewed. As a tool to reduce stress, a relaxation exercise (based on progressive muscle-relaxation) is practised. Homework assignments consist of filling out ABC worksheets related to stressful situations during the next week, keeping records of blood glucose values in stressful situations and daily practising of relaxation techniques.

Session 3: complications and the future

The third session starts with a review of homework assignments, in the same way as described in Session two. The theme *'complications and worries about the future'* is introduced after the break. First, it is explained that fear and anxiety are 'normal' and adaptive, i.e. protect us from harm. Several ways to cope with fear and worries are discussed, with two ends of the continuum being: from not thinking about it at all, i.e. trying to push away anxious thoughts whenever they surface, to actual confrontation, i.e. 'thinking through' anxiety provoking thoughts. The latter approach involves reflection on 'how realistic are my fears?' 'What can I do when my fears become truth?' By doing so, the thought loses much of its threat, while pushing anxious thoughts away usually is not effective in reducing fear and takes a lot of energy. An anxiety-exploration exercise is performed individually, where participants indicate what fears they have (see Table 8.1). This is used to start group discussion, focusing on how fear can be a motivation to develop an active coping style.

As a homework assignment, participants are asked to fill out ABC worksheets in situations in which worries and apprehension about complications and the future arise. A typical activating event that gave rise to a considerable amount of distress and worry was brought in by one of the participants:

Table 8.1. Exercise—exploration of anxiety

1. In what situation do you experience excessive anxious thoughts about your future?
   - What are you afraid of?
   - How can you tell that you're afraid?
   - Can other people see that you're afraid?
   - When does it happen?
   - What do you do about it (do you talk to someone?) when the fear increases?
   - What does the fear look like in daily life?
   - How does this fear affect your life and your diabetes?
2. What is the worst that could happen to you?
3. How bad would this be for you? (rate from 1 to 100)
4. How likely is it that this will happen?
5. What can you do to make excessive fear manageable/functional?

'I see someone in a wheelchair in the doctor's waiting room'. Thoughts causing the distress were explored (e.g. 'Surely there's no escape from complications for me'; 'My life will be worthless if I end up in a wheelchair'), and disputed by asking questions like: 'What's the proof for what I'm thinking?'; 'Does it help me to achieve my goals and to avoid unpleasant emotions?'. Rational alternatives were formulated for irrational, negative thoughts.

Session 4: social relationships

In session four, ABC worksheets are reviewed to identify and challenge irrational beliefs that give rise to fear and hamper adequate self-care behaviour. The theme of *'diabetes and social relationships'* is introduced. In group discussion, several topics are discussed—What are reasons (not) to tell others about your diabetes (e.g. in relationships, at work)? What positive and negative experiences did you have, and how do you deal with the positive and negative reactions of others? Suggestions are exchanged on how to increase positive and reduce negative experiences.

An example, contributed by one of the participants, involved a situation in which she feared experiencing a hypoglycaemic episode in public. In exploring her beliefs ('They should not notice something is wrong, otherwise they'll think I'm pathetic'. 'I'll have to explain myself, and I don't want to. What will they think of me?' 'I have to get out of this as soon as possible!'), it became apparent that the underlying core-belief was one of self-demandingness: 'I must, under all circumstances, perform well and have the approval of others; if not, I'm incompetent and unworthy!' This belief triggered anxiety and made her tense, resulting in 'acting as if nothing was wrong', i.e. not testing her blood glucose.

The session is followed by a short formative evaluation.

SELECTION OF PATIENTS

Participants in CBGT were recruited from the Diabetes Outpatient Clinic of the Vrije Universiteit Hospital. Potential candidates were approached either in the department of Medical Psychology or during their routine visit to their diabetologist or diabetes educator. Patients showing interest received a leaflet explaining the goal and procedures of CBGT.

Included were patients between 18 and 50 years of age, with type 1 diabetes diagnosed at least 12 months before. Other criteria for inclusion were poor glycaemic control (HbA1c over 8%) and on intensive therapy, i.e. multiple (two or more) daily injections of insulin or pump therapy. Excluded were patients with a severe medical illness other than diabetes, or severe disabling complications of diabetes. Also, for obvious reasons, patients unable to speak or read Dutch, abusing alcohol or drugs, being mentally retarded or currently under treatment for a severe mental disorder were excluded from the study.

From October 1997 to November 1998, a total of 24 patients participated in CBGT, in four groups of five to seven participants. Approximately two-thirds of the patients that were approached declined from participation. The main reasons for not participating were: a lack of time, or not being able to assure attendance at all four meetings (due mainly to work or holidays). Four patients enrolled in this pilot despite the fact that they did not meet inclusion criteria (one participant with insulin-dependent type 2 diabetes, two participants with HbA1c values under 8%, and one patient with severe complaints of neuropathy). Most participants were already familiar with psychological treatment or counselling: ten participants had received psychological help at our hospital, four others had received counselling by a social worker in the past. Sociodemographic and medical characteristics of participants at baseline are shown in Table 8.2.

Prior to CBGT, 'readiness to change' and motivation for participation were checked in an interview, conducted by a psychologist. Patients were also asked what they thought was the cause of not achieving tight control, and what they experienced as the most burdensome feature of living with diabetes. Some patients did not express explicit worries about their regulation, and had no specific ideas about the causes of their poor control: 'I have no idea, I guess I'm just used to high blood glucose'. More explicit named causes were: an irregular lifestyle, and not monitoring blood glucose as often as they should: 'I guess I haven't accepted it, I can't seem to fit it into my life. Having to monitor my blood glucose is a great burden'. Food, especially eating too much and not adjusting food properly, was also mentioned by some patients. A few participants had more specific ideas about their own

Table 8.2. Characteristics of participants at baseline

Sex	Male	9
	Female	15
Age	(years)	35.17 (±11.13; 20–58)
Education	High school or less	12
	College or more	12
Duration of diabetes	(years)	17.62 (±9.35; 3–40)
Insulin therapy	Conventional (two injections)	2
	Intensive (> three injections)	17
	CSII	5
HbA1c		9.22 (±1.19; 7.10–12.80)

CSII: Continuous subcutaneous insulin infusion (pump therapy)

role: 'There is a direct relation between my regulation and me being actively involved in it or pushing it aside. I can see a direct result of my own efforts'.

Aspects of diabetes that were experienced as most burdensome were: hypoglycaemia, the risk of late complications, weight problems, over-eating in case of hypoglycaemia, blood glucose monitoring, blood glucose fluctuations, and having to deal with diabetes every day. Some statements: 'I worry most about the large fluctuations in daily measurements. Being forced to pay constant attention, especially when I can't get my glucose under control'. 'The most burdensome is not being able to take a break. Monitoring your blood glucose is like being graded at school. You're constantly wondering: how did I do?'

The primary expectation most participants had of CBGT was 'lowering my HbA1c'. The way in which they hoped to achieve this differed, however. Most participants entered CBGT with an open mind and an expectant attitude, saying 'I hope to learn something, although I'm not quite sure what'. Some were somewhat sceptical: 'I'm very curious what you [the therapists] can do about it in four meetings'. Others hoped to gain more motivation or 'Get clear what I can do myself to keep my glucose in a good range'. Sharing experiences with others was also an important motive: 'Meeting people that are seriously working at it, to learn from them'.

OUTCOMES OF CBGT

In this section, the effects of CBGT will be described in terms of changes in diabetes-related psychological functioning (emotional distress, coping behaviour), perceived barriers, self-care, glycaemic control and emotional well-being. At this moment, data are available for 16 participants (the first three groups of CBGT) at 3 months follow-up. One participant did not complete questionnaires in time, and was excluded from the analyses.

PSYCHOLOGICAL ASSESSMENT

To assess psychological characteristics and self-care behaviours of participants, several self-report questionnaires (see Table 8.3) were administered. These assessments (with the exception of the SCL-90) were done before, and 3 and 6 months after the intervention. High scores on these scales indicate more distress, barriers or worries.

Table 8.3. Assessment measures

Measure	Items	Subscales	Scoring range	
			Items	Total
SCL-90	90	Anxiety/Agoraphobia/Somatic complaints/Depression/ Insufficient thinking or behaviour/Suspicion or interpersonal sensitivity/ Hostility/Sleep disturbances	1–5	90–450
HFS-worry	13	Fear of hypoglycaemia	1–5	13–65
BDQ	25	Attitude towards SMBG and advice from care providers (6)/Perceived difficulties in injecting, SMBG, self-regulation (6)/Perceived difficulties in self-regulation in specific situations (9)	1–5	25–125
WBQ-12	12	Positive well-being (4)/Negative well-being (4)/Energy (4)	0–3	0–36
PAID	20	Diabetes-specific emotional distress	1–6	0–100
DSCI-1	12	(a) SMBG/Physical exercise/Mild hypoglycaemia	(a) Frequency/week	
		(b) Omitting insulin-injections/Injecting less insulin than needed/ Skipping meals/Foot-inspection/Not reacting to high blood glucose/Severe hypoglycaemia/Drinking too much alcohol	(b) Frequency/mth	
		(c) Smoking	(c) Yes/no	
		(d) Taking diabetes into account when eating/ drinking	(d) 1–5	

Psychological profile

Current psychological functioning was assessed following the interview, using the Symptom Checklist-90 (SCL-90)[90]. SCL-90 scores show elevated levels of psychological dysfunctioning among the participants. On every subscale as well as on the total scale, eight to 12 participants have scores up to or above the 80th percentile, compared to a normal population. Only five participants with high scores had received treatment at the department of Medical Psychology, and one patient had started antidepressant medication recently. Others had not received any psychological or psychiatric treatment.

Diabetes-related distress

Diabetes-related distress was assessed using a Dutch version of the Problem Areas In Diabetes (PAID) questionnaire[91]. As we expected, feelings of distress regarding diabetes are very distinct in this group. The amount of distress varies greatly, with PAID scores ranging from 16 to 76. Four patients reported before the intervention that they did not experience any problems, while six patients indicated that they experienced serious problems (defined as an item score $\geqslant 5$ on a scale of 1–6) in a lot (6–11) of areas. Compared to a sample of insulin-dependent type 1 and type 2 patients[92], a vast majority of patients reported experiencing one or more serious problems in living with diabetes (83.3% vs. 60.2%). The mean PAID score of 37.93 (± 15.07) is also higher than mean scores reported for unselected IDDM outpatients (32.9 ± 20.2)[91].

Individual PAID items endorsed as serious problems ($\geqslant 5$ on a scale of 1–6) by at least 25% of the participants were: 'Not knowing whether moods or feelings are related to blood glucose levels', 'Worrying about low blood sugar reactions', 'Worrying about the future and the possibility of serious complications', 'Coping with complications of diabetes', 'Uncomfortable interactions around diabetes with family or friends', 'Feeling guilty or anxious when getting off-track with diabetes management' and 'Not accepting diabetes'.

After CBGT, the mean PAID score ($n = 16$) decreased significantly from 41.64 (± 15.67) to 33.14 (± 12.08; $p = 0.007$). The mean number of problems decreased from 4.44 to 2.25 ($p = 0.005$). Of the six participants that experienced six or more serious problems, four improved considerably.

Perceived barriers

Barriers to self-management were assessed using the Perceived Barriers in Diabetes Self-care scale (BDQ)[93]. The mean score at baseline (61.04 ± 13.50) indicates that participants do not report greater barriers in performing self-care behaviours than a sample of 240 type 1 and type 2 diabetic outpatients[93]. Individual BDQ items that are endorsed as a serious barrier most often (scoring more then two standard deviations above normal scores) are items concerning self-monitoring of blood-glucose, difficulties in maintaining normal blood-glucose levels in special situations (on weekends, when under stress) and items concerning hypoglycaemia.

Scores varied greatly between participants: 14 patients did not experience any barriers, seven patients experienced some barriers (one to three high scores), three patients reported many barriers (seven to eight high scores).

At 3 months follow-up, there were slight decreases on all subscales (mean total score dropped from 65.44 ± 13.97 to 61.19 ± 13.51). The attitude towards SMBG and advice given by care providers became more positive (from 17.94 ± 5.08 to 15.63 ± 4.69; $t = 2.23$, $p = 0.04$).

Fear of hypoglycaemia

Another potential barrier to good glycaemic control, fear of hypoglycaemia, was measured by the worry scale of the Hypoglycaemia Fear Survey (HFS)[94,95]. Fear of hypoglycaemia is not prominent in the group as a whole (mean score 29.78 ± 11.07). However, looking at individual scores, two participants appeared to score far above the range.

At 3 months follow-up, no significant changes in fear of hypoglycaemia were found for the group as a whole. However, one participant had an increased worry-score (29–42), without an increase in hypoglycaemic episodes, while two others had considerably lower scores (drops from 26 to 17 and from 61 to 54). Alhough this last change may be an important improvement clinically, it still indicates a high level of fear.

Emotional well-being

Changes in emotional well-being were evaluated using the short form of the Well-Being Questionnaire (WBQ-12)[96,97] with a higher total score indicating greater well-being. Mean total score (23.86 ± 5.47) and subscale scores are comparable to those found in a large sample of Dutch diabetic patients and a sample of 464 Japanese type 1 and type 2 patients[98]. At follow-up, mean total score on the WBQ increased slightly (22.6 ± 5.83 to 24.0 ± 1.09; $n = 15$). Positive well-being even increased significantly (6.94 ± 2.41 to 7.63 ± 2.55; $t = -2.42$; $p = 0.029$), indicating that improvement of HbA1c did not occur at the cost of well-being.

SELF-CARE BEHAVIOUR

Self-management behaviours over the past month and frequency of mild and severe hypoglycaemia were assessed using a short adapted form of the Diabetes Self-Care Inventory-1 (DSCI-1)[99] (see Table 8.3).

As with psychological parameters, self-reported self-care behaviour varied greatly among participants. Five participants adhered to practically every aspect of self-care as measured in our survey, while others deviated from most recommendations. The degree of non-adherence varied from participants not inspecting their feet to not performing SMBG at all. Given this large inter-individual variation, the effects of CBGT are likely to be differential: every participant has his/her own areas of potential improvement. Alhough a detailed description of individual patterns goes beyond the scope of this chapter, some points will be highlighted:

- *Self-monitoring of blood glucose (SMBG)*, in our view a central component of self-management, was performed two to four times daily—as recommended—by half the participants. Eight participants measured their blood glucose three times a week at the most. Three patients measured blood glucose five to eight times a day (n = 23). Alhough we expected participants to improve their adherence, at follow-up this was true for only one out of seven non-adherers.
- *Omission of insulin injections* was reported by nine patients; seven skipped injections two to three times a month; two patients even two to four times a week. All others reported sticking to their recommended number of insulin injections.
- *Injecting less insulin than needed* once a week or more often was reported by 11 patients.
- *Taking diabetes into account when eating or drinking* was reported by seven patients to be the case some of the time, while five patients never or rarely took their diabetes into consideration when eating/drinking. Only one of them improved this behaviour at follow-up.
- *Skipping meals* occasionally occurred in nine patients, while four people skipped meals at least every other day (two of whom also reported skipping insulin injections).
- *Not taking any action while being aware of high blood glucose* was reported by 10 patients, varying from one to eight occasions in the past month. One participant wrote that this might happen to her every day, because she never measured her blood glucose. At follow-up, she reported monitoring her blood glucose occasionally.
- *Not doing any physical exercise* was reported by nine patients.
- *Drinking too much alcohol* in the past month was reported by six participants.

GLYCAEMIC CONTROL

As parameters for glycaemic control, HbA1c values (4.3–6.1%) and self-reported frequency of mild and severe hypoglycaemia were obtained.

HbA1c

At baseline, nine participants were in moderately poor control (HbA1c 8–9%), nine were in poor control (HbA1c 9–10%), four were in very poor control (HbA1c >10%). Two participants appeared to be in fairly good glycaemic control when their most recent HbA1c was checked. They were included in the study based on their own conviction and that of their doctors that they were poorly controlled.

HbA1c at baseline and follow-up is shown in Table 8.4. At 3 months follow-up, mean HbA1c improved from 9.57 (±1.22) to 8.86 (±1.38; $t = 1.83$, $p = 0.088$). Table 8.4 shows that substantial changes in HbA1c (over 0.5%) occurred for 12 participants. Nine of them improved, three had higher HbA1c after CBGT. Of interest is that all participants in very poor control (group 3) improved, some even drastically. In group 2, results varied; in the group with lowest initial HbA1c, three participants improved. Also shown are HbA1c values available at 6 months follow-up. Mean HbA1c for these 14 participants improved from 9.50 (±1.23) to 8.61 (±0.99; $t = 3.63$, $p = 0.003$). Table 8.4 shows that two participants who did not benefit at 3 months improved eventually.

Hypoglycaemia

Episodes of severe hypoglycaemia (requiring the assistance of others) in the month prior to CBGT were reported by three participants. Two of them experienced one episode, one participant, already mentioned for her fear of hypoglycaemia, reported three episodes. At follow-up, she did not report

Table 8.4. HbA1c at baseline, 3 months and 6 months follow-up

Baseline	3 month follow-up	6 month follow-up
Group 3—very poor control		
12.8	9.7 (−3.1)	10.1 (−2.7)
11.1	7.4 (−3.7)	–
10.4	9.8 (−0.6)	10.1 (−0.3)
10.3	8.9 (−1.4)	8.9 (−1.4)
Group 2—poor control		
9.9	9.2 (−0.7)	8.7 (−1.2)
9.6	7.1 (−2.5)	7.5 (−2.1)
9.6	11.8 (+2.2)	9.4 (−0.2)
9.5	9.7 (+0.2)	8.4 (−1.1)
9.5	10.9 (+1.4)	8.7 (−0.8)
9.2	9.9 (+0.7)	10.0 (+0.8)
9.0	8.6 (−0.4)	–
Group 1—moderately poor control		
8.9	7.2 (−1.7)	7.3 (−1.6)
8.7	8.2 (−0.5)	8.5 (−0.2)
8.6	7.6 (−1.0)	7.9 (−0.7)
8.6	7.9 (−0.7)	7.6 (−1.0)
7.4	7.8 (+0.4)	7.5 (+0.1)

any episodes. Another participant, however, reported three episodes after the intervention.

The mean number of mild hypoglycaemic episodes before intervention was 2.87 (range 0.5–10.5 ± 2.38) a week, with most patients reporting one or two reactions a week (n = 13), which is common. Three patients reported more then five episodes a week. At 3 months follow-up, one participant reported an enormous increase of mild hypoglycaemic episodes (from 2 to 28 per week). Even without this extreme increase, the mean number of episodes doubled (from 2.07 ± 1.32 to 4.17 ± 3.47; n = 15).

As is shown by the PAID scores, low blood glucose is a matter of concern for many patients. The increase of hypos may be directly related to the observed improvement in glycaemic control. Also, it is likely that participants have become more aware of hypoglycaemia.

FORMATIVE EVALUATION

At the end of the last session, CBGT was evaluated by means of anonymous evaluation forms regarding appreciation of content and format of CBGT.

CBGT was appreciated by all 21 participants who filled out the form, rated 7.6 on a scale from 1 to 10. Three-quarters would 'absolutely' recommend others to participate in CBGT. Difficulty and pace of the sessions were adequate for practically all participants. The duration of the programme (4 weeks) and the length of the sessions (2 hours) was considered as too short by half the participants and exactly right by the other half.

The content of CBGT was rated as reasonably clear and appealing to most patients. What they found most useful was exchanging experiences with other group-members, followed by practising RET principles. This is especially interesting, since many patients stated in the interview that they were reluctant about participating in a group. The theme that was most appreciated was 'the effect of cognitions on emotions and behaviour'.

It was stated by most patients that they had learned most from the experiences of others: 'Experiences of others, who have different feelings and behaviours in comparable situations, taught me that certainties I had about myself are not always true'. They also indicated that CBGT helped them to put things into perspective: 'I encountered other insights, different views. I'm not using them yet, but I know I could look at it differently'. Other remarks were related to the specific content of RET: 'More understanding of the how and why of my actions'. Some participants had a feeling of more control: 'Being more aware that I am in control, or at least can strive for more control'; 'Don't ask *why*, but *how* can I do better!'

More than half of the participants indicated they felt that CBGT had changed them, in particular towards being more open, confident and at ease.

They also took their diabetes more seriously: 'I have come to accept diabetes as being a part of me, rather than a series of lab-results'.

IMPLICATIONS AND FUTURE DIRECTIONS

Based on our preliminary results, we can conclude that CBGT is feasible and appreciated by the patients. Moreover, CBGT appears to be successful in improving HbA1c while reducing diabetes-related distress and preserving well-being.

An important question to ask is who benefits most and who least. Interestingly, HbA1c of patients with relatively high SCL-90 scores at baseline seems to improve even more than that of patients with low to normal SCL-90 scores. The five participants who did not profit from CBGT, in terms of lowering HbA1c, could not be characterized as a group in terms of sociodemographic characteristics, psychological functioning, perceived barriers, well-being or self-care behaviour. Changes on these measures were similar to those in other participants.

While HbA1c improves, preliminary results do not show consistent improvements in self-care behaviour, although some patients show a remarkable change. Further research into the mediating factors in improving glycaemic control is therefore warranted.

Although homogeneity of groups is often advocated in group therapy, differences in age, duration of diabetes and other characteristics in the groups had no observable adverse effect. Living with diabetes apparently provided sufficient 'common ground'. What did become clear to us, is that it is crucial to pay ample attention to the patients' motivation for participation and 'readiness to change' prior to CBGT. Patients in persistent poor control who indicate that they do not experience any specific areas of distress should perhaps first be assisted in identifying their specific problem areas before participating in a CBGT programme.

It has been decided to add two classes to CBGT, extending CBGT from four to six sessions. These sessions will involve the themes of 'goal setting' and 'how to be a patient'. The first theme will be added to focus more on self-care behaviour, to help patients set out individual, realistic goals for the intervention. These goals will be monitored and adapted during sessions if necessary. The combination of goal setting and feedback should be especially effective in facilitating the mastery of new skills[100], and may help to heighten motivation and increase the amount of time invested in homework assignments.

The session on 'how to be a patient' will focus on adopting an assertive, active attitude, to get the most out of contacts with health care providers. In our experience, education and information are widely available in The Netherlands, but are not always extensively used.

Adding two sessions will increase the amount of time and effort participants will have to invest in CBGT, and may negatively impact attendance. But we have reason to believe that the extended programme will prove to be more effective in terms of glycaemic control and emotional well-being.

CBGT seems highly cost-effective, especially considering that most participants had been in persistent poor control for quite some time and are therefore prone to developing complications that would lead to high costs in terms of medical care in the future. Delivering a programme like CBGT requires the availability of a skilled diabetes educator and a psychologist during the sessions, and a psychologist to interview patients prior to participation.

Considering the observed beneficial effects of CBGT, dissemination of CBT in diabetes care deserves to be promoted. This can be achieved by training diabetes educators and psychologists in the principles of CBT, and by protocolizing and transferring CBGT programmes to other centres and health care professionals. The 6-week CBGT programme will be studied in a randomized, controlled trial, and new research projects studying the efficacy of CBGT in adolescents with diabetes and type 2 patients are under way.

REFERENCES

1. DCCT Research Group. The effect of intensive treatment of diabetes on the development and progression of long-term complications in insulin-dependent diabetes mellitus. *N Engl J Med* 1993; **329**(14): 977–86
2. Ruggiero L, Glasgow RE, Dryfoos JM, Rossi JS, Prochaska JO, Orleans CT, Prokhorov AV, Rossi SR, Greene GW, Reed GR, Kelly K, Chobanian L, Johnson S. Diabetes self-management. Self-reported recommendations and patterns in a large population. *Diabet Care* 1997; **20**(4): 568–76
3. Lazarus RS, Folkman S. *Stress, Appraisal and Coping*. New York: Springer, 1984
4 Becker MH. The health belief model and personal health behaviour. *Health Educ Monogr* 1974; **2**: 324–473
5. Becker MH, Janz NK. The Health Belief Model applied to understanding diabetes regimen compliance. *Diabet Educ* 1985; **11**(1): 41–7
6. Bandura, A. Self-efficacy: toward a unifying theory of behavioral change. *Psychol Rev* 1977; **84**(2): 191–215
7. Rotter JB. Generalised expectancies for internal versus external control of reinforcement. *Psychol Monogr* 1966; **80**: 1–28
8. Wallston KA, Wallston BS, De Vellis R. Development of the multidimensional health locus of control (MHLC) scales. *Health Educ Monogr* 1978; **6**: 160–70
9. Weiner B. A theory of motivation for some classroom experiences. *J Educ Psychol* 1979; **71**: 3–25

10. Bradley C. Measures of perceived control of diabetes. In Bradley C (ed) *Handbook of Psychology and Diabetes*. Amsterdam: Harwood Academic, 1994
11. Leventhal H, Nerenz DR, Steele DJ. Illness representations and coping with health threats. In Baum A, Taylor SE, Singer JE (eds) *Handbook of Psychology and Health*, vol 4. Hillsdale NJ: Erlbaum, 1984
12. Hampson SE. Illness representations and the self-management of diabetes. In Petrie KJ, Weinman JA (eds) *Perceptions of Health and Illness*. Amsterdam: Harwood Academic, 1997
13. Rosenstock IM. Understanding and enhancing patient compliance with diabetic regimens. *Diabet Care* 1985; **8**(6): 610–16
14. Alogna M. Perception of severity of disease and health locus of control in compliant and noncompliant diabetic patients. *Diabet Care* 1980; **3**(4): 533–4
15. Bloom Cerkoney KA, Hart LK. The relationship between the Health Belief Model and compliance of persons with diabetes mellitus. *Diabet Care* 1980; **3**(5): 594–8
16. Lockington TJ, Meadows KA, Wise PH. Compliant behaviour: relationship to attitudes and control in diabetic patients. *Diabet Med* 1986; **4**: 56–61
17. Wilson W, Ary DV, Biglan A, Glasgow RE, Toobert DJ, Campbell DR. Psychosocial predictors of self-care behaviors (compliance) and glycemic control in non-insulin dependent diabetes mellitus. *Diabet Care* 1986; **9**(6): 614–22
18. Hampson SE, Glasgow RE, Toobert DJ. Personal models of diabetes and their relations to self-care activities. *Health Psychol* 1990; **9**(5): 632–46
19. Weerdt I De, Visser AP, Kok G, van der Veen EA. Determinants of active self-care behaviour of insulin treated patients with diabetes: implications for diabetes education. *Soc Sci Med* 1990; **30**(5): 605–15
20. Jacobson AM, Adler AG, Derby L, Anderson BJ, Wolfsdorf JI. Clinic attendance and glycemic control. Study of contrasting groups of patients with IDDM. *Diabet Care* 1991; **14**(7): 599–601
21. Bond GG, Aiken LS, Somerville SC. The health belief model and adolescents with insulin-dependent diabetes mellitus. *Health Psychol* 1992; **11**(3): 190–98
22. Hampson SE, Glasgow RE, Foster LS. Personal models of diabetes among older adults: relationship to self-management and other variables. *Diabet Educ* 1995; **21**(4): 300–307
23. Aalto AM, Uutela A. Glycemic control, self-care behaviors, and psychosocial factors among insulin treated diabetic: a test of an extended health belief model. *Int J Behav Med* 1997; **4**(3): 191–214
24. Glasgow RE, Hampson SE, Strycker LA, Ruggiero L. Personal-model beliefs and social-environmental barriers related to diabetes self-management. *Diabet Care* 1997; **20**(4): 556–61
25. Palardy N, Greening L, Ott J, Holderby A, Atchison J. Adolescents' health attitudes and adherence to treatment for insulin-dependent diabetes mellitus. *J Dev Behav Pediat* 1998; **19**(1): 31–7
26. Sjöberg S, Carlson A, Rosenqvist U, Ostman J. Health attitudes, self-monitoring of blood glucose, metabolic control and residual insulin secretion in type I diabetic patients. *Diabet Med* 1988; **5**: 449–53
27. Lewis KS, Jennings AM, Ward JD, Bradley C. Health belief scales developed specifically for people with tablet-treated type 2 diabetes. *Diabet Med* 1990; **7**(2): 148–55
28. Harris R, Linn MW. Health beliefs, compliance, and control of diabetes mellitus. *South Med J* 1985; **78**(2): 162–6
29. Brownlee-Duffeck M, Peterson L, Simonds JF, Kilo C, Goldstein D, Hoette

S. The role of health beliefs in the regimen adherence and metabolic control of adolescents and adults with diabetes mellitus. *J Consult Clin Psychol* 1987; **55**(2): 139–44

30. Polly RK. Diabetes health beliefs, self-care behaviors and glycemic control among older adults with non-insulin-dependent diabetes mellitus. *Diabet Educ* 1992; **18**(4): 321–7
31. McCaul KD, Glasgow RE, Schafer LC. Diabetes regimen behaviors. Predicting adherence. *Med Care* 1987; **25**(9): 868–81
32. Padgett DK. Correlates of self-efficacy beliefs among patients with non-insulin dependent diabetes mellitus in Zagreb, Yugoslavia. *Patient Educ Counsel* 1991; **18**: 139–47
33. Hurley CC, Shea CA. Self-efficacy: strategy for enhancing diabetes self-care. *Diabet Educ* 1992; **18**(2): 147–50
34. Littlefield CH, Craven JL, Rodin GM, Daneman D, Murray MA, Rydall AC. Relationship of self-efficacy and bingeing to adherence to diabetes regimen among adolescents. *Diabet Care* 1992; **15**(1): 90–94
35. Kavanagh DJ, Gooley S, Wilson PH. Prediction of adherence and control in diabetes. *J Behav Med* 1993; **16**(5): 509–22
36. Grossman HY, Brink S, Hauser ST. Self-efficacy in adolescent girls and boys with insulin-dependent diabetes mellitus. *Diabet Care* 1987; **10**(3): 324–9
37. Bradley C, Lewis KS, Jennings AM, Ward JD. Scales to measure perceived control developed specifically for people with tablet-treated diabetes. *Diabet Med* 1990; **7**: 685–94
38. Peyrot M, Rubin R. Structure and correlates of diabetes-specific locus of control. *Diabet Care* 1994; **17**(9): 994–1001
39. Day JL, Bodmer CW, Dunn OM. Development of a questionnaire identifying factors responsible for successful self-management of insulin-treated diabetes. *Diabet Med* 1996; **13**: 564–73
40. StenstrÖm U, Wikby A, Andersson PO, Ryden O. Relationship between locus of control beliefs and metabolic control in insulin-dependent diabetes mellitus. *Br J Health Psychol* 1998; **3**: 15–25
41. McNabb WL. Adherence in diabetes: can we define it and can we measure it? *Diabet Care* 1997; **20**(2): 215–8
42. Bradley C, Gamsu DS, Moses JL, Knight G, Boulton AJM, Drury J, Ward JD. The use of diabetes-specific perceived control and health belief measures to predict treatment choice and efficacy in a feasibility study of continuous subcutaneous insulin infusion pumps. *Psychol Health* 1987; **1**: 133–46
43. Bradley C. Health beliefs and knowledge of patients and doctors in clinical practice and research. *Patient Educ Counsel* 1995; **26**: 99–106
44. Lazarus RS. Progress on a cognitive–motivational–relational theory of emotion. *Am Psychol* 1991; **46**(8): 819–34
45. Beck AT, Rush AJ, Shaw BF, Emery G. *Cognitive Therapy of Depression*. Chichester: Wiley, 1980
46. Beck AT, Emery G. *Anxiety Disorders and Phobias: a Cognitive Perspective*. New York: Basic Books, 1985
47. Salkovskis PM (ed). *Frontiers of Cognitive Therapy.* New York: Guilford, 1996
48. Beck AT. Beyond belief: a theory of modes, personality, and psychopathology. In Salkovskis PM (ed) *Frontiers of Cognitive Therapy.* New York: Guilford, 1996
49. Epictetus. *The Collected Works of Epictetus*. Boston: Little, Brown, 1890
50. Ellis A. *Reason and Emotion in Psychotherapy* (revised and updated edn). New York: Birch Lane Press, 1994

51. Rubin RR, Peyrot M. Psychosocial problems and interventions in diabetes. A review of the literature. *Diabet Care* 1993; **15**(11), 1640–57
52. Fosbury JA, Bosley CM, Ryle,A, Sonksen PH, Judd, SL. A trial of cognitive analytic therapy in poorly controlled type 1 patients. *Diabet Care* 1997; **29**(6): 959–64
53. Lustman PJ, Griffith LS, Freedland KE, Kissel SS, Clouse RE. Cognitive behavior therapy for depression in type 2 diabetes mellitus. A randomized, controlled trial. *Ann Intern Med* 1998; **129**(8): 613–21
54. Lustman PJ, Freedland KE, Griffith LS, Clouse RE. Predicting response to cognitive behavior therapy of depression in type 2 diabetes. *Gen Hosp Psychiat* 1998; **20**: 302–6
55. Gavard JA, Lustman PJ, Clouse RE. Prevalence of depression in adults with diabetes: an epidemiologic evaluation. *Diabet Care* 1993; **16**: 1167–78
56. Citrin WS, Furman SG, Girden E. Diabetes in adolescence: group assertiveness training and the traditional "Rap" group. *Diabetes* 1983; **32**(37A, suppl 1)
57. Follansbee DJ, La Greca AM, Citrin WS. Coping skills training for adolescents with diabetes. *Diabetes* 1983; **32**(37A, suppl 1)
58. Smith KE, Schreiner B, Jackson C, Travis LB. Teaching assertive communication skills to adolescents with diabetes: evaluation of a camp curriculum. *Diabet Educ* 1993; **19**(2): 136–41
59. Smith KE, Schreiner B, Brouhard BH, Travis LB. Impact of a camp experience on choice of coping strategies by adolescents with insulin-dependent diabetes mellitus. *Diabet Educ* 1991; **17**(1): 49–53
60. Marrero DG, Myers GL, Golden MP, West D, Kershnar A, Lau N. Adjustment to misfortune: the use of a social support group for adolescent diabetics. *Pediat Adolesc Endocrinol* 1982; **10**: 213–18
61. Kaplan RM, Chadwick MW, Schimmel LE. Social learning intervention to promote metabolic control in type I diabetes mellitus: pilot experiment results. *Diabet Care* 1985; **8**(2): 152–5
62. Gross AM, Heimann L, Shapiro R, Schultz RM. Children with diabetes. Social skills training and HbA1c levels. *Behav Modification* 1983; **7**(2): 151–64
63. Boardway RH, Delamater AM, Tomakowsky J, Gutai JP. Stress maangement training for adolescents with diabetes. *J Pediat Psychol* 1993; **18**(1): 29–45
64. Grey M, Boland EA, Davidson M, Yu C, Sullivan-Bolyai S, Tamborlane WV. Short term effects of coping skills training as adjunct to intensive therapy in adolescents. *Diabet Care* 1998; **21**(6): 902–8
65. Mendez FJ, Belendez M. Effects of a behavioral intervention on treatment adherence and stress management in adolescents with IDDM. *Diabet Care* 1997; **20**(9): 1370–75
66. Rabin C, Amir S, Nardi R, Ovadia B. Compliance and control: issues in group training for diabetics. *Health Soc Work* 1986; 141–51
67. Zettler A, Duran G, Waadt S, Herschbach P, Strian F. Coping with fear of long-term complications in diabetes mellitus: a model clinical program. *Psychother Psychosom* 1995; **64**: 178–84
68. Rubin RR, Peyrot M, Saudek CD. Effect of diabetes education on self-care, metabolic control, and emotional well-being. *Diabet Care* 1989; **12**(10): 673–9
69. Rubin RR, Peyrot M, Saudek CD. The effect of a diabetes education program incorporating coping skills training on emotional well-being and diabetes self-efficacy. *Diabet Educ* 1993; **19**(3): 210–14
70. Anderson RM, Funnell MM, Butler PM, Arnold MS, Fitzgerald JT, Feste

CC. Patient empowerment. Results of a randomized controlled trial. *Diabet Care* 1995; **18**(7): 943–9

71. Emmelkamp PMG, van Oppen P. Cognitive interventions in behavioral medicine. *Psychother Psychosom* 1993; **59**: 116–30
72. Newton-John TR, Spence SH, Schotte D. Cognitive-behavioural therapy versus EMG biofeedback in the treatment of chronic low back pain. *Behav Res Ther* 1995; **33**(6): 691–7
73. Basler HD, Rehfisch HP. Follow-up results of a cognitive-behavioural treatment for chronic pain in a primary care setting. *Psychol Health* 1990; **4**(4): 293–304
74. Vlaeyen JW, Haazen IW, Schuerman JA, Kole-Snijders AM, van Eek H. Behavioural rehabilitation of chronic low back pain: comparison of an operant treatment, an operant-cognitive treatment and an operant-respondent treatment. *Br J Clin Psychol* 1995; **34**(1): 95–118
75. Goossens ME, Rutten-van Molken MP, Leidl RM, Bos SG, Vlaeyen JW, Teeken-Grubben NJ. Cognitive–educational treatment of fibromyalgia: a randomized clinical trial. Economic evaluation. *J Rheumatol* 1996; **23**(7): 1246–54
76. Vlaeyen JW, Teeken-Grubben NJ, Goossens ME, Rutten-van Molken MP, Pelt RA, van Eek H, Heuts PH. Cognitive-educational treatment of fibromyalgia: a randomized clinical trial. Clinical effects. *J Rheumatol* 1996; **23**(7): 1237–45
77. Arathuzik D. Effects of cognitive-behavioral strategies on pain in cancer patients. *Cancer Nurs* 1994; **17**(3): 207–14
78. Evans RL, Connis RT. Comparison of brief group therapies for depressed cancer patients receiving radiation treatment. *Publ Health Rep* 1995; **110**(3): 306–11
79. Lutgendorf SK, Antoni MH, Ironson G, Starr K, Costello N, Zuckerman M, Klimas N, Fletcher MA, Schneiderman N. Changes in cognitive coping skills and social support during cognitive behavioral stress management intervention and distress outcomes in symptomatic human immunodeficiency virus (HIV)-seropositive gay men. *Psychosom Med* 1998; **60**(2): 204–14
80. Toner BB, Segal ZV, Emmott S, Myran D, Ali A, DiGasbarro I, Stuckless N. Cognitive-behavioral group therapy for patients with irritable bowel syndrome. *Int J Group Psychother* 1998; **48**(2): 215–43
81. Vollmer A, Blanchard EB. Controlled comparison of incividual versus group cognitive therapy for irritable bowel syndrome. *Behav Ther* 1998; **29**(1): 19–33
82. Kraaimaat FW, Brons MR, Geenen R, Bijlsma JWJ. The effect of cognitive behavior therapy in patients with rheumatoid arthritis. *Behav Res Ther* 1995; **33**(5): 487–95
83. Dworkin SF, Turner JA, Wilson L, Massoth D, Whitney C, Huggins KH, Burgess J, Sommers E, Truelove E. Brief group cognitive behavioral intervention for temporomandibular disorders. *Pain* 1994; **59**(2): 175–87
84. Turk DC, Rudy TE, Kubinski JA, Zaki HS, Greco CM. Dysfunctional patients with temporomandibular disorders: evaluating the efficacy of a tailored treatment protocol. *J Consult Clin Psychol* 1996; **64**(1): 139–46
85. Johansson C, Dahl J, Jannert M, Melin L, Andersson G. Effects of a cognitive-behavioral pain management program. *Behav Res Ther* 1998; **36**: 915–30
86. Moorey S, Greer S, Bliss J, Law M. A comparison of adjuvant psychological therapy and supportive counselling in patients with cancer. *Psycho-Oncol* 1998; **7**(3): 218–28
87. Snoek FJ, van der Ven NCW, Lubach C. Cognitive behavioral group training (CBGT) for poorly controlled type 1 diabetic patients—a psychoeducational approach. *Diabet Spectrum* 1999; **12**(3): 147–52

88. Rubin RR, Walen SR, Ellis A. Living with diabetes. *J Rational Emotive Cogn Behav Ther* 1990; **8**(1): 21–39
89. Snoek FJ, Ven NCW van der, Heine RJ. Improving glycaemic control and well-being: a cognitive behavioural based group training for poorly controlled type 1 diabetes patients. *Diabetes* 1999; **48**(suppl 1): A9 (0037)
90. Arrindell WA, Ettema JHM. SCL-90. Handleiding bij multi-dimensionele psychopathologie indicator [Manual for a multi-dimensional indicator of psychopathology]. Lisse: Swets en Zeitlinger, 1986
91. Welch GW, Jacobson AM, Polonsky WH. The Problem Areas in Diabetes Scale. An evaluation of its clinical utility. *Diabet Care* 1997; **20**(5): 760–66
92. Polonsky WH, Anderson BJ, Lohrer PA, Welch G, Jacobson AM, Aponte JE, Schwartz CE. Assessment of diabetes-related distress. *Diabet Care* 1995; **18**(6): 754–60
93. Mollema ED, Snoek FJ, Heine RJ. Assessment of perceived barriers in self-care of insulin-requiring diabetic patients. *Patient Educ Counsel* 1996; **29**: 277–81
94. Irvine A, Cox DJ, Gonder-Frederick LA. The Fear of Hypoglycaemia Scale. In Bradley C (ed) *Handbook of Psychology and Diabetes*. Chur, Switzerland: Harwood Academic, 1994
95. Snoek FJ, Pouwer F, Mollema ED, Heine RJ. De Angst voor Hypoglycemie Vragenlijst (AHV). Interne consistentie en validiteit [The Fear of Hypoglycaemia Scale. Internal consistency and validity]. *Gedrag Gezondheid* 1996; **24**(5): 287–92
96. Bradley C. The Well-being Questionnaire. In Bradley C (ed) *Handbook of Psychology and Diabetes*. Chur, Switzerland: Harwood Academic, 1994
97. Pouwer F, van der Ploeg HM, Adèr HJ, Heine RJ, Snoek FJ. The 12-Item Well-being Questionnaire: An evaluation of its validity and reliability in Dutch people with diabetes. *Diabet. Care* 1999; **22**(12): 2004–10.
98. Bradley C. Well-being questionnaire (W-BQ): translation and development of a Japanese version, the W-BQ12 [in Japanese]. Unpublished manuscript, 1996
99. Pennings-van der Eerden, LJM. Self-care behaviour in the treatment of diabetes mellitus: theory, assessment and determinants of self-care behaviour and diabetes education. Amsterdam: Thesis, 1992
100. Bandura A. *Social Foundations of Thought and Action: A Social Cognitive Theory.* Englewood NJ: Prentice-Hall, 1986

9

Psychotherapy and Counselling in Diabetes Mellitus

RICHARD R. RUBIN
Johns Hopkins University School of Medicine, Baltimore, MD, USA

INTRODUCTION

The importance of emotional issues in diabetes mellitus has been recognized for centuries. In 1679, Thomas Willis, the British physician who was the first person to recognize the presence of glucose in the urine of people with diabetes, wrote, 'The cause of diabetes is an emotional state I will call extreme sorrow'. Until the past 20 years, those studying the role of psychosocial issues in diabetes concentrated, as Willis had, on psychological *causes* of diabetes. More recently, researchers and clinicians have turned their attention to psychological issues which affect diabetes self-management, and to the sequelae of living with diabetes. This chapter deals with counselling and psychotherapeutic inverventions intended to relieve psychological distress in people with diabetes. Psychological or emotional distress in people with diabetes takes two forms: coping difficulties, which arise as a consequence of the daily stress and hassles of living with the disease; and frank psychopathology[1].

Psychology in Diabetes Care. Edited by Frank J. Snoek and T. Chas Skinner.

COPING PROBLEMS

WHY ARE COPING PROBLEMS SO COMMON?

Coping problems are common among people with diabetes largely because the demands of diabetes management are so substantial and unremitting. Specifically, the regimen is demanding and unpleasant, factors outside the patient's control often affect glycaemic control, and the avoidance of diabetes-related complications can not be guaranteed. Each of these points deserves elaboration. There are no vacations from diabetes. Diabetes management is a 24-hour-a-day, 365-day-a-year proposition. Thus, diabetes affects every aspect of a person's life, including job, social life, recreation and family life. My son, who has had diabetes for 20 years, recently told me that he has had to think about his diabetes at least once every 15 minutes every day for the past two decades. At least that often he stops to ponder how he feels, and what he must do to avoid high or low blood glucose levels. Another thing that makes the diabetes regimen so demanding is the fact that many of its requirements are unpleasant. Few people relish the prospect of sticking themselves with sharp objects four to eight or more times a day, as many people with diabetes must do. And almost everyone feels that diabetes-related dietary restrictions are a major burden.

In addition, my patients often remind me that even when they manage their diabetes by the book, their blood glucose levels are still sometimes unpredictable. Many of these individuals are stress-responsive, and the release of stress-induced counter-regulatory hormones can dramatically affect their glycaemic control. Finally, while the benefits of good glycaemic control are now beyond debate following the release of the results of several large-scale randomized clinical trials[2–5], we can not assure our patients that good glycaemic control offers an absolute guarantee that they will not suffer from diabetes-related complications.

'DIABETES OVERWHELMUS' AND ITS CONSEQUENCES

What is common to all the demands of diabetes which I have just noted is the fact that they can leave a person feeling overwhelmed and unable to cope, a state inimical to an effective effort to manage diabetes and to the achievement of optimal glycemic control.

This sense of being overwhelmed, which I call *'diabetes overwhelmus'*, to parallel diabetes mellitus, the technical name for the disease which affects our patients, is one important factor leading to the low levels of diabetes self-care we see reported in the literature. Robiner and Keel[6] reviewed studies of medication taking, self-monitoring of blood glucose (SMBG), diet, weight management and exercise among people with diabetes, and Ruggiero and colleagues[7] described self-reported self-management patterns in a large sample of people with diabetes. Both studies reported a wide range of findings, with medication taking adherence highest and life-style behaviour adherence lowest. The difficulty most people with diabetes report in their efforts to manage their diabetes effectively is illustrated by my experience at a recent lecture. When I asked the audience of over 2000 people with diabetes to raise a hand if they felt they did everything they should do to manage their disease, two hands were raised. One of these individuals had been diagnosed with diabetes for 1 week and the other for 2 weeks!

THE VAST MAJORITY OF DIABETES CARE IS *SELF*-CARE

Self-care is a critical issue in diabetes because more than 99% of diabetes care is self-care. The vast majority of diabetes care takes place not 2–4 times a year in the health care provider's office, but literally countless times each day in the places where people with diabetes live, work, eat and play.

Levels of self-care and glycaemic control among people with diabetes in the USA are not good. The average HbA1c of a person with type 2 diabetes is 9.5%, representing an average blood glucose level of about 250 mg/dl or about 14 mmol/l. It is apparent that one essential goal of diabetes care is to improve diabetes-related coping skills among people with diabetes and, as a consequence, to improve self-care behaviour, metabolic outcomes and quality of life as well. Quality of life is affected by improved coping skills, both directly, through reduced emotional distress, and indirectly, through the effects of coping skills on self-care, glycaemic control and long-term health outcomes.

RELAXATION TRAINING CAN IMPROVE GLUCOSE TOLERANCE AND REDUCE LONG-TERM HYPERGLYCAEMIA

A variety of studies over the past two decades support the notion that improving stress management or coping skills can improve self-care, metabolic outcomes and quality of life. For example, several studies of people with type 2 diabetes generally report improved glucose tolerance and reduced long-term hyperglycaemia following biofeedback-assisted relaxation training (BART)[8–10]. Evidence for the effectiveness of BART in people with type 1 diabetes is less conclusive. While several studies[11,12] reported positive effects of BART and related treatments for those with type 1 diabetes, others[13–15] found no such benefits. Surwit and Feinglos[15] suggest that sympathetic nervous system activity may be altered only in those with type 2 diabetes, making these individuals more sensitive than those with type 1 diabetes to the effects of stress on glucose metabolism. Elsewhere[16], the same authors suggest that there is probably a subpopulation of type 1 individuals who are stress-responsive and who could benefit from BART, as most people with type 2 diabetes would.

GROUP COPING SKILLS TRAINING CAN IMPROVE COPING, SELF-CARE BEHAVIOUR AND GLYCAEMIC CONTROL

In addition, a wide range of interventions including therapy groups, self-help groups, support groups and diabetes camps have been employed to promote more effective coping with the day-to-day hassles of diabetes. Most of this reseach, which was designed to improve the ability of children and adolescents to use social skills and assertive behaviour for coping effectively with diabetes-related interpersonal situations, involved small numbers of subjects and did not include either a control group or follow-up measures. Most interventions used peer modelling and role-play techniques and took place in group settings. These studies reported benefits such as greater emotional well-being[17–20], enhanced coping skills[21,22], better regimen adherence[23,24] and improved glycaemic control[18,23,24]. Diabetes camps usually include formal or informal interventions designed to enhance the coping skills of young campers. Reported benefits of diabetes camps include shifts in health locus of control orientation toward internal locus of control (i.e. the belief that one's own actions affect health outcomes[25–27]. The effects of a camp may be short-lived, and the two studies that incorporated control groups reported no differences in psychosocial adjustment between campers and non-campers[28,29].

Marrero and colleagues[19] found that adolescents who participated in a series of sessions designed to improve diabetes-related coping skills were less depressed, and also tended to have higher self-esteem and more often used emotion-based coping skills, when compared with a control group. Mendez and Belendez[30] evaluated the effects of a behavioural programme designed to increase treatment adherence and stress management skills in adolescents with type 1 diabetes. This invervention incorporated a variety of procedures, including instruction, blood glucose discrimination training, role playing, relaxation exercises and problem-solving strategies, among others. Improvements that were maintained at 13-month follow-up included reduced barriers to adherence and reduced severity of daily diabetes-related hassles, as well as less uneasiness in diabetes-related interpersonal situations. Anderson and colleagues[23] provided separate group sessions for adolescents and their parents as a supplement to regular diabetes clinic visits. The goal of the adolescent sessions was to increase skill in using SMBG data for regimen adjustments; the goal of the parent sessions was to develop strategies for negotiating appropriate levels of parental involvement in the adolescents' diabetes care. Eighteen months after completion of the 12-session group intervention, adolescents in the treatment group had significantly lower HbA1c and reported significantly more use of SMBG data for selected regimen adjustments than adolescents in a control group.

Group psychosocial interventions have also been employed with adults who have diabetes. These groups generally addressed coping difficulties rather than frank psychopathology. Reported benefits of these interventions, which often lacked control groups, statistical power, or follow-up measures, include increases in: emotional well-being[31–35]; coping skills[33–35]; regimen adherence[33]; and glycaemic control[31]. The only controlled study in this area found an increase in psychological well-being and social function-ing, but these improvements did not differ significantly from those achieved by a lecture control group[35]. Neither group improved in glycaemic control.

SEEING DIABETES CARE THROUGH NEW EYES

If improving coping skills is a key to improving other diabetes-related outcomes, as some of the research cited here suggests, we must attempt to identify critical elements of coping for translation to clinical practice. At the outset, health care providers must recognize the need to see their patients with diabetes through new eyes, and we must help our patients see us and themselves in a different light, as well[36]. Through these new eyes, we must all see diabetes care and our roles in providing it as they really are not as we have been trained to see them. Health care providers are trained to deliver care and education, and many of us are pretty good at doing this. Unfortunately, delivering care to people with diabetes does not fit the realities of diabetes management. As I mentioned earlier, the vast majority of diabetes care is self-care. It takes place countless times each day in our patients' homes, in the places where they work and play, and even in the endless hours many spend talking—or trying to talk—to health care plan representatives.

The fact is, nothing we offer a patient, no matter how brilliant or potentially effective it might be, will do any good unless it makes sense to that patient in the real context of his/her daily life. The longer I work, the clearer it is to me that the best solutions to the myriad day-to-day problems my patients face almost always come from the patients themselves, and not from me. I can help my patients uncover these solutions, and it is my responsibility to do so, but I can not come up with them on my own. I simply do not know enough about my patients' lives to do this. They are the only ones who do. Thus, the principal job of the health care provider is to recognize the essential nature of the patient's expertise and to help the patient apply this expertise to the ongoing task of enhancing coping skills.

KEY ELEMENTS OF DIABETES-SPECIFIC COPING SKILLS TRAINING

The counselling process by means of which the health care provider facilitates the development of diabetes-related coping skills in people with diabetes involves a number of specific techniques. These techniques are designed to help patients identify problematic diabetes-related issues, identify thoughts and feelings associated with these issues, identify attitudes and beliefs underlying the problem and establish self-care goals, and develop and commit to a plan for achieving the goal. These coping skills training techniques, designed to facilitate patients' self-awareness about the cognitive, emotional, social and spiritual components of their lives as they relate to the daily decisions about diabetes care, are described below, and more fully elsewhere[37,38].

Ask questions

While history-taking questions such as, 'Have you been having any low blood sugars lately?' or 'How often are you testing your blood sugar these days?' are important, they are not particularly effective in facilitating diabetes coping and self-management. Questions like 'What's the hardest thing for you right now about dealing with your diabetes?' are more likely to generate the kind of information the health care provider and patient will need to generate a self-care plan which will actually work for a given patient. It is a waste of precious time when the health care provider attempts, visit after visit, to offer recommendations without knowing what is actually bothering the patient most. The provider will end up making suggestions that have no meaning for the patient, and both the provider and patient end up frustrated. Thus, asking questions which facilitate the development of coping and problem-solving skills can actually save valuable time for the health care provider and the patient.

Start with the patient's agenda

Health care providers often feel they know the things their patients need to do to improve their health, as well as the order in which these things need to be done. Unfortunately, operating as if patients will follow the agenda a health care provider sets almost never works. Patients simply veto any suggestions that don't make sense to them. Veto power is rarely expressed directly in words. More often, patients express this veto power by simply not doing what their providers have recommended. Starting with the patient's agenda actually increases the likelihood that the health care provider will accomplish his/her goals for the patient, because when patients see that their needs are the provider's primary concern, openness to the provider's suggestions will likely grow.

Individualize the treatment plan for each patient

Everybody is different, so there is no one-size-fits-all plan that works for every person with diabetes. The key to successful individualization is that fundamental tool: good questions. If the patient's goal is weight loss, for example, the health care provider might ask how much weight the person wants to lose, what success the patient has had losing weight in the past, what facts of life will facilitate and hinder weight loss efforts, and what the patient would like the health care provider to do when it comes to facilitating the weight loss process.

Be as specific as possible in defining the problem you're dealing with

The more specifically the health care provider and patient define a problem, the more likely it is that they will solve it. Once again, questions are the key to success. If a patient complains of difficulties with his/her diet, for example, the educator should help the patient define the problem more specifically. The specific 'sticking point' might turn out to be a problem in resisting late-night snacks, for instance. Most patients have specific sticking points, and identifying these sticking points has two benefits. First, it helps both patient and provider to see that the problem they face is more manageable than they originally believed (i.e. snacking after dinner is less overwhelming than overall dietary failure). Thus, motivation is greater to make necessary changes. Second, identifying ways to cope successfully with specific problem is usually much easier than identifying ways to cope with general problems.

Take a step-by-step approach

Problems no-one could solve all at once, many people can solve one-step-at-a-time. Most diabetes-related problems are daunting. Health care providers can help their patients cut a problem down to size by taking a step-by-step approach. Take establishing an exercise programme, for instance. The health care provider knows that a healthy exercise regimen for most people would involve a minimum of activity equivalent to three brisk 30 minute walks a week. Yet many patients who want to start exercising would feel overwhelmed starting at this level. The health care provider should help the patient identify the first step in initiating the programme. Even if this first step is a modest one, walking for 15 minutes twice a week, for example, the health care provider should try to enthusiastically support the patient's proposal. This support has three benefits. First, it establishes a cooperative working relationship between the health care provider and patient in dealing with a goal the patient has chosen to work on. Second, the first step the patient has suggested is a meaningful one. Walking twice a week for 15 minutes each time is better than not walking at all. Third, a patient who succeeds in taking a first step is likely to have the confidence to take a second step, and a third.

Focus on behaviours, not outcomes

When a health care provider helps a patient work on health behaviours, the outcomes they both seek are more likely to be attained. It is easier to achieve goals such as improved blood sugar control, reduced weight and similar outcomes when both provider and patient focus on the *behaviours* required to reach these goals. Behaviour is something the patient can work on and ultimately control directly, while outcomes such as blood sugar levels are often influenced by factors outside the person's control. Focusing on medical outcomes can lead to feelings of frustration, and even of helplessness. Focusing on behaviour, while not a panacea, increases the patient's sense of control.

Use contracts

Formally contracting with patients to specify what they will do to reach mutually agreed-upon goals can facilitate self-management. A useful behavioural contract should begin with a statement of the patient's goal, stated in specific, measurable, behavioural terms. The goal should be both ambitious and realistic; the contract should also identify the rewards the patient will get for achieving the goal. These rewards may be anything the patient chooses, ranging from sleeping through the night (with improved blood sugar control lessening the need to awaken and urinate), to being alive to see a grandchild graduate from high school, to feeling good about oneself for improved self-care. A final element of the contract is a statement of to whom the patient will turn at the first sign of slipping in efforts to achieve the goal. The patient could identify the health care provider or any other appropriate person for this role.

Involve the family in your patient's care

Diabetes is a family disease. It is powerful enough to affect the lives of everyone who loves, lives with, or cares for a person with diabetes. Family members also significantly affect the way a person with diabetes lives with his/her disease. Involving the family may take several forms. If at all possible (and with the patient's permission), include important family members in office visits. Getting the perspective of family members can be helpful to the health care provider and the patient. When it is not possible to include family members in office visits, the health care provider should ask questions about the involvement of family members in diabetes care. These questions include queries concerning what family members do to facilitate and to hinder self-care, and what the patient would like to see family members do differently to make life with diabetes easier.

Maintain contact with patients between visits

This can be difficult for many health care providers, but research and clinical experience show that even brief, occasional contact with a health care provider can powerfully affect people struggling with a chronic disease. Some effective approaches to maintaining contact include: phone calls, postcards, newsletters, e-mail messages and office-based support groups. Maintaining contact not only helps patients feel cared for, which enhances motivation, it also provides the health care provider with an invaluable early-warning system for problems that might get much worse before the patient calls about them.

Facilitate problem-solving skills

Living well with diabetes requires a high level of problem-solving skill. Diabetes makes life more complicated, so people with diabetes have more problems to solve day-to-day than people who do not have diabetes. Patients develop diabetes-related problem-solving skills through trial and error and continuous practice. As one young man said, 'I hate having diabetes, but it's forced me to be a really good problem-solver, and I wouldn't give that up for anything in the world'.

Nourish emotional coping skills

One of the things people with diabetes need most is a strong emotional foundation. One of the things those who educate and care for people with diabetes need most is skill in helping their patients deal with emotional issues. Resources to help people with diabetes cope with the emotional side of their disease include *Psyching Out Diabetes*[37]. Resources to help health care providers cope with these issues include *Practical Psychology for Diabetes Clinicians*[39].

Get help

The health care provider often needs help because caring for diabetes can be as hard as living with it, although in different ways. Getting help may mean consulting with a colleague to get suggestions for dealing with a difficult issue. Sometimes just talking things out or getting someone else's perspective can help. Getting help may also mean referring a patient for specialized services that the provider is not trained, or does not have the time, to provide.

CASE EXAMPLE OF INDIVIDUAL DIABETES-SPECIFIC COPING SKILLS TRAINING

I have employed this model for coping skills training in my private counselling practice, and I offer here a case example to illustrate its application. Fred, was a 55 year-old man who had been diagnosed with type 2 diabetes 7 years prior to his consultation with me. I began our interview by asking Fred what was the hardest thing for him about his life with diabetes. Fred's response, 'Everything!' immediately identified him as a man suffering from 'diabetes overwhelmus'. I told Fred that if he was like most people with diabetes I had treated he could, with some thought, identify a more specific problem in his diabetes management. Fred pondered this notion, then responded that eating properly was the hardest issue for him. I encouraged Fred to think more deeply and be even more specific, recommending that he consider an image I have found helpful: If one is able to identify a 'sticking point', a problem so specific and concrete that one could take a photograph of it, paint a picture of it, or make a videotape of it, finding a solution to the problem becomes much easier. Fred found this suggestion helpful, and applying himself to the question I'd posed, he responded with his typical humour, 'I'm a grazer; every night between dinner and bed time I'm like a cow, "munch munch here, munch munch there". By the time I'm ready to sleep I feel guilty and sick. Then I'm up half the night urinating'.

Once Fred had identified his sticking point, he felt an immediate sense of relief because he now had a specific problem to work on and because he realized for the first time that he was actually doing quite well with many aspects of his regimen. Now we set to work helping Fred identify the solution to his problem. I began this phase of the work by asking Fred if there was ever a time he did not graze. He answered that there were such times, specifically those occasions when he had stuffed himself so full at dinner that he could not fit in another bite before bed, and those occasions (about once every 2 weeks) when he went to an evening activity at his church. No food was served at these meetings, and Fred said he returned home feeling full spiritually, which sufficed to keep him from grazing before he went to sleep. Since Fred did not want to stuff himself at dinner and his church only held infrequent meetings, we had to search elsewhere for a solution to his problem. I asked Fred if there was ever a time when he didn't stuff himself at dinner and didn't go to church, yet still did not graze. Fred responded that there were such times, but that they were 'once in a blue moon.' I told Fred that even if he had avoided grazing only once under these circumstances it would provide us with guidance. I pointed out that when something has never happened the critical question is whether it could happen. If something has happened even once, this question is no longer valid. Now the question is *how* it happened. And it was this question which we now set out to answer.

I asked what was the difference between those many times when Fred grazed, and those rare occasions when he was not stuffed from dinner, did not go to church, and still did not graze. After thinking a moment, Fred said that the difference was, "something about by attitude, my frame of mind, something I say to myself'. Fred had identified the critical role of cognitions in influencing emotions and behaviour, and he went on to identify the specific thoughts which triggered his grazing. They included the following: 'I've had a hard day; I deserve to eat when I want' or (after his second snack of the evening), 'I've had more to eat this evening than I should; I've already ruined things so it doesn't matter how much more I eat now'. Fred was also able to identify his thoughts on the infrequent occasions when he didn't graze. Fred's first grandchild had been born a few months earlier, and Fred realized that on those occasions when he resisted the urge to graze he said to himself, 'I want to be alive to see that boy walk across the stage and get his high school diploma'. Thus, Fred was able to identify his sticking point and his way to avoid getting stuck.

When I asked Fred how he felt about what we had discovered he said, 'I'm not sure. I see that my thoughts trigger my behaviour, but most of the time by thoughts are negative and so is my behaviour. How does that help me?' I pointed out to Fred that the thoughts that triggered his abstention from grazing, just like those that triggered his grazing, were not thoughts he had been born with. Nor were they thoughts that he had to accept as random events. Thinking in ways that trigger constructive behaviour is a skill, and just like any skill, thinking positively could be learned through persistent practice. Fred decided to practise keeping his grandson in mind by putting pictures of the boy on his refrigerator, on his kitchen cabinets and, eventually, on his bathroom mirror and the headboard of his bed as well. Through this effort Fred reduced his rate of grazing from almost every night to about three nights a week. While this was not a perfect result, it did represent a marked improvement.

COPING SKILLS TRAINING AS AN ELEMENT OF COMPREHENSIVE GROUP DIABETES PSYCHO-EDUCATION

An intervention based on the diabetes-specific coping skills training model I have just described has also been incorporated into the comprehensive 5 day (37 hour) outpatient education programme offered by the Johns Hopkins Diabetes Center at the Johns Hopkins Hospital in Baltimore. Over 3000 participants have completed this programme since its inception in 1984. The programme is taught by a multidisciplinary team of health care providers, including mental health professionals who offer diabetes-specific coping skills training.

As noted earlier, diabetes coping skills training is designed to help people overcome barriers to successful application of new knowledge and skills. The approach used in this programme, a cognitive-behavioural psycho-educational group intervention, focusing on beliefs and attitudes that underlie patterns of self-care, has been described in detail elsewhere[37,40,41]. The training is active and individualized; participants begin the process by identifying their own regimen barriers or 'sticking points'. The more specifically the problem is defined, the easier it is to solve. Even with common issues such as diet adherence, one person's sticking point might be an irrepressible sweet tooth, while another's might be an overpowering urge to 'graze', or continuously snack, after dinner.

Once a personal sticking point has been identified, a problem-solving orientation is invoked. Potential solutions are inventoried, with special attention to those the person has used successfully in the past. This process helps patients learn that certain thoughts or attitudes trigger non-constructive behaviour. The group then works together to identify thoughts or attitudes that have triggered their own pattern of response. Patients learn that the ability to achieve a positive attitude is a skill that they can develop if they practice patiently and persistently. Next, patients are taught how to implement this procedure, how to note successful and less-than-successful outcomes, and how to continuously adapt their approach based on the results.

A final element of the coping skills training intervention is relapse prevention[42]. Since perfect self-care is an ideal no-one can realize, people

Table 9.1. Coping skills training example

First Session (90 minutes)
- *Identify specific regimen problem:* 'grazing' (continuous nibbling) after dinner
- *Identify 'trigger' thoughts for failure:* 'I've already blown my diet (after the first nibble) so it makes no difference what I do now
- *Identify 'trigger' thoughts for success (personal or generated by the group):* 'I've done pretty well with my diet all day. If I stop after the first nibble I can still feel good about myself and I won't be up all night going to the toilet'
- *Practice 'trigger' thoughts for success:* based on a common problem, group participants visualize the problem situation and rehearse solutions

Between Sessions
- *Implement coping skills:* at home, implement approaches learned in first session
- *Identify successful and less-than-successful outcomes:* 'I grazed less than usual, but I did not stop altogether'

Second Session (60 minutes)
- *Refine coping approaches:* add coping tactics, e.g. preparing acceptable snack and then not re-entering kitchen for the rest of the evening, identifying non-food treats (music, social contacts) and incorporate them into evening routine
- *Develop relapse prevention techniques:* 'contracts for change' are completed by all participants. Contracts include cognitive elements ('Remember, everybody slips; your goal is to keep a lapse from becoming a collapse') and behaviour ('When you lapse, use your support network—family, friends, medical staff, and especially other group members'). Group participants are provided with a list of members' phone numbers and encouraged to call when in need of support

must have strategies for coping with inevitable lapses and failures. Patients are helped to develop specific techniques for coping with slips when they occur, in order to prevent lapses from becoming full-blown collapses. A case example of the coping skills training process is described in Table 9.1. The first coping skills training session is held on the morning of the second day of the group education programme, and the second coping skills training session is held on the afternoon of the fourth day of the programme.

BENEFITS OF GROUP PSYCHO-EDUCATION INCORPORATING COPING SKILLS TRAINING

The benefits of the educational programme, which incorporates the coping skills training intervention I have just described, are wide-ranging and robust. Six months after the educational intervention, programme participants improved significantly on: several measures of emotional well-being (including self-esteem, diabetes self-efficacy, depression, and anxiety); several measures of self-care behaviour (including SMBG frequency, medication adherence and adjustment, diet and exercise); and glycaemic control (assessed by HbA1c assay), as compared with their levels at the outset of the program[43]. Improvements in glycaemic control and self-regulation behaviours (SMBG and medication adherence and adjustment) were maintained at 12 month follow-up, as were improvements in all measures of emotional well-being except for depression[40,44].

The Johns Hopkins Diabetes Center educational programme is integrated and multi-faceted, so it is impossible to determine which aspects of the intervention, alone or in combination, were responsible for the benefits I have just noted. The coping skills training component could have contributed to these outcomes in several ways. Diabetes self-efficacy could have been affected directly, and other outcomes such as self-esteem, depression, anxiety, self-care behaviour, and glycaemic control could have been affected indirectly. It is also possible that the programme's benefits flow from other aspects of the intervention, from enhanced self-care skills or changes in medication regimens, for example. A conclusive determination of the benefits of coping skills training will require controlled clinical trials. I look forward to studies in which the control group receives traditional diabetes education and the intervention group receives traditional education supplemented by coping skills training.

The addition of coping skills training seems financially feasible for most diabetes education programmes. Costs for adding this component are relatively low ($35 per patient for the Hopkins programme), and the additional patient time required is relatively small ($2\frac{1}{2}$ hours during the 37 hour educational programme). The most difficult obstacle for establishing any coping skills training programme may be identifying a professional who is sufficiently experienced in diabetes-specific coping skills training. If such a professional is not available, two approaches should be considered. It may be possible to identify a mental health professional who is interested in developing expertise in working with people who have diabetes. Alternatively, diabetes health care providers who are not mental health specialists may be interested in developing expertise in coping skills training. This approach is teachable, and I have had success in training professionals to implement this intervention. Given the apparent benefits of this intervention, I think a strong case can be made for incorporating coping skills training into diabetes education programmes.

PSYCHOPATHOLOGY

The relationship between diabetes and clinical psychiatric disorders has received increased attention over the past 15 years. According to some estimates, almost half of all people with diabetes have a diagnosable psychiatric disorder at some point during their lifetimes[45]. Depression and anxiety disorders are the most common diagnoses and occur far more often in people with diabetes than in the general US population[46]. These disorders can result in glycaemic disregulation directly via alterations in neurochemical and neurotransmitter functioning, and indirectly via disruption of diabetes self-care.

The number of documented cases of eating disorders among people with diabetes appears to be growing[47,48]. While it is not clear whether these disorders are more prevalent among people with diabetes than they are in the general population[49], eating disorders have been associated with poor glycaemic control and an increased risk for retinopathy[48]. Depression, anxiety disorders and eating disorders can be treated effectively, but all tend to recur and require repeated treatment. A detailed discussion of depression, anxiety disorders and eating disorders among people with diabetes follows, along with counselling and psychotherapeutic treatment modalities for each disorder.

DEPRESSION IS COMMON, SEVERE, AND HAS ESPECIALLY ADVERSE CONSEQUENCES AMONG PEOPLE WITH DIABETES

Depression appears to be more common among people with diabetes than it is in the general population. While estimates of the prevalence of depression vary, it likely affects at least one of every five people with diabetes[46]. Some studies suggest that approximately 40% of people with diabetes have significantly elevated levels of depressive symptomatology, although they are not all diagnosably clinically depressed[45]. In a study of 634 people with diabetes, higher rates of depression were found in women, those who were unmarried, and those with lower levels of education—findings commonly reported in studies of depression in the general population—and in people who had three or more diabetes-related complications. In this study, age, type of diabetes and duration of diabetes were not significantly associated with depression, and the association between depression and HbA1c levels did not reach significance, although there was a tendency for higher levels of depression to be associated with higher levels of HbA1c[45]. Other studies[50–54] have found that HbA1c levels were significantly higher in patients with depression than in those who were not depressed. Levels of diagnosable depression among people with diabetes are about three times the estimated prevalence in the population at large[54].

The course of depression may be more chronic and severe in people with diabetes. Depression is a recurring condition for many such people. Only about 20% of diabetic patients who recover from an episode of depression remain well for more than 5 years. These patients averaged 4.2 episodes of depression over this period.[50] For people with diabetes, individual depressive episodes may be more severe as well as more common. The symptoms of depression and diabetes may exacerbate one another at a neuroendocrine level. For example, hormonal disregulation associated with depression may contribute to glycaemic disregulation (and vice versa)[55].

Depression has especially adverse effects for people with diabetes. Clinical depression can severely hamper the medical management of diabetes. Feelings of helplessness and hopelessness often associated with depression may contribute to a disastrous cycle of poor self-care, worsened glycaemia and deepened depression[56]. Depression has also been associated with increased rates of smoking and substance abuse. Even subclinical depression (i.e. persistent depression symptoms that fall short of the criteria for diagnosing depression) appears to be associated with diminished functioning and increased medical morbidity[57]. All of these studies strongly suggest that effective treatment of depression in people with diabetes can prevent or delay diabetes complications, both macrovascular and microvascular.

DEPRESSION IN DIABETES IS UNDERDIAGNOSED AND UNDERTREATED

Depression remains unrecognized and untreated in a majority of cases, despite its specific relevance to diabetes[54]. Most estimates suggest that only about one-third of people with diabetes and major depression are recognized and treated[58]. Reasons for under-diagnosis of depression in people with diabetes include: the perception that depression in the medically ill is secondary to the medical condition, and thus not of independent importance; and concerns about the accuracy of the diagnosis of depression in persons with diabetes. Some of the symptoms of depression, such as fatigue, or changes in libido, appetite and weight, are also symptoms of hyperglycaemia[51]. Current diagnostic approaches are relatively sensitive in their ability to detect depression in a person with diabetes, even when the patient is chronically hyperglycaemic. The health care provider can screen patients for depression using criteria-based diagnostic techniques, such as those specified in the DSM-IV[59]. Clinical depression is diagnosed when a person has five or more specific symptoms for a period of at least 2 weeks. These symptoms are listed in Table 9.2.

Psychometric instruments like the Center for Epidemiologic Studies Depression Scale[60], the Beck Depression Inventory[61], and the Zung Self-rating Depression Scale[62] are also effective tools for detecting depression in people with diabetes.

EFFECTIVE TREATMENT FOR DEPRESSION IN DIABETES

While there are almost no systematic data available concerning the treatment of depression in people with diabetes, it appears that depression in diabetes

Table 9.2. Symptoms of clinical depression

1. Depressed mood (feeling sad or empty) most of the day, nearly every day
2. Significant weight loss when not dieting, or weight gain (e.g. a change of more than 5% of body weight in a month), or decrease or increase in appetite nearly every day
3. Trouble sleeping or sleeping too much nearly every day.
4. Feeling really agitated or really sluggish physically nearly every day
5. Fatigue or loss of energy nearly every day
6. Markedly diminished interest or pleasure in all, or almost all, activities most of day, nearly every day
7. Feeling worthless or excessively or inappropriately guilty nearly every day
8. Diminished ability to think or concentrate, on indecisiveness, nearly every day
9. Recurrent thoughts of death (not just fear of dying), recurrent thoughts of suicide, or a suicide attempt or a specific plan to commit suicide

may be responsive to psychotherapy. Interpersonal therapy and cognitive-behavioural therapy are both proven treatments for depression in people who have no other medical conditions[63,64]. According to the model from which interpersonal therapy (IPT) is derived, stressful and conflicted relationships cause, maintain and exacerbate depression. IPT helps patients to develop and refine specific skills in communication and social interaction, and it may be particularly useful for those with diabetes, because so many stressful treatment-related situations involve interactions with other people.

Cognitive-behavioural therapy (CBT) is based on the observation that depressed people tend to think in negative, stereotypical ways ('Nobody likes me; I'm a failure'; 'I'll never be able to control by diabetes'). CBT involves a structured programme of cognitive modification or reframing and behavioural activation, which I have already described. Negative, self-defeating thoughts and actions are identified and efforts are made to replace them with more accurate and constructive thoughts and behaviours[41]. Preliminary findings from a controlled study suggest that CBT is robustly effective in the treatment of depression in diabetes[65] Both IPT and CBT help patients build skills for coping better with stressful life circumstances. This may provide these patients some advantage over treatment with antidepressant medication in terms of more lasting relief from depression, a significant advantage given the recurrent feature of depression in diabetes[3].

Based largely on studies of people who do not have diabetes, it can be said that depression in diabetes is probably also treatable with psychopharmacological agents. While a full discussion of this modality is beyond the scope of this chapter, it should be mentioned that Lustman and colleagues[54] recently demonstrated that depression in diabetes could be treated successfully with antidepressant medication. In the first placebo-controlled trial with diabetes patients, 60% of those treated with nortriptyline (a member of the tricyclic class of antidepressants) had a complete remission of their depression, while only 35% of those treated with a placebo were free of depression at the end of the study. This study yielded other important findings. It showed that a complete remission of depression among study participants was associated with a 0.8–1.2% reduction in glycohaemoglogin (GHb) levels over the 8-week study period. As the authors point out, sustained reductions in GHb of this magnitude could decrease the progression of retinopathy by as much as one-third. This study was initiated before newer classes of antidepressant medication, such as the selective serotonin uptake inhibitors (SSRIUs) were widely available. These medications are now probably the most common agents used in treating depression in people with diabetes, as they are for the treatment of depression in the general population. SSRIUs also have advantages for many people with diabetes when compared with the older tricyclic agents, as they tend to have fewer of the anticholinergic, central nervous system, cardiovascular, appetite stimulating, and weight gain side effects than the tricyclics.

ANXIETY DISORDERS ARE COMMON AMONG PEOPLE WITH DIABETES

While little is known about the rate of anxiety disorder among people with diabetes, one study[45] suggests that people who have diabetes may suffer from this disorder as frequently as they do from depression, and at much higher rates than people who do not have diabetes. This study of over 600 people with diabetes found that women, African–Americans, and those with less education were more likely to report symptoms consistent with a clinically significant anxiety disorder. The only diabetes-related predictor of significant anxiety disorder symptons was the presence of two or more long-term diabetes complications. Type of diabetes, duration of diabetes, and glycohaemoglobin level were not associated with an increased risk for anxiety symptomatology. Prevalence studies using structured diagnostic interviews have reported an increased incidence of anxiety disorders, especially generalized anxiety disorder and simple phobia, in people with diabetes[53,66].

The health care provider can screen patients for anxiety by asking a series of simple questions concerning symptoms. Clinical anxiety disorder is diagnosed when a person has been uncontrollably anxious for at least 6 months about a number of events and activities, and during that period has had five or more specific symptoms for more days than not. These symptoms are listed in Table 9.3.

Some of the symptoms of anxiety disorder overlap with those of clinical depression. This is because some psychological problems share similar symptoms and because some people suffer from more than one clinical psychological disorder.

Table 9.3. Symptoms of clinical anxiety disorder

1. Restlessness or feeling keyed up or on edge
2. Being easily fatigued
3. Difficulty concentrating or mind going blank
4. Irritability
5. Muscle tension
6. Sleep disturbance (difficulty falling or staying asleep, or restless, unsatisfying sleep)

Anxiety disorders may be more prevalent among people with diabetes because of additional stresses. Anxiety disorders are an exaggerated emotional response to the normal fears most people have, and people with diabetes often live with sources and levels of fear greater than those most people experience. Fear of hypoglycaemia, complications, and the effects of diabetes on day-to-day life are some of the more common fears reported by people who have diabetes.

Anxiety disorders, like depression, remain largely undiagnosed and untreated in patients with diabetes. In addition, little is known about the effects of anxiety on metabolic control in people with diabetes. It is reasonable to assume that severe anxiety affects quality of life and may affect metablic control indirectly by interfering with diabetes self-care. Unfortunately no research has been conducted to test this hypothesis. The direct effects of anxiety (often conceived of as stress) on glycaemia in people with diabetes has been the subject of numerous studies[67]. The results of this research have been contradictory, as noted earlier in this chapter, with some studies reporting hyperglycaemia responses to stress, while others found no such response.

EFFECTIVE TREATMENT FOR ANXIETY DISORDERS IN PEOPLE WITH DIABETES

Anxiety disorders in some people with diabetes may be responsive to psychotherapy and related treatments. Studies[10] of people with type 2 diabetes report improved glucose tolerance and reduced long-term hyperglycaemia after biofeedback-assisted relaxation training (BART). The effectiveness of BART for those with type 1 diabetes is less clear-cut, although some studies[68] have reported positive findings.

Based largely on studies of people who do not have diabetes, anxiety disorders in diabetes are probably treatable with psychopharmacological agents. Unfortunately, very little information is available on the use of these drugs in people with diabetes. Lustman[69] reported improved glycaemic control in patients treated with alprazolam (Xanax), regardless of whether or not they had a formal diagnosis of anxiety disorder. Treatment with fludiazepam (Erispan), a benzodiazepine, in a small group of patients with type 2 diabetes, resulted in decreased anxiety ratings as well as an increase in high-density lipoproteins[70].

EATING DISORDERS

The problem of eating disorders in people with diabetes has received increased attention in the past few years. Eating disorders appear to be more common in people who have diabetes than they are in the general population, at least in the USA. In contrast, a recent publication[49] reported that in a German multi-centre study, prevalence rates for clinical eating disorders (anorexia nervosa and bulimia nervosa) were not considerably higher for patients with either type of diabetes than they were for the general population.

Eating disorders come in two forms. One, *anorexia nervosa,* involves a severe self-imposed restriction of caloric intake, often combined with extremely high levels of exercise. The other *bulimia nervosa,* involves binge eating followed by purging, usually by means of vomiting or the use of diuretic medications or laxatives. While some young men suffer from eating disorders, the condition is about 10 times more common among young women. This is probably because of the far more intense pressure young women in our society experience to be thin.

The health care provider can screen patients for eating disorders by asking a series of simple questions concerning symptoms. Keep in mind that it may be difficult for a patient to acknowledge an eating disorder. One of the reasons it is difficult to estimate the actual prevalence of eating disorders in people with diabetes is the fact that in this population it is often hard to distinguish between a normal (and even positive) focus on food and body image, which are a part of life with diabetes, and the abnormal concerns and behaviour that indicate the presence of an eating disorder. A clinical eating disorder is diagnosed when a person has any of the signs and symptoms listed in Table 9.4. Some[71] have suggested the concept of an eating continuum with normal at one end, clinical eating disorders at the other end, and subclinical aspects at points in between, as a useful way to view this problem.

Although there is no clear agreement in the literature concerning the prevalence of eating disorders in those who have diabetes, a meta-analysis of the existing data suggests a prevalence 1 to 1.5 times that found in the general population of those the same gender and similar age and educational level[72]. Women who have type 1 diabetes are about 10 times more likely than men with the same diagnosis to have an eating disorder.

Table 9.4. Signs and symptoms of clinical eating disorder

1. Weighs less than 85% of normal for height, body frame and age
2. Has an intense fear of gaining weight or becoming fat, even though underweight
3. Sees self as fat when others say too thin
4. Exercises far more than is necessary to stay fit
5. Misses at least three consecutive menstrual cycles
6. Denies the seriousness of low body weight
7. Binge eats (eats very large amounts of food at a single sitting), at least twice a week for 3 months
8. Feels unable to stop eating or control what or how much is eaten

Eating disorders in diabetes may be particularly devastating

There are some indications that eating disorders in patients with diabetes are more severe than these same disorders in those without diabetes. Hillard and Hillard[73] note many similarities in the eating-disordered behaviours and aetiology of people with type 1 diabetes and people who do not have diabetes. These similarities include the type and symptoms of their eating disorder, underlying personality structure, family history of eating disorder, and other psychiatric diseases. In the same article[73] however, Hillard and Hillard point out a unique and uniquely troubling feature of eating-disordered behaviour common to many young people with diabetes: insulin purging. Recent research[48] suggests that between one-third and one-half of all young women with type 1 diabetes frequently take less insulin than they need for good glycaemic control in order to control their weight.

Eating disorders have especially devastating consequences for a person with diabetes. Eating disordered behaviour, including manipulation of insulin dosage to control weight, can severely compromise diabetes self-care, glycaemic control and medical management. A relationship has been reported between eating problems (especially bulimia) and poor adherence to non-diet aspects of the diabetes regimen[74,75], poor glycaemic control[74,76] and complications[77,78]. Even subclinical disorders can interfere with glycaemic control. Several researchers found that insulin manipulation *per se* was associated with an increased risk for poor metabolic control[80] and microvascular complications[48,78,81,82]. Hepertz and colleagues[49], on the other hand, found that in the German population they studied neither the presence of eating disorders nor insulin omission-influenced glycaemic control.

Eating disorders in people with diabetes are often unrecognized and untreated. As previously noted, differentiating between normal concerns with food and body image and pathological ones can be difficult in patients with diabetes. Those suffering from eating disorders are often resistant to acknowledging the problem. For many of these patients controlling eating feels crucially important, and they are terrified at the prospect of giving up this control, which they feel they will be pressured to do if they acknowledge their disorder. For these reasons, the health care provider must be alert to signs that a patient may be suffering from an eating disorder, especially when the patient is a young woman. These signs include frequent diabetic ketoacidosis (DKA), elevated glycohaemoglobin levels in a knowledgeable patient, anxiety about or avoidance of being weighed, frequent and severe hypoglycaemia, bingeing with alcohol, or severe stress in the family.

Effective treatment for eating disorders in people with diabetes

Eating disorders may be responsive to psychotherapy. Once again, the number of published intervention studies is small, and several of the studies which have been published lack rigour, statistical power, control groups and follow-up measures. With these caveats in mind, one finds in the literature some evidence that psycho-education directed toward specific cognitive distortions may be effective for individuals with mild to moderate eating disorders in the early stages[83]. Psycho-educational therapy is a highly structured treatment programme in which therapeutic milieu and didactic instruction are used to help patients understand the nature, aetiology and complications of disordered eating behaviours. The purpose of this intervention is to foster attitudinal and behavioural change in the patient.[84] Psychotherapeutic interventions should address the complex of underlying issues which often cause and sustain eating-disordered behaviour. These issues include depression, diminished self-esteem and excessive dependence. Risk-taking behaviour, such as substance abuse and sexual acting out, should also be addressed[72]. Boehnert and colleagues[85] described strategies for the management of patients with diabetes and eating disorders who are severely non-compliant with the medical regimen. These strategies include: (a) The specific monitoring of provider countertransference; (b) the development of a careful working alliance with the patient and his/her family; (c) careful limit setting; and (d) dealing with the patient's frustrated dependency needs. These authors caution that patients must be dealt with honestly, directly and proactively. They suggest that therapy address denial, magical thinking and enhanced vulnerability secondary to diabetes, depression and demoralization.

Given the tremendous difficulties inherent in treating established eating disorders in people with diabetes, health care providers should be familiar with strategies for primary prevention for young female patients who have diabetes. These strategies, discussed fully elsewhere[71] include: addressing the drive for thinness and associated body dissatisfaction; de-emphasizing dieting; counselling patients about the need to express negative feelings about diabetes management; helping the patient with conflict over normal developmental struggles; addressing metabolic reactivity during adolescence; and involving the family.

Pharmacotherapy may benefit some patients with eating disorders. Since many patients suffering from eating disorders are also depressed, treatment with any of the antidepressants discussed earlier in this chapter should be considered. Some antidepressants in the SSRI class may positively affect compulsive behaviour, including eating disordered behaviour, as well as depression. Prozac has been used successfully for this purpose, and other agents in the same class may provide similar benefits.

PSYCHOPATHOLOGY PRESENTING AS MEDICAL CRISIS

In many cases a medical crisis may be the first sign that a patient is suffering from a psychiatric disorder. Such medical crises include: RDKA; frequent, severe hypoglycaemic and hyperglycaemic episodes (sometimes called 'brittle diabetes'); and severe non-compliance with the treatment regimen, especially insulin administration. These destructive behaviours frequently coincide with severe psychological disturbance, including individual psychopathology[86], family dysfunction[85] or both[87]. The literature contains several studies indicating that these disturbances may be effectively treated by intensive individual[88] and family therapy, often conducted at least partly in residential or inpatient settings[89]. Unfortunately, the fact that in all studies cited the psychological intervention was only one element of a comprehensive (and substantially undocumented) treatment makes it impossible to estimate the contribution of the psychological treatment *per se* to the benefit reported.

SUMMARY AND CONCLUSIONS

In this chapter I have reviewed counselling and psychotherapeutic interventions for patients with diabetes who are having difficulties coping with the day-to-day demands of life with diabetes, and for patients with diabetes who suffer from frank psychopathology, specifically depression, anxiety disorder or eating disorder. Since the effects of coping problems and psychological disorders may be especially malevolent for people with diabetes, effective psychological treatment is especially important for these individuals. Psychological problems of any magnitude may affect metabolic control directly via the neuroendocrine and physiological effects of stress, or indirectly via a cascade of events, including worsened self-care and deteriorating metabolic control, which may in turn exert a negative reciprocal effect on emotional well-being. This downward spiral can lead to acute life-threatening medical crises, and may also accelerate the long-term complications of diabetes. Thus, psychological problems represent a clear and present danger to many people with diabetes, and the need to effectively address these problems in susceptible individuals is equally clear.

Unfortunately, the literature offers a few unequivocal treatment guidelines. The number of published intervention studies is small, and many studies which have been published utilized small or unrepresentative samples, and therefore lack rigour and statistical power. Many studies do not include a control group or follow-up measures, so we can not say with confidence that the intervention was effective or enduring. Studies often describe comprehensive interventions which incorporate a variety of medical and psychological components. While this approach maximizes the likelihood of effective treatment, it makes the attribution of observed benefits to particular components of the intervention impossible.

Despite these limitations, the existing literature does provide some guidance for clinicians treating coping difficulties and psychological disorders in people with diabetes. We find some evidence for the benefits of formal and informal coping skills training, utilized as a unique intervention[21,30,31,35] or as part of a comprehensive psycho-educational program[40,43,44]. We also find some evidence that BART may facilitate stress management and glycaemic control in those with type 2 diabetes[8–10] and in some stress-responsive individuals with type 1 diabetes[11,12,16]. Recent studies suggest that psychotherapy (and pharmacotherapy) may relieve emotional distress in people with diabetes who suffer from depression and anxiety disorder, just as these treatments relieve symptoms in those who do not have diabetes[54,65,69]. Finally, we find some evidence for the effectiveness of comprehensive approaches to treating acute medical crises and eating disorders in young people with diabetes[84–86,89]. These approaches generally incorporate individual psychotherapy, family counselling and intensive medical management.

One can only hope that the growing awareness of the critical connection between diabetes and emotional distress will lead to the development of a more adequate research base than the one to which we must currently turn for guidance. Clinicians and researchers in a wide variety of settings can contribute to this development. As we prepare for the kind of clinical trials which are likely to provide definitive answers to our questions about the problem-specific effectiveness of various psychotherapeutic and psycho-educational interventions, small-scale research will continue to play a critical role in advancing our understanding. Health care providers who treat patients with diabetes might consider creating clinical dabatabases. These databases could include information about patients, such as demographic and disease-specific characteristics and presenting problems, a description of the treatment employed, and treatment duration and outcomes. Providers could supplement this information with the results of pre- and post-treatment psychological assessments, using available standardized self-report measures. Over time, such a database could be large enough to use for designing more effective interventions, or even for publication.

It is also clear that we need studies involving larger numbers of patients. Many potentially effective interventions are probably going unrecognized because the studies describing them lack the statistical power to confirm their benefits. Current research has demonstrated the need for counselling and psychotherapy and the potential efficacy of these interventions for people with diabetes, and it has done so with relatively small amounts of research funding. Research of the kind required to more conclusively answer the critical questions in this area require an increased commitment to funding psychosocial intervention studies on the part of governmental and other large grantors. Funding policy is one important frontier for psychosocial research in the near future.

REFERENCES

1. Rubin RR, Peyrot M. Psychological problems and interventions in diabetes: A review of the literature. *Diabet Care* 1992; **15**: 1640–57
2. Diabetes Control and Complications Trial Research Group. The effect of intensive treatment of diabetes on the development and progression of long-term complications in insulin-dependent diabetes mellitus. *N Engl J Med* 1993; **329**: 977–86
3. Okubo Y, Kishikawa H, Araki E *et al.* Intensive insulin therapy prevents the progression of diabetic microvascular complications in Japanese patients with non-insulin-dependent diabetes mellitus: a randomized prospective 6-year study. *Diab Res Clin Pract* 1995; **28**: 103–17
4. UK Prospective Diabetes Study Group. Intensive blood-glucose control with sulfonylureas or insulin compared with conventional treatment and risk of complications with type 2 diabetes (UKPDS 33). *Lancet* 1998; **352**: 837–53
5. UK Prospective Diabetes Study Group. Effects of intensive blood-glucose control with metformin on complications with type 2 diabetes (UKPDS 34). *Lancet* 1998; **352**: 854–65
6. Robiner W, Keel PK. Self-care behaviors and adherence in diabetes mellitus. *Sem Clin Neuropsychiat* 1997; **2**: 40–56
7. Ruggiero L, Glasgow RE, Dryfoos JM *et al.* Diabetes self-management: self-reported recommendations and patterns in a large population. *Diabet Care* 1997; **30**: 568–76
8. Surwit RS, Feinglos MN. The effects of relaxation on glucose tolerance in non-insulin-dependent diabetes mellitus. *Diabet Care* 1983; **6**: 176–9
9. Lammers CA, Naliboff BD, Straatmeyer AJ. The effects of progressive relaxation on stress and diabetes control. *Behav Res Ther* 1984; **22**: 641–50
10. Surwit RS, Ross SL, McCaskill CC *et al.* Does relaxation therapy add to conventional treatment of diabetes mellitus? (abstract). *Diabetes* 1989; **38** (suppl 1): 9A

11. McGrady A, Bailey BK, Good MP. Controlled study of biofeedback-assisted relaxation in type 1 diabetes. *Diabet Care* 1991; **14**: 360–65
12. Rosenbaum L, Tannenberg RJ. Differential glucose responses to biofeedback in IDDM (abstract). *Diabetes* 1985; **34** (suppl 1): 209A
13. Bradley C, Moses JL, Gamnsu DS *et al.* The effects of relaxation on metabolic control of type 1 diabetes: a matched controlled study (abstract). *Diabetes* 1985; **34** (suppl 1): 17A
14. Landis B, Jovanovic L, Landis E *et al.* Effect of stress reduction on daily glucose range in previously stabilized insulin-dependent diabetic patients. *Diabet Car* 1985; **8**: 624–6
15. Surwit RS, Feinglos MN. Stress and autonomic nervous system in type 2 diabetes: a hypothesis. *Diabet Care* 1988; **11**: 83–5
16. Feinglos MN, Hastedt P, Surwit RS. Effects of relaxation therapy on patients with type 1 diabetes mellitus. *Diabet Care* 1987; **10**: 72–5
17. Follansbee DJ, LaGreca Am, Citrin WS. Coping skills training for adolescents with diabetes (abstract). *Diabetes* 1983; **32** (suppl 1): 37A
18. Shalom R, Ryan J. Support and education groups for type 1 diabetics in a college campus (abstract). *Diabetes* 1987; **36** (suppl 1): 210A
19. Marrero DG, Meyers GL, Golden MP *et al.* Adjustment to misfortune: the use of a social support group for adolescent diabetics. *Pediat Adolesc Endocrinol* 1982; **10**: 213–18
20. Boardway RH, Delameter AM, Tomakowsky J *et al.* Stress management training for adolescents with diabetes. *J Pediat Psychol* 1993; **18**: 29–45
21. Gross AM, Heimann L, Shapiro R *et al.* Children with diabetes: social skills training and hemoglobin A1c levels. *Behav Modification* 1983; **7**: 151–64
22. Smith KE, Schreiner BJ, Brouhard BH *et al.* Impact of camp experience on choice of coping strategies for adolescents with insulin-dependent diabetes mellitus. *Diabet Educ* 1991; **17**: 49–53
23. Anderson BJ, Wolf FM, Burkhart MT *et al.* Effects of peer-group interventions on metabolic control of adolescents with IDDM: randomized outpatient study. *Diabet Care* 1989; **12**: 179–83
24. Chadwick MW, Kaplan RM, Schimmel LE. Social learning intervention improves metabolic control in type 1 diabetic teenagers (abstract). *Diabetes* 1984; **33**: 69A
25. Sandor J. The effect of diabetic summer camp on locus of control (abstract). *Diabetes* 1981; **30**: 49A
26. Lipets MS. The effects of juvenile diabetic camping on self-esteem and locus of control. St. Louis, MO: Washington University, PhD thesis, 1983
27. Moffatt MEK, Pless IB. Locus of control in juvenile diabetic campers: changes during camp and relationship to staff assessments. *J Pediat* 1983; **103**: 146–50
28. Scharf LS, Leach DC, Adams KM. Diabetes camp as a psychological intervention: some findings (abstract). *Diabetes* 1987; **36**: 109A
29. McCraw RK, Travis LB. Psychological effects of a special summer camp on juvenile diabetics. *Diabetes* 1973; **22**: 275–8
30. Mendez FJ, Melendez M. Effects of a behavioral intervention on treatment adherence and stress management in adolescents with IDDM. *Diabet Care* 1997; **20**: 1370–75
31. Warren-Boulton E, Anderson BJ, Schwartz NL *et al.* A group approach to the management of diabetes in adolescents and young adults. *Diabet Care* 1981; **4**: 620–23
32. Dupuis A. Assessment of the psychological factors and responses in self-managed patients. *Diabet Care* 1980; **3**: 117–20

33. Rabin C, Amir S, Nardi R *et al.* Compliance and control: issues in group training for diabetics. *Health Soc Work* 1986; **11** 141–51
34. Cain C, Childs C. Development of a peer support group for patients using a subcutaneous insulin infusion pump (abstract). *Diabetes* 1982; **31** (suppl 1): 18A
35. Aveline MO, McCulloch DK, Tattersall RB. The practice of group psychotherapy with adult insulin-dependent diabetics. *Diabet Med* 1985; **2**: 275–82
36. Rubin RR. The challenges of the millenium: are we ready or not? *Diabet Spectrum* 1998; **11**: 121–3
37. Rubin RR, Biermann J, Toohey B. *Psyching Out Diabetes*, 2nd edn. Los Angeles, CA: Lowell House, 1997
38. Rubin RR. Behavior change. In Funnell MM *et al.* (eds) *Core Curriculum for Diabetes Education*, 3rd edn. Chicago, IL: American Association of Diabetes Educators, 1998
39. Anderson BJ, Rubin RR (eds). Practical psychology for diabetes clinicians: how to deal with the key behavioral issues faced by patients and health care teams. Alexandria, VA: American Diabetes Association, 1996
40. Rubin RR, Peyrot M, Saudek CS. The effect of a diabetes education program incorporating coping skills training on emotional well-being and diabetes self-efficacy. *Diabet Educ* 1993; **19**: 210–14
41. Rubin RR, Walen SR, Ellis A. Living with diabetes. *J Rational–Emotive Cogn Behavior Ther* 1990; **8**: 21–39
42. Marlatt GA, Gordon JR. *Relapse Prevention: a Self-Control Strategy for the Maintenance of Behavior Change*. New York: Guilford, 1985
43. Rubin RR, Peyrot M, Saudek CS. Effect of diabetes education on self-care, metabolic control, and emotional well-being. *Diabet Care* 1989; **12**: 673–9
44. Rubin RR, Peyrot M, Saudek CS. Differential effect of diabetes education on self-regulation and life style behaviours. *Diabet Care* 1991; **14**: 335–8
45. Peyrot M, Rubin RR. Levels and risk of depression and anxiety symptomatology among diabetic adults. *Diabet Care* 1997; **20**: 585–90
46. Gavard JA, Lustman PJ, Clouse RE. Prevalence of depression in adults with diabetes: an epidemiological evaluation. *Diabet Care* 1993; **16**: 1167–78
47. Pevelier RC, Boller I, Fairburn CG *et al.* Eating disorders in adolescents with IDDM. *Diabet Care* 1992; **15**: 1356–60
48. Rydall AC, Rodin GM, Olmsted MP *et al.* Disordered eating behavior and microvascular complications in young women with insulin-dependent diabetes mellitus. *N Engl J Med* 1997; **336**: 1849–54
49. Hepertz S, Albus C, Wagener R *et al.* Comorbidity of diabetes and eating disorders: does diabetes control reflect disturbed eating behavior? *Diabet Care* 1998; **21**: 1110–16
50. Lustman PJ, Griffith LS, Clouse RE. Recognizing and managing depression in patients with diabetes. In Anderson BJ, Rubin RR (eds) *Practical Psychology for Diabetes Clinicians: How to Deal with the Key Behavioral Issues Faced by Patients and Health Care Teams*. Alexandria, VA: American Diabetes Association, 1996; 143–54
51. Lustman PJ, Griffith LS, Clouse RE. Depression in adults with diabetes. *Sem Clin Neuropsychiat* 1997; **2**: 15–23
52. Mazze RS, Lucido D, Shamoon H. Psychological and social correlates of glycemic control. *Diabet Care* 1984; **7**: 360–66
53. DeGroot M, Jacobson AM, Samson JA. Psychiatric illness in patients with type 1 and type 2 diabetes mellitus. *Psychosom Med* 1994; **56**: 176A
54. Lustman PJ, Clouse RE, Alrakawi A *et al.* Treatment of major depression in adults with diabetes: a primary care perspective. *Clin. Diabet* 1997; **15**: 122–6

55. Lustman PJ, Griffith LS, Clouse RE. Depression in adults with diabetes: results of a 5-year follow-up stiudy. *Diabet Care* 1988; **11**: 605–12
56. Rubin RR, Peyrot M. Psychosocial problems in diabetes treatment: impediments to intensive self care. *Pract Diabetol* 1994; **13**: 8–14
57. Frasure-Smith N, Lesperance F, Talajic M. Depression and 18-month prognosis after myocardial infarction. *Circulation* 1995; **91**: 999–1005
58. Lustman PJ, Harper GW. Nonpsychiatric physicians' identification and treatment of depression in patients with diabetes. *Compr Psychiat* 1987; **28**: 22–7
59. American Psychiatric Association. *Diagnostic and Statistical Manual of Mental Disorders*, 4th edn. Washington, DC: American Psychiatric Association, 1994
60. Radloff L. The CES-D scale: a self-report depression scale for research in the general population. *Appl Psychol Meas* 1977; **1**: 385–401
61. Beck AT, Beck RW. Screening depressed patients in family practice: a rapid technique. *Postgrad Med* 1972; **52**: 81–5
62. Zung WW, Richards CB, Short MJ. Self-rating depression scale in an outpatient clinic. *Arch Gen Psychiat* 1965; **13**: 508–15
63. Rush AJ, Beck AT, Kovacs M *et al.* Comparative efficacy of cognitive therapy and pharmacotherapy in the treatment of depressed patients. *Cogn Ther Res* 1977; **1**: 17–37
64. Frank E, Kupfer DJ, Wagner EF *et al.* Efficacy of interpersonal psychotherapy as a maintenance treatment for recurrent depression. *Arch Gen Psychiat* 1991; **48**: 1053–9
65. Lustman PJ, Griffith LS, Clouse RE *et al.* Efficacy of cognitive therapy for depression in NIDDM: results of a controlled clinical trial (abstract). *Diabetes* 1997; **46** (suppl 1): 13A
66. Popkin MK, Callies AL, Lentz RD *et al.* Prevalence of major depression, simple phobia, and other psychiatric disorders in patients with long-standing type 1 diabetes mellitus. *Arch Gen Psychiatr* 1988; **45**: 64–8
67. Barglow P, Hatcher R, Edidin DV. Stress and metabolic control in diabetes: psychosomatic evidence and evaluation of methods. *Psychosom Med* 1984; **46**: 127–44
68. McGrady A, Bailey BK, Good MP. Controlled study of biofeedback-assisted relaxation in type 1 diabetes. *Diabet Care* 1991; **14**: 360–65
69. Lustman PJ, Griffith LS, Clouse RE *et al.* Effects of alprazolam on glucose regulation in diabetes. *Diabet Care* 1995; **18**: 1133–9
70. Okada S, Ichiki K, Tanokuchi S *et al.* Effects of an anxiolytic on lipid profile in non-insulin-dependent diabetes mellitus. *J Int Med Res* 1994; **22**: 338–42
71. Rapaport WS, LaGreca AM, Levine P. Preventing eating disorders in young women with type 1 diabetes. In Anderson BJ, Rubin RR (eds) *Practical Psychology for Diabetes Clinicians: How to Deal with the Key Behavioral Issues Faced by Patients and Health-care Teams*. Alexandria, VA: American Diabetes Association, 1996; 133–42
72. Hall RCW. Bulimia nervosa and diabetes mellitus. *Sem Clin Neuropsych* 1997; **2**: 24–30
73. Hillard JR, Hillard PJA. Bulimia, anorexia, and diabetes: deadly combinations. *Psychiat Clin N Am* 1984; **7**: 367–79
74. LaGreca A, Schwartz L, Satin W *et al.* Binge eating among women with IDDM: associations with weight dissatisfaction, adherence, and metabolic control. *Diabetes* 1990; **39** (suppl 1): 164A
75. Pollock M, Kovacs M, Charon-Prochownik D. Eating disorders and maladaptive dietary/insulin management among youths with childhood-onset insulin-dependent diabetes mellitus. *J Am Acad Child Adolesc Psychiat* 1995; **34**: 291–6

76. Stancin T, Link DL, Reuter JM. Binge eating in young women with IDDM. *Diabet Care* 1989; **12**: 601–3
77. Steel JM, Young RJ, Lloyd GG *et al.* Abnormal eating attitudes in young insulin-dependent diabetics. *Br J Psychiat* 1989; **155**: 515–21
78. Rodin G, Rydall A, Olmstedt M *et al.* A four-year follow-up study of eating disorders and medical complications in young women with insulin dependent diabetes mellitus. *Psychosom Med* 1994; **56**: 179
79. Wing RR, Norwalk MP, Marcus MD *et al.* Subclinical eating disorders and glycemic control in adolescents with type 1 diabetes. *Diabet Care* 1986; **9**: 162–7
80. LaGreca A, Schwartz L, Satin W. Eating patterns in young women with IDDM: another look (letter). *Diabet Care* 1987; **10**: 659–60
81. Polonsky W, Anderson BJ, Lohrer P *et al.* Insulin omission in women with IDDM. *Diabet Care* 1994; **17**: 1179–84
82. Biggs MM, Basco MR, Patterson G *et al.* Insulin withholding for weight control in women with diabetes. *Diabet Care* 1994; **176**: 1186–9
83. Olmsted MP, Davis R, Rockert W *et al.* Efficacy of a brief group psychoeducational intervention for bulimia nervosa. *Behav Res Ther* 1991; **29**: 71–83
84. Davis R, Dearing S, Faulkner J *et al.* The road to recovery: a manual for participants in the psychoeducation group for bulimia nervosa. In Harper-Giuffre H, MacKenzie KR (eds) Washington, DC: American Psychiatric Press, 1992; 281–341
85. Boehnert CE, Popkin MK. Psychological issues in treatment of severely noncompliant diabetics. *Psychosomatics* 1986; **27**: 11–20
86. Gill G, Robinson M, Marrow J. Hypoglycemic brittle diabetes successfully managed by social worker intervention. *Diabet Med* 1989; **6**: 448–50
87. Coyne JC, Anderson BJ. The 'psychosomatic family' reconsidered: II. Recalling a defective model and looking ahead. *J Marital Fam Ther* 1989; **15**: 139–48
88. Follansbee DJ, LaGreca AM, Citrin WS. Coping skills training for adolescents with diabetes. *Diabetes* 1983; **32**: (suppl 1) 37A
89. Moran G, Fonagy P, Kurtz A *et al.* A controlled study of psychoanalytic treatment of brittle diabetes. *J Am Acad Child Adolesc Psychiat* 1991; **30**: 926–35

INDEX

Page numbers in **bold** refer to figures, and those in *italics* to tables.

Index compiled by Elisabeth Pickard

THE DIABETES IN PRACTICE SERIES .....

☐

PSYCHOLOGY IN DIABETES CARE

Edited by: FJ Snoek and TC Skinner

Bridging the gap between psychological research on self-care and management of diabetes, and the delivery of care and services provided by the diabetes care team, this book provides a background and practical guidelines on behavioural issues much needed by health care professionals.

0471 97703 9 approx 279pp 2000

☐

EXERCISE AND SPORT IN DIABETES

Editors: Bill Burr and Dinesh Nagi

A rare look at the benefits and risks of strenuous and easy exercise for people with diabetes. Accessible to all diabetes patient carers, it allow the reader to fully understand the issues, and brief patients accordingly:

- accumulating the most up-to-date information
- exploring issues with a practical outlook

0471 98496 5 194pp 1999

☐

HYPOGLYCAEMIA IN CLINICAL DIABETES

Editors: Brian M Frier and B Miles Fisher

An up-to-date and accessible publication, covering a very common problem in the clinical management of diabetes. It discusses risk factors and treatment regimes, while concentrating on the clinical and practical aspects of hypoglycaemia.

0471 98264 4 301pp 1999

☐

CHILDHOOD AND ADOLESCENT DIABETES

Editors: Simon Court and Bill Lamb

The management of diabetes in children and young people continues to develop in important areas, including self-monitoring, insulin delivery, dietary prescription, concept of control and the early identification of complications. This book is practical and invaluable to all members of the diabetes specialist team working with children.

0471 97003 4 384pp 1997

☐

DIABETES AND PREGNANCY

An International Approach to Diagnosis and Management

Editors: Anne Dornhorst and David R Hadden

A comprehensive and practical guide to the present state of knowledge regarding diabetic pregnancy. It summarises published literature, and offers clear and valuable information on the practicalities of providing special care, before, during and after pregnancy.

0471 96204 X 424pp 1996